Memorix Pe

JOIN US ON THE INTERNET VIA WWW, GOPHER, FTP OR EMAIL:

WWW: http://www.thomson.com
GOPHER: gopher.thomson.com
FTP: ftp.thomson.com
EMAIL: findit@kiosk.thomson.com

A service of I(T)P

Memorix

The *Memorix* series consists of easy to use pocket books in a number of different medical and surgical specialities. They contain a vast amount of practical information in very concise form through the extensive use of tables and charts, lists and hundreds of clear line diagrams, often in two colors.

Memorix will give students, junior doctors and some of their senior colleagues a handy and comprehensive reference in their pockets.

Titles in the series include:

Clinical Medicine
Conrad Droste and Martin von Planta

Emergency Medicine
Sönke Müller

Gynecology
Thomas Rabe

Neurology
Peter Berlit

Obstetrics
Thomas Rabe

Pediatrics
Dieter Harms and Jochem Scharf

Physiology
Robert Schmidt, W.D. Willis and L. Reuss

Surgery
Jürgen Hussmann and Robert Russell

Memorix

Pediatrics

Dieter Harms and Jochem Scharf

Translated by Albert Davis MD and Renate Davis MB

With additional material by Gerald Graham MD

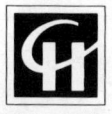

CHAPMAN & HALL MEDICAL

London · Weinheim · New York · Tokyo · Madras

Published by Chapman & Hall, 2–6 Boundary Row, London SE1 8HN, UK

Chapman & Hall, 2–6 Boundary Row, London SE1 8HN, UK

Chapman & Hall GmbH, Pappelallee 3, 69469 Weinheim, Germany

Chapman & Hall USA, 115 Fifth Avenue, New York, NY 10003, USA

Chapman & Hall Japan, ITP-Japan, Kyowa Building, 3F, 2-2-1 Hirakawacho, Chiyoda-ku, Tokyo 102, Japan

Chapman & Hall India, R. Seshadri, 32 Second Main Road, CIT East, Madras 600 035, India

English language edition 1997

© 1997 Chapman & Hall

Original German language edition – Memorix Spezial – Pädiatrie © 1993, VCH Verlagsgesellschaft mbH, D-6940 Weinheim, Germany

Typeset in Times by Best-set Typesetter Ltd., Hong Kong

Printed and bound in Hong Kong

ISBN 0 412 73830 9

Apart from any fair dealing for the purposes of research or private study, or criticism or review, as permitted under the UK Copyright Designs and Patents Act, 1988, this publication may not be reproduced, stored, or transmitted, in any form or by any means, without the prior permission in writing of the publishers, or in the case of reprographic reproduction only in accordance with the terms of the licences issued by the Copyright Licensing Agency in the UK, or in accordance with the terms of licences issued by the appropriate Reproduction Rights Organization outside the UK. Enquiries concerning reproduction outside the terms stated here should be sent to the publishers at the London address printed on this page.

The publisher makes no representation, express or implied, with regard to the accuracy of the information contained in this book and cannot accept any legal responsibility or liability for any errors or omissions that may be made.

A catalogue record for this book is available from the British Library

Library of Congress Catalog Card Number: 96-86261

CONTENTS

Contents

Preface xviii

Symbols used in the book xix

Abbreviations xx

Basics/normal values/diagnostic methods 2

Body surface 2
Conversion tables: normal ranges 3
SI units: conversion, conventional and SI units 5
Basic and derived SI units 6
Reference values for blood, plasma, serum, CSF, urine, feces and sweat 8
Catheter sizes 18
Calculation of drip speed for infusions 19
Prefixes for decimal units 20
Diagnostic principle of ELISA 21
DNA, RNA and protein analysis by the blot technique 22
Principle of the polymerase chain reaction (PCR) 24
International double-digit dental chart 25
Sequence of dentition 26
Epidemiological definitions 27
Assessment of diagnostic tests 28
Morphological terminology of developmental disorders 29
Symbols for documentation of a family tree 30
Indications for chromosome analysis in children 31
Group classification of chromosomes on morphological criteria 31
X-chromosomal inherited diseases 32
Cytogenetic nomenclature 34
DNA diagnosis 40
Organ development: sensitive periods 41
Early prenatal development 42
Thoracic suction drainage 44
Thoracic puncture 45
Pleural puncture 46
Puncture of the abdominal cavity 47
Venepuncture: central venous catheter 47
Venepuncture: epicutaneous catheter 49
Arterial puncture and catheterization 50
Establishment of brain death 51
X-ray investigations 52
X-ray diagnosis 54

v

CONTENTS

Thoracic imaging	57
Computed tomography (CT): window technique	58
CT characteristics	59
CT imaging topography	60
Topography of space-occupying structures in the mediastinum	63
Space-occupying structures in the abdomen	64
Nuclear medicine diagnosis	65
Changes in radioiodine uptake	66
Magnetic resonance imaging (MRI)	67
MRI: signal intensity of tissues and fluids	67
MRI: interpretation/indications	68
Intracranial MRI	68
Ultrasound diagnosis	70
Ultrasound diagnosis: organs	71
Ultrasound, normal values: spleen	77
Ultrasound, normal values: kidneys	78
Intracranial hemorrhage	79

Cardiology   80

Color-coded Doppler ultrasonography	80
Principle of Doppler ultrasonography	81
Doppler ultrasound	82
Ultrasound measurement of normal flow velocities in the heart and great vessels	82
M-mode echocardiography	83
Measurements with M-mode echocardiogram	84
M-mode echocardiogram measuring sites	84
One-dimensional (M-mode) echocardiography	85
Cardiac cycle	86
Normal values for cardiovascular pressures and O_2 saturation	87
Arterial pulse types – diagnostic significance	88
Normal values for heart rate	88
Heart murmurs – grades of intensity	89
Auscultation points in congenital heart defects	89
Congenital defects: glossary (heart and great vessels)	90
Pressures and oxygen saturation in congenital heart defects	92
Possible recurrence risk (%) for congenital defects	95
Hemodynamic degrees of severity of congenital heart disease	112
Guidelines for hemodynamic assessment of operative results in congenital heart defects	113
Recommendations for participation in school sports	114
Shunt-dependent congenital heart defects	115
ECG: electrode positions	116

CONTENTS

RS patterns of electrical axis positions/deviations	117
Cabrera circle	118
Age-dependent normal ranges for different ECG measurements	119
ECG: relative and rate-corrected QT interval	120
ECG: normal values for R : S ratio and R and S amplitudes	121
ECG: signs of hypertrophy	122
ECG: right-sided hypertrophy	123
ECG: left-sided hypertrophy	124
ECG: criteria of atrial hypertrophy	125
Sequence in the ECG diagnosis of cardiac arrhythmias	126
Causes of arrhythmias	127
Sympathomimetics	130
Anti-arrhythmic drugs: indications and dosages	132
Digitalis treatment	134
Digitalis poisoning	135
ECG changes in electrolyte disorders	138
Cardiomyopathies	139
Synopsis of idiopathic forms in children and adolescents	140
Indirect blood pressure measurement	141
Blood pressure percentiles	142
Hypertension	145
Checklist of the underlying diseases in hypertension	146
Diagnosis of hypertension	147
Antihypertensive treatment: three-stage program	149
Treatment of hypertensive crises	150
Antihypertensive medication for long-term treatment	151
Hypotension: active orthostatic test	152
Indications for endocarditis prophylaxis according to degree of risk	153
Antibacterial dosages for the prophylaxis of endocarditis	154
Cardiac failure: principles of treatment	156
Hypoxemic attack: pathophysiology and treatment	157

Pulmonology 158

Morphology of lung development	158
Differential diagnosis of rhythmic respiration	159
Oxyhemoglobin binding: partial pressure profile	160
Differential diagnosis of cyanosis	161
Bronchial segments: anatomy	162
X-ray diagnosis: schema of lung segments	163
X-ray diagnosis: appearance of lobar atelectasis/pleurisy	164
Types of pleurisy in the A-P X-ray film	164

CONTENTS

X-ray diagnosis: appearance of pulmonary vessels   **165**
X-ray diagnosis: appearance of different forms of thymus hyperplasia   **166**
Pleuromediastinal lines in chest film   **166**
Differential diagnosis of stridor   **167**
Parameters of lung function   **168**
Normal lung volumes/O_2 treatment   **169**
Lung function diagnosis   **170**
Disorders of lung function   **171**
Bronchial asthma: symptom scores for calculating grade of severity of an asthma attack   **172**
Grading of bronchial asthma   **172**
Drug treatment   **173**
Anti-asthmatic drugs   **174**

Nephrology/urology   **176**

Renal function   **176**
Renal function tests: distal tubular function   **178**
Renal tubular acidosis (RTA)   **179**
Renal tubular acidosis: diagnostic plan   **180**
Causes of renal tubular acidosis/tubulopathy   **181**
Potter's pathological classification of cystic kidney diseases   **182**
Characteristics of cystic nephropathies   **183**
Hematuria   **185**
Proteinuria   **186**
Renal diagnosis/renal biopsy   **187**
Nephritic syndrome: morphological description   **188**
Glomerulonephritis   **189**
Nephrotic syndrome: definitions   **190**
Nephrotic syndrome: checklist of causes   **191**
Nephrotic syndrome: treatment   **192**
Grading of vesicoureteral reflux   **194**
Urinary tract infection: diagnostic algorithm   **195**
Urine bacterial count   **196**
Schema of bladder function   **196**
Pharmacological treatment of micturition disorders   **197**
Classification of neurogenic disorders of micturition   **198**
Urinary stones   **199**
Urinary stones: diagnostic aids   **200**
Hypercalciuria: calcium loading test   **201**
Electrolyte disturbances   **202**
Hyperkalemia   **202**
Hypokalemia   **203**

CONTENTS

Metabolism — 204

- Blood gases – normal levels — 204
- Buffering — 204
- Acidosis/alkalosis: pathophysiology — 205
- Acid–base disorders — 206
- Causes of disorders in acid–base equilibrium — 207
- Anion gap — 208
- Congenital lactacidosis — 209
- Metabolic acidosis — 210
- Diagnosis of ketoacidosis — 211
- Congenital defects of energy metabolism — 212
- Enzyme defects — 212
- Model of pyruvate metabolism — 213
- Schema of the enzyme complex of the mitochondrial respiratory chain — 213
- Clinical symptoms of respiratory chain defects — 214
- Hyperammonemia: diagnostic plan — 215
- Hypoglycemia — 218
- Hypoglycemia: diagnostic substances and tests — 220
- Glycogen metabolic defects — 221
- Diabetes mellitus — 222
- Insulin therapy — 224
- Biphasic insulins — 225
- Diabetes: daily energy requirement — 226
- Mucopolysaccharidoses — 231
- Lipid storage diseases — 232
- Synopsis of lipid storage diseases — 233
- Properties of serum lipoproteins — 234
- Function of the apoproteins — 234
- Hypercholesterolemia: diagnosis and screening according to history — 235
- Lipoprotein analysis — 236
- Percentiles of normal lipid and lipoprotein levels — 236
- Familial hyperlipoproteinemia — 237
- Familial hypolipoproteinemia — 238
- Functions of the peroxisomes — 239
- Synopsis of peroxisomal diseases — 240

Endocrinology/growth — 241

- Calcium phosphate metabolism: hormone regulation — 241
- Parathormone: regulation/disorders — 243
- Vitamin D metabolism and rachitogenic disorders — 243

CONTENTS

Calcium phosphate metabolic diseases	244
Growth	245
Dwarfism: history/investigation	246
Skeletal development	247
Growth: estimation of final height	248
Growth and weight percentile curves (girls)	249
Growth and weight percentile curves (boys)	251
Typical growth curves	253
Causes of short stature	254
Causes of tall stature	254
Developmental stages of secondary sex characteristics	255
Pubertal development and age of onset	257
Phenotypical course of puberty	258
Onset of puberty	259
Causes of delayed puberty	259
Synopsis of premature puberty	260
Normal sexual development	261
Disorders of masculine differentiation and development	262
Congenital disorders of steroid biosynthesis	263
Adrenogenital syndrome	264
Steroid biosynthesis: enzyme defects	265
Treatment of undescended testis	266
Causes of hypothyroidism	267
Screening for hypothyroidism	268
Aftercare program in congenital hypothyroidism	269
Stages of goiter	270
Growth function tests	271
TRH test	273
LHRH test	274
HCG test	274
Dexamethasone test	275
ACTH test	276
Metyrapone test	276
Test combinations for the multiple diagnosis of pituitary functions	277
Vasopressin (desmopressin) test	278

Gastroenterology/nutrition 280

Peptide hormones in the gastrointestinal tract	280
Hypertrophic pyloric stenosis	281
Intestinal innervation	282
Megacolon	282

Disease stages of mucoviscidosis	283
Hyperbilirubinemia	284
Biliary atresia	284
Cholelithiasis in childhood and adolescence	285
Differential diagnosis of vomiting	286
Indigestion/malabsorption: function tests	288
Pathogenic (enterovirulent) *Escherichia coli* (EVEC)	289
Diagnosis of dehydration	290
Oral rehydration	291
Parenteral rehydration	292
Nutrition in the first year of life	293
Nutritional energy	294
Nomogram for estimating potassium imbalance	294
Parenteral nutrition	295
Breast milk: nutrition in prematures	297
Special nutrition in metabolic defects	299

Infections/immunology/rheumatology 300

Fever types	300
Bacteriology	301
Diagnostic bacterial microscopy	302
Differentiation of human pathogenic organisms by Gram staining	303
Ziehl–Neelsen staining	303
Meningitis: diagnosis of cerebrospinal fluid	304
Treatment of bacterial meningitis	305
Tuberculosis: contacts, diagnosis and treatment	306
Toxoplasmosis	307
Serodiagnosis of prenatal infection	307
Diagnosis of postnatal toxoplasmosis infection	308
Identification of parasites in blood	308
Syphilis: serodiagnosis of infection with treponemes pathogenic in humans	309
Notification of infectious diseases	310
Immunization schedule	312
Indications for immunization	313
Incomplete immunization	314
Immunization in pregnancy	315
Immunization: special indications	316
Schedule for rabies immunization	317
Vaccine data	318
Recommendations for hepatitis B prophylaxis after exposure	319

CONTENTS

Schedule for travelers' immunization ... 320
Immunization in allergy, or suspected allergy/combined immunization ... 321
Course of serology in acute and chronic hepatitis B ... 322
Controlled hepatitis B immunization ... 322
Diagnostic components of the hepatitis B virus ... 323
Antigen–antibody pattern for the assessment of hepatitis B infectivity ... 323
Course of serology in hepatitis A ... 323
Early summer meningoencephalitis (ESME) ... 324
Classification of herpes viruses ... 324
Diagnostic survey of the commonest viral diseases ... 325
Human enteroviral diseases ... 327
Malaria prophylaxis/recommendations ... 329
Kawasaki's syndrome ... 330
Sequence of immunological findings after HIV infection ... 331
HIV infection: definitions ... 332
HIV infection: Centers for Disease Control classification ... 333
Biological properties of the immunoglobulins ... 335
Allergies: types of allergic reaction ... 336
Immunodeficiency syndrome ... 337
Primary immune defects: WHO classification ... 338
Complement defects and associated diseases ... 340
Complement activation (schematic) ... 341
Diagnosis of primary and secondary immune defects ... 342
Immune defect: step-by-step diagnosis ... 343
Cell–cell interactions: synopsis of cytokines ... 344
Synopsis of juvenile chronic arthritis (JCA) ... 345
American Rheumatism Association criteria for classification of chronic rheumatoid arthritis ... 346
Selection of antibiotics ... 347
Antibiotics against rarer organisms ... 349
Antibiotic treatment ... 350

Hematology/hemostasis/oncology ... 353

Schema of the coagulation system ... 353
Differential diagnosis of the commonest coagulation disorders ... 354
Diseases with thrombocytosis ... 354
Synopsis of von Willebrand's disease ... 355
Causes of thrombophilia ... 355
Diagnosis of anemia: erythrocyte forms in blood smears ... 356
Microscopy of erythrocytes: staining variants ... 357

CONTENTS

Definitions of automatic blood cell analysis	358
Morphological differentiation of the anemias	359
Pathophysiological differentiation of the anemias	360
Hemoglobin development	361
Exchange transfusions	362
Blood transfusion: reactions	363
Diagnosis of leukemia	364
FAB classification of the acute leukemias	365
FAB classification of ANLL	366
Classification of the histiocytoses in childhood	367
Schema of lymphocytopoiesis and phenotypical classification of the leukemias	368
Schema for hematopoiesis and classification of acute nonlymphocytic leukemias (ANLL) according to the FAB classification	369
CD antigens on normal and neoplastic leukocytes	370
TNM classification	371
TN classification of neuroblastoma	372
pTN classification of neuroblastoma	372
TN classification of nephroblastoma (Wilms' tumor)	373
pTN classification of nephroblastoma (Wilms' tumor)	373
TN classification of soft tissue sarcoma	374
pTN classification of soft tissue sarcoma	374
Lymphoma	375
Risk grouping of the B cell lymphomas	375
Stages of Burkitt's lymphoma	375
Stages of Hodgkin's disease	376
Stages of non-Hodgkin's lymphoma	376
Stages of neuroblastoma	377
Neuroblastoma	378
Staging of Wilms' tumor (nephroblastoma)	378
Postoperative stages of Wilms' tumor	379
Stages of ovarian tumors (intraoperative classification)	379
Histopathological stages of testicular tumors	379
Revised WHO classification of brain tumors in childhood	380
Stages of cerebral medulloblastoma	386
MAPS classification of PNET of the posterior cranial cavity	387
Tumors as a complication of diseases and syndromes	388
Stages of retinoblastoma	390
Cytostatic agents/antimetabolites	391
Overview of cytostatic agents	392

xiii

CONTENTS

Neonatology — 394

- Definitions of dysmaturity — 394
- Evaluation of newborn: Apgar score — 395
- Assessment of fetal maturity of neonates — 396
- Neuromuscular signs or maturity — 397
- Testing for neuromuscular signs of maturity — 398
- Finnström method of calculating fetal maturity from external characteristics — 399
- Intrauterine growth in body length and weight — 400
- Intrauterine head circumference — 401
- Infant respiratory distress syndrome (IRDS) — 401
- Differential diagnosis of neonatal jaundice — 402
- Hyperbilirubinemia — 403
- Umbilical vein catheter — 404
- Umbilical artery catheter — 405
- Neonatal ventilation: masks, endotracheal tubes and laryngoscopes — 406
- Test to distinguish HbA from HbF — 407
- Neonatal seizures — 408
- Nutrition of the premature infant — 409
- Exclusively parenteral nutrition — 410
- Drug dosages for immature and mature neonates — 412
- Antibiotics in the neonatal period — 413

Neuropediatrics — 414

- Approximate timetable for motor development — 414
- Neurological investigation in neonates and infants — 415
- Milestones in motor development — 423
- Motor development: erect gait — 424
- Motor development: grasp — 426
- Diagnostic EEG — 427
- Stages of sleep in the EEG — 428
- Pathological EEG variations — 429
- Pathological EEG patterns — 430
- Evoked potentials — 431
- Visual evoked potential — 432
- Acoustic evoked potential (AEP) — 432
- Electroretinogram (ERG) — 434
- Retinopathies — 435
- Somatosensory evoked potential (SSEP) — 435
- Electromyography (EMG) — 436
- Clinical forms of myasthenia gravis — 437

CONTENTS

Hereditary sensorimotor neuropathies (HSMN)	438
Summary of the hereditary sensory neuropathies (HSN)	439
Percentile growth curves for head circumference: boys 0–6 years	440
Percentile growth curves for head circumference: girls 0–6 years	441
Macrocephaly/megaloencephaly: differential diagnosis	442
Classification of the clinical types and diagnostic criteria of the neurofibromatoses	443
Encephalofacial angiomatosis (Sturge–Weber syndrome)	443
CSF–blood barrier	444
International classification of epileptic seizures	445
International classification of epilepsies and epileptic syndromes	446
Febrile convulsions	448
Treatment of epilepsy	449
Antiepileptics	450

Emergencies 452

List of aids to resuscitation	452
Ventilation	453
Frequently used types of ventilation	454
Effects of mechanical ventilation	455
Indications for mechanical ventilation	456
Guidelines for the initial setting of the ventilator when ventilating children	456
Neonatal ventilation	457
Criteria of acute respiratory failure	458
Complications of assisted ventilation	459
Resuscitation	460
Disorders of consciousness: diagnostic procedures	463
The Glasgow Coma Scale and age-related modifications	465
Intracranial pressure	466
Burns	467
Status epilepticus	469
Types of shock	470
Pulmonary edema	473
Status asthmaticus	474
Diabetic coma	475
Poisoning: common symptoms	476
Antidotes to poisoning and overdosage	478

CONTENTS

Poisons information services in the UK and the Republic of Ireland	479
Reye's syndrome	480
Acute renal failure (ARF)	481
Drug dosages in impaired renal function	485

Pediatric surgery/orthopedics — 487

Degrees of pain	487
Treatment of pain: WHO step schema for analgesic therapy	488
Diagnosis of appendicitis	489
Differentiation of types of ileus	490
Types of esophageal atresia	491
Midfacial fractures (Le Fort's classification)	492
Hip joint sonography	492
Sonographic determination of maturation of the hip joint	493
X-ray diagnosis of the hip joint	494
Diagnosis: hip joint dysplasia/pes adductus	495
Aseptic osteochondronecrosis	496
Quantification of leg malposition	498
Testing for joint mobility	498
Neutral–zero method of testing joint mobility	499

Ophthalmology/otology — 501

Measurement of visual acuity	501
Normal function of the ocular muscles	501
Strabismus	502
Nystagmus	502
Types of nystagmus	503
Diseases associated with congenital cataracts	504
Gaze paresis	505
Pharmocodynamics of pupil size	505
International classification of retinopathy of prematurity (retrolental fibroplasia)	506
Normal speech development	507
Effect of hearing impairment on speech development	508
Assessment of the tympanogram	509
Congenital hearing disorders	510

Clinical pharmacology — 515

Drugs during lactation	515

xvi

CONTENTS

Comparative pharmacological data for glucocorticoids 516
Action of the glucocorticoids 517

References 518

Index 525

PREFACE

Preface

The commencement of medical practice is invariably accompanied by the acquisition of a notebook that fits into the pocket of the new doctor's white coat. Initially small, it rapidly expands as the doctor's field of activity increases, to include a wide collection of data, useful but haphazardly noted and time-consuming to search through later for specific items as they are needed.

Considering the size of the field of pediatric medicine, the *Memorix* concept represents an interesting new approach. This book gives, in a concise but comprehensive format, most of the details required in daily practice, including normal values and levels, diagnostic criteria, dosages and clinical directions and instructions, all readily accessible. The practical facts contained in this book include developmental data, flowcharts, checklists, recommended diagnostic procedures, laboratory tests and the indicators for differential diagnoses and treatments. The Memorix concept thus acts as a constant touchstone of basic specialist knowledge.

The size constraints on a pocket-book prevent repetition but have not been allowed to restrict the basics to any great extent. Any such loss is more than compensated for by the saving of time and effort in accessing the information provided.

The usefulness of a personal notebook is compromised by the sporadic nature of the entries and the difficulty of retrieving the information in it. With its classified and authoritative format this book supplies the answers to questions that may arise during examinations or consultations, giving advice on symptoms, diagnosis and therapuetic measures.

We hope that the detailed but concise information given in this book will prove of value to students and experienced practitioners alike.

Dieter Harms and Jochem Scharf

SYMBOLS USED IN THE BOOK

Symbols used in the book

n/N	normal (unchanged)
+/++/+++	positive, present (also, increasing)
(+)	stimulation
−[ø]	negative, not present, not tested
(−)	inhibition
( )	questionable, unclear findings, rare
$\updownarrow/\approx$	variable findings, approximate value
$\nearrow$	moderately raised, upward tendency
$\searrow$	moderately reduced, downward tendency
< ≪	smaller than, younger than (also falling)
> ≫	greater, older than (also rising)
↑ ↑↑ ↑↑↑	raised, increased (also rising)
↓ ↓↓ ↓↓↓	reduced, lowered
→	directional (causal, timed, logical), relationship, pointer
←X	number (amount) decreasing/removed

ABBREVIATIONS

Abbreviations

AB	antibody
AD	autosomal dominant
ADH	antidiuretic hormone
AG	antigen
AR	autosomal recessive
B	blood
BM	bone marrow
BP	blood pressure
BS	blood sugar
CNS	central nervous system
CSF	cerebrospinal fluid
d	day(s)
ECG	electrocardiogram
EEG	electroencephalogram
EMG	electromyogram
h	hour(s)
HBa	adult hemoglobin
HIV	human immunodeficiency virus
i.c.	intracutaneous
Ig	immunoglobulin
i.m.	intramuscular
i.v.	intravenous
min	minute(s)
P	plasma
s	second(s)
S	serum
s.c.	subcutaneous
XR	X chromosomal recessive
y	year(s)

The dosages given in this book have been checked with great care. However, the authors and publishers take no responsibility for the accuracy of the dosages printed here.

It is recommended that before any drug administration is made the reader should familiarize him- or herself with the indications, contraindications, dosage and any other relevant information from the manufacturers regarding the drug instructions.

SHORT CONTENTS

Basics/normal values/diagnostic methods	2
Cardiology	80
Pulmonology	158
Nephrology/urology	176
Metabolism	204
Endocrinology/growth	241
Gastroenterology/nutrition	280
Infections/immunology/rheumatology	300
Hematology/hemostasis/oncology	353
Neonatology	394
Neuropediatrics	414
Emergencies	452
Pediatric surgery/orthopedics	487
Ophthalmology/otology	501
Clinical pharmacology	515
Index	525

MEMORIX PEDIATRICS

Body surface: Nomogram for calculating body surface from length and weight

(After Du Bois and Du Bois from Crawford, Terry, and Rourke (1950).)

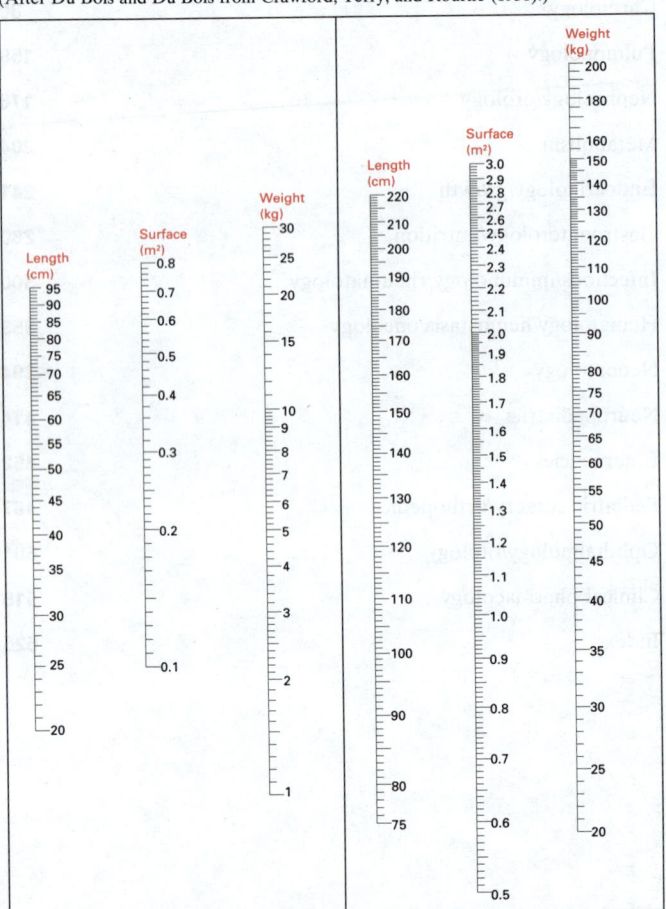

BASICS/NORMAL VALUES/DIAGNOSTIC METHODS

Conversion tables: normal ranges

For rapid orientation, draw pencil lines from scale to red column to demarcate normal ranges as obtained at your particular laboratory.

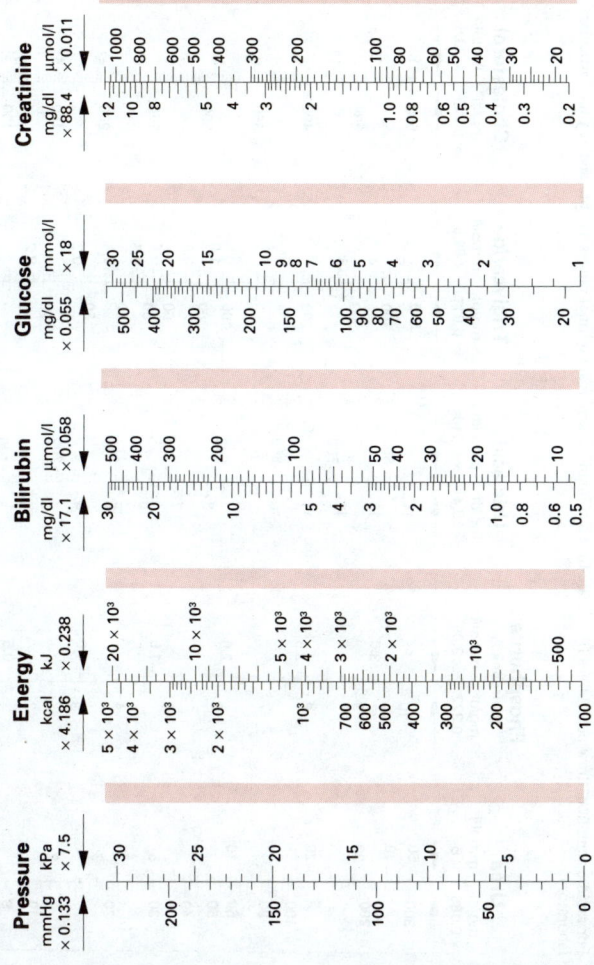

MEMORIX PEDIATRICS

For rapid orientation, draw pencil lines from scale to red column to demarcate normal ranges as obtained at your particular laboratory.

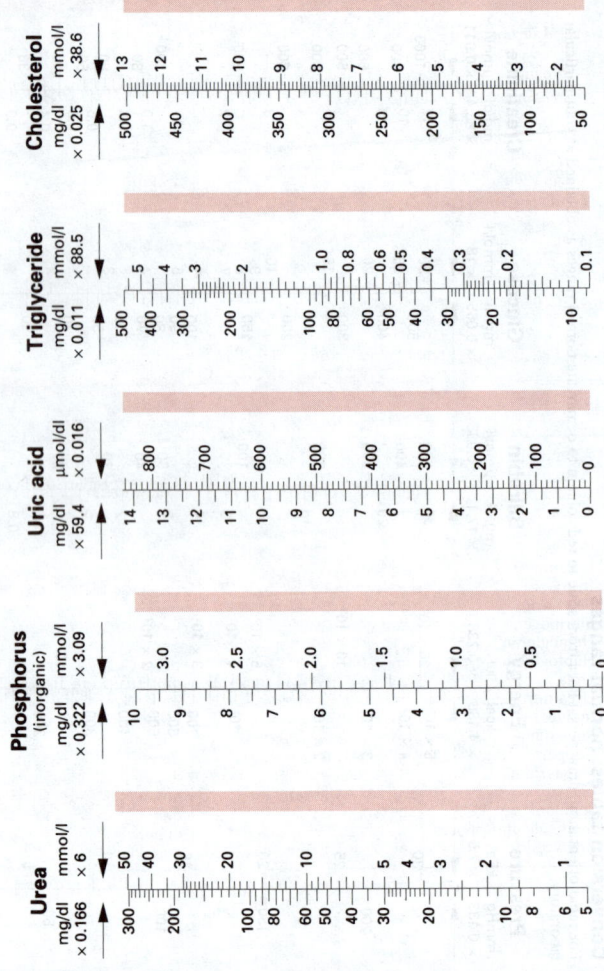

BASICS/NORMAL VALUES/DIAGNOSTIC METHODS

SI units: conversion of conventional and SI units

General formulas

$$\frac{\text{Weight (g, mg, µg, ng, pg)}}{\text{Atomic or molecular weight (MW)}} = \text{Mol (mol, nmol, µmol, pmol)}$$

$$\text{mol (or subunits)} \times \text{MW} = \text{g (or subunits)}$$

$$\frac{(\text{mg/dl}) \times 10}{\text{Atomic or molecular weight}} = \text{mmol/l} \qquad \frac{(\text{mmol/l}) \times \text{atomic or molecular weight}}{10} = \text{mg/dl}$$

$$\frac{\text{mval/l}}{\text{Valency}} = \text{mmol} \qquad \begin{array}{l} \text{single valency: Na, K, Cl, socium bicarbonate} \\ \text{double valency: Ca, Mg} \end{array}$$

$$\text{mg/dl} \times 0.01 = \text{g/l} \qquad \text{g/l} \times 100 = \text{mg/dl} \qquad \text{mg/dl} = \text{mg\%}$$

Individual conversions

Substance	Multiplication factor to convert old units to SI units	Multiplication factor to convert SI units to old units
Albumin	g% × 144.9 = µmol/l	µmol/l × 0.0069 = g%
Ammonia	µg% × 0.5872 = µmol/l	µmol/l × 1.703 = µg%
Ceruloplasmin	mg% × 0.0625 = µmol/l	µmol/l × 16 = mg%
Calcium	mg% × 0.2495 = mmol/l	mmol/l × 4.008 = mg%
Chloride	mg% × 0.2821 = mmol/l	mmol/l × 3.545 = mg%
Cortisol	µg% × 27.59 = nmol/l	nmol/l × 0.03625 = µg%
Creatinine	mg% × 88.4 = µmol/l	µmol/l × 0.01131 = mg%
Iron	µg% × 0.1791 = µmol/l	µmol/l × 5.585 = µg%
Fatty acids	mg% × 0.0354 = mmol/l	mmol/l × 28.25 = mg%
Fibrinogen	mg% × 0.02941 = µmol/l	µmol/l × 34 = mg%
Hemoglobin	g% × 0.6206 = mmol/l	mmol/l × 1.611 = g%
Haptoglobin	mg% × 0.1176 = µmol/l	µmol/l × 8.5 = mg%
Urea	mg% × 0.1665 = mmol/l	mmol/l × 6.006 = mg%
Urea nitrogen	mg% × 0.357 = mmol/l	mmol/l × 2.801 = mg%
Iodine	µg% × 78.8 = nmol/l	nmol/l × 0.01269 = µg%
Potassium	mg% × 0.2557 = mmol/l	mmol/l × 3.91 = mg%
Copper	µg% × 0.1574 = µmol/l	µmol/l × 6.355 = µg%
Magnesium	mg% × 0.4114 = mmol/l	mmol/l × 2.431 = mg%
Lactate	mg% × 0.111 = mmol/l	mmol/l × 9.008 = mg%
Sodium	mg% × 0.435 = mmol/l	mmol/l × 2.299 = mg%
Inorganic phosphorus	mg% × 0.3229 = mmol/l	mmol/l × 3.097 = mg%
Triglyceride	mg% × 0.01129 = mmol/l	mmol/l × 88.54 = mg%

MEMORIX PEDIATRICS

Basic and derived SI units

SI = International system of units. The appropriate symbols are printed in red. Old units are included, for conversion, in the 'Equivalent units and conversions' column.

Measurement (Symbol)	Name of unit	Abbreviation of unit name	Equivalent units and conversions	Subunits
Time (t)	second	s		ks, ms, µs, a, d, h, min
Mass (m)	kilogram	kg		g, mg, µg, ng, pg
Mass concentration		kg/l		g/l, mg/l, µg/l, ng/l
Volume (V)	cubic metre litre	m^3 l	1 m^3 = 1000 l	mm^3, $µm^3$, nm^3, ml, µl, nl, pl, fl
Quantity	mole	mol		mmol, µmol, nmol
Molarity	mole/cubic metre	mol/m^3	1 mol/l = 10^3 mmol/l	
Molality	mole/kilogram	mol/kg		mmol/kg, µmol/kg
Force (F)	newton	N		
Pressure (p), sonic pressure	pascal megapascal	Pa MPa	1 Pa = 1 N/m^2 10^6 Pa = 10 bar (Bar) 1 mmHg = 133.32 Pa 1 Torr = 133.32 Pa	
	physical atmosphere	atm	1 atm = 760 Torr = 10 1325 Pa	
Surface tension (σ)		N/m	1 N/m = 10^3 dyn/cm	
Dynamic viscosity (η)	pascal second	Pa × s	Liquidity 1 Pa × s	
Kinematic viscosity (v)		m^2/s	Compressed 1 kg/m^3	
Work, energy, heat, radiation	joule	J	J × 0.2388 → cal J ← cal × 4.1868	
Performance, heat-current, energy-current (P)	watt	W	= J/s = N m s^{-1}	
Action	joule second	Js	= J × s	

BASICS/NORMAL VALUES/DIAGNOSTIC METHODS

Thermodynamic temperature (T)	Kelvin	K	$1\,K = 1\,°C = \frac{9}{5}\,°F$ $273.15\,K = 0\,°C$ $K = °C + 273.15$ $°C = K - 273.15$ $°Fahrenheit = \frac{9}{5}\,°C + 32$ $°C = \frac{5}{9}(°F - 32)$
Magnetic induction flow (φ)	weber	Wb	= volts × seconds (V s)
Magnetic induction (B)	tesla	T	= Wb/m²
Electric tension (U)	volt	V	
Electric current strength (I)	ampere	A	
Electric loading (Q)	coulomb	C	= A s
Electrical resistance	ohm	Ω	= V/A
Electrical conductance	siemens	S	= A/V
Light current	lumen	lm	
Light power	candela	cd	
Light strength	lux	lx	lx = lm/m²
Frequency	hertz	Hz	
Sound level	decibel	dB	
Activity (radioactivity)	becquerel	Bq	$3.7 \times 10^{10} = 1\,Ci$ (Curie)
Absorbed (energy) dose Equivalent dose	gray	Gy J/kg	$1\,Gy = 100\,rd$ (rad) $1\,Gy = 1\,J/kg$
Absorbed energy dose performance, absorbed energy dose rate, equivalent dose performance, equivalent dose rate dose rate		Gy/s	= 100 rd/s
Ionic dose	coulomb/kg	C/kg	$2.58\,C/kg = 10^4\,R$ (roentgen)
Ion dose performance, ion dose rate	ampere/kg	A/kg	$2.58\,A/kg = 10^4\,R/s$

MEMORIX PEDIATRICS

Reference values for blood (B), plasma (P), serum (S), CSF, urine, feces and sweat
(From Dörner (1990); Nathan and Oski (1981); Thomas (1988); Sitzmann (1976).)

Substance/cells (Material) Method	Age group	Reference values (x̄ + 2 SD) SI units	Conventional units	Remarks and clinical value
Acetylsalicylic acid (ASA) (S) Salicylic acid (SA) (S)		1.1–2.2 mmol/l	15–30 mg/dl	ASA: ASA → SA SA: Steady state after 1–5 d, blood taken 1–3 h after oral dosage
Adrenaline (24 h urine) HPLC*	3–6 y	13.1 (4.9–27.3) nmol/d 6.6 (2.9–13.1) µmol/mol Creatinine	2.4 (0.9–5.0) µg/d 9.2 (4.1–18.3) µg/g Creatinine	
	6–10 y	22.4 (10.9–53.5) nmol/d 6.4 (2.0–11.9) µmol/mol Creatinine	4.1 (2.0–9.8) µg/d 9.0 (4.1–16.6) µg/g Creatinine	
	10–16 y	26.2 (8.7–51.3) nmol/d 4.7 (1.3–8.7) µmol/mol Creatinine	4.8 (1.6–9.4) µg/d 6.5 (1.8–12.2) µg/g Creatinine	
Aldolase (S)	4–8 d 2–3 months 4–12 months 2–6 y 7–15 y		6.4 (0.6–12.2) U/l 3.8 (→ 7.7) U/l 3.1 (0.6–5.6) U/l 2.4 (0.6–4.2) U/l 2.4 (1.0–3.8) U/l	
Ammonia (EDTA, heparin, P)*	1 d 5–6 d Schoolchildren	97 (30–144) µmol/l 67 (53–144) µmol/l 36 (24–48) µmol/l	165 (51–245) µg/dl 114 (53–144) µg/dl 61 (41–82) µg/dl	NB: ammonia released in clotting
Amylase (S)	Infants Older children	→ 40 U/l → 50 U/l		
Anion gap (P)		7–16 mmol/l		
Antithrombin III (Citrate, P) Immunodiffusion			♀ 28.6 (21–57) mg/dl ♂ 34.2 (26–53) mg/dl	
Alpha, antitrypsin (S) Nephelometry	0–7 d 8 d–12 months >1 y		200–400 mg/dl 130–240 mg/dl 130–300 mg/dl	
Apolipoprotein A I Apolipoprotein A II Apolipoprotein B	1–7 d Older children Children 1–7 d Older children		76 (22–130) mg/dl 118 (42–194) mg/dl 44 (18–70) mg/dl 53 (9–90) mg/dl 86 (74–98) mg/dl	
Bilirubin (S)	Infants Older Children	4.89 (1.73–13.8) µmol/l 6.05 (1.7–21.5) µmol/l	0.3 (0.1–0.8) mg/dl 0.4 (0.1–1.3) mg/dl	} Direct bilirubin negative
Blood volume	Neonates 10–18 y	**Plasma volume** 41 ml/kg 51 ml/kg	**Total erythrocyte volume** 43 ml/kg 26 ml/kg	

* HPLC, high pressure liquid chromatography; EDTA, ethylenediamine tetra-acetic acid.

BASICS/NORMAL VALUES/DIAGNOSTIC METHODS

Substance/cells (Material)* Method	Age group	Reference values ($\bar{x} \pm 2$ SD) SI units	Reference values ($\bar{x} \pm 2$ SD) Conventional units	Remarks and clinical values
Calcium (S)	Neonates	2.27 (1.76–2.78) mmol/l	9.1 (7.1–11.1) mg/dl	
	Infants	2.39 (2.04–2.73) mmol/l	9.6 (8.2–10.9) mg/dl	
	Older children	2.35 (2.09–2.61) mmol/l	9.4 (8.4–10.5) mg/dl	
Ionized calcium (S)	3 d	1.10 (1.03–1.17) mmol/l	4.42 (4.14–4.70) mg/dl	
	3 months	1.15 (1.07–1.24) mmol/l	4.62 (4.28–4.96) mg/dl	
	6 months–6 y	1.15 (1.06–1.24) mmol/l	4.60 (4.24–4.96) mg/dl	
	6–16 y	1.14 (1.04–1.25) mmol/l	4.58 (4.16–5.00) mg/dl	
	16–20 y	1.10 (1.00–1.20) mmol/l	4.40 (4.0–4.80) mg/dl	
Calcium (urine)	Schoolchildren	116 (14–492) µmol/mol Creatinine	41 (5–174) µg/mg Creatinine	Morning urine (8 h)
Chloride (S)	Neonates	105 (95.2–116) mmol/l		
	Infants	103 (92.9–112) mmol/l		
	Older children	103 (94.5–111) mmol/l		
(CSF)	→ 3 months	108–123 mmol/l		
	→ 1 y	113–127 mmol		
	→ 12 y	117–131 mmol		
(Urine)	1 d	0.43 (0.07–0.79) mmol/kg × d		
	7 d	0.44 (0.08–0.8) mmol/kg × d		Breast milk
		2.99 (1.25-4.73) mmol/kg × d		Cows' milk
	Infants	1.61 (0.53–2.69) mmol/kg × d		
	2 y	3.49 (1.59–5.39) mmol/kg × d		
	4–5 y	3.26 (0.28–6.24) mmol/kg × d		
	6–10 y	73.3 (61.7–84.9) mmol/kg		♂
		40.8 (32.6–49.0) mmol/kg		♀
	10–14 y	120 (104–136) mmol/d		♂
		105 (80.6–129) mmol/d		♀
(Sweat)	Infants	12.3 (2.5–22.1) mmol/l		
	1–10 y	15.3 (0–31.5) mmol/l		
	10–16 y	19.9 (1.5–38.3) mmol/l		
Cholesterol (total) (S) (Enzymatic)	Neonates	1.94 (0.97–3.63) mmol/l	75 (38–140) mg/dl	
	Infants	3.52 (2.34–4.98) mmol/l	136 (90–193) mg/dl	
	2–5 y	4.31 (1.95–6.3) mmol/l	167 (75–244) mg/dl	
	6–9 y	4.54 (3.1–6.63) mmol/l	176 (120–246) mg/dl	
	10–12 y	4.47 (2.66–6.25) mmol/l	173 (103–242) mg/dl	
	>12 y	4.18 (2.57–5.79) mmol/l	162 (99–224) mg/dl	
HDL cholesterol (S) Electrophoresis	Neonates	0.78 (0.34–1.37) mmol/l	30 (13–53) mg/dl	
	5–18 y	1.22 (0.57–2.3) mmol/l	47 (22–89) mg/dl	
LDL cholesterol (S)	Neonates	2.07 (1.16–3.03) mmol/l	80 (45–117) mg/dl	
	5–18 y	3.4 (1.53–5.61) mmol/l	132 (59–217) mg/dl	
Cholinesterase (S)	1–15 y		5.8 (3.5–8.5) kU/l	
Chymotrypsin (feces)	Children Youths		20.8 (4.5–43.5) U/g	
Ceruloplasmin (S)	Neonates		14 (6–20) mg/dl	
	Schoolchildren		31 (23–43) mg/dl	
C-reactive protein (S) Nephelometry	1–3 d		≤1.2 mg/dl	
	≥4 d		← 0.6 mg/dl	
Dopamine (24 h urine) HPLC	3–6 y	1.06 (0.25–1.31) µmol/d	163 (38–309) µg/d	
		516 (205–852) µmol/mol Creatinine	603 (239–995) µg/g Creatinine	
	6–10 y	1.31 (0.28–2.22) µmol/d	200 (43–340) µg/d	
		410 (73.7–690) µmol/mol Creatinine	479 (86–806) µg/g Creatinine	
	10–16 y	1.91 (1.41–2.62) µmol/d	292 (216–401) µg/d	
		339 (200–586) µmol/mol Creatinine	396 (234–684) µg/g Creatinine	

* B, blood; P, plasma; S, serum.

MEMORIX PEDIATRICS

Substance/cells (Material)* Method	Age group	Reference values ($\bar{x} \pm 2$ SD) SI units	Conventional units	Remarks and clinical values
Iron (S)	14 d	11–36 µmol/l	63–201 µg/dl	
	6 months	5–24 µmol/l	28–135 µg/dl	
	1 y	6–28 µmol/l	35–155 µg/dl	
	2–12 y	4–24 µmol/l	22–135 µg/dl	
Iron binding capacity (S)	14 d	34 (18–50) µmol/l	191 (105–277) µg/dl	
	6 months	58 (40–76) µmol/l	321 (219–423) µg/dl	
	1 y	64 (50–78) µmol/l	358 (282–434) µg/dl	
	Older children	59 (43–76) µmol/l	331 (239–423) µg/dl	

Protein electrophoresis (S) Ponceau S stain (S) (If amido black 10 B stain is used, values are higher)			Albumin	α_1-globulin	α_2-globulin	β-globulin	γ-globulin
	Neonates	(g/l, rel. %)	37.1 (32.7–45.3) 68.1%	1.7 (1.1–2.5) 3.1%	4.2 (2.6–5.7) 7.7%	4.2 (2.5–5.6) 7.6%	7.4 (3.9–11.0) 13.5%
	Infants		49.2 (35.7–51.3) 69.6%	1.7 (1.3–2.5) 2.7%	6.2 (3.8–10.8) 10.0%	5.3 (3.5–7.1) 8.7%	5.6 (2.9–11.0) 9.0%
	1–2.5 y		45.1 (36.5–53.3) 67.0%	1.9 (1.1–2.9) 2.8%	6.9 (4.9–9.4) 10.3%	5.9 (4.3–7.9) 8.7%	7.5 (4.7–11.8) 11.2%
	2.5–6 y		45.6 (33.1–52.2) 67.4%	1.9 (0.9–2.9) 2.7%	6.6 (4.3–9.5) 9.7%	5.9 (3.5–7.6) 8.8%	7.7 (4.5–12.1) 11.4%
	Schoolchildren		46.0 (40.0–52.5) 67.4%	1.8 (1.2–2.5) 2.6%	6.4 (4.3–8.6) 8.4%	5.7 (4.1–7.9) 8.3%	8.4 (5.9–13.7) 12.3%

CSF protein electrophoresis	Children		(g/l, rel. %)	
		Pre-albumin	8 (3–13)%	
		Albumin	59 (40–70)%	
		α_1-globulin	4 (2–9.5)%	
		α_2-globulin	6.5 (3.5–12)%	
		β-globulin	10 (7–14.5)%	
		τ-globulin	4 (2–7)%	
		$\beta + \tau$-globulin	14 (9–21.5)%	
		γ-globulin	7.5 (3–13)%	

Total protein (S) Biuret reaction	Neonates		5.69 (4.52–6.86) mg/dl	
	Infants		5.95 (4.57–7.33) mg/dl	
	Older children		6.93 (5.85–8.01) mg/dl	
(24 h urine)	All ages		≤150 mg/1.73 m² · d	
CSF	All ages		≤40 mg/dl	

Erythrocyte fragility (Osmotic resistance) Heparin, blood	All ages		0.46–0.42% NaCl 0.34–0.30% NaCl	Early lysis Complete lysis

Erythrocyte parameters (EDTA, blood)		No. × 10⁶/µl	MCV (µm³)*	MCH (pg)*	MCHC (g/dl)*
	Birth	3.9–6.5	98–118	31–37	30–36
	1–3 d	4–6.6	95–121	31–37	29–37
	7 d	3.9–6.2	88–126	28–40	28–38
	14 d	3.6–6.2	86–119	28–40	28–38
	1 month	3.0–5.4	85–123	28–40	29–37
	2 months	2.7–4.9	77–118	26–34	29–37
	3–6 months	3.1–4.5	74–108	25–35	30–36
	0.5–2 y	3.7–5.3	70–86	23–31	30–36
	2–6 y	3.9–5.3	75–87	24–30	31–37
	6–12 y	4.0–5.2	77–95	25–33	31–37
	♀ 12–18 y	4.1–5.1	78–102	25–35	31–37
	♂ 12–18 y	4.5–5.3	78–98	25–35	31–37

Ferritin (S)	14 d		23.8 (9–62.8) µg/dl	
	1 month		24.0 (14.4–39.9) µg/dl	
	2 months		19.4 (8.7–43.0) µg/dl	
	4 months		9.1 (3.7–22.3) µg/dl	
	6 months		5.1 (1.9–14.2) µg/dl	
	9 months		3.9 (1.4–10.3) µg/dl	
	12 months		3.1 (1.1–9.1) µg/dl	
	1–10 y		4.3 (1.5–11.9) µg/dl	

* B, blood; P, plasma; S, serum; EDTA, ethylenediamine tetra-acetic acid; MCV, mean corpuscular volume; MCH, mean corpuscular hemoglobin; MCHC, mean corpuscular hemoglobin concentration.

BASICS/NORMAL VALUES/DIAGNOSTIC METHODS

Substance/cells (Material)* Method	Age group	Reference values ($\bar{x} \pm 2$ SD) SI units	Conventional units	Remarks and clinical values
α₁ Fetoprotein (S) Radioimmunoassay Enzyme immunoassay	Prematures Neonates → 14 d 14–28 d 6 months		13.4 (9.0–21.8) mg/dl 4.8 (2.0–11.8) mg/dl 3.3 (1.0–9.8) mg/dl 0.95 (0.05–3.5) mg/dl 1.3 (0.5–3.2) µg/dl	
Fat excretion (Feces)			<4.5 g/d	5 day feces after 5 g/kg fat
Fatty acids (free) (P)	Neonates 4 months–10 y	435–1375 µmol/l 500–900 µmol/l		14 h fasting
Folic acid (P), (S) Radioimmunoassay		4.3–23.6 nmol/l	1.9–14.0 ng/ml	
Fructose (B) (Urine)	Neonates Infants Older children	<10 mg/dl → 3.9 mmol/l → 1.1 mmol/l → 0.06 mmol/l	<0.6 mmol/l → 70 mg/d → 20 mg/d → 10 mg/d	Fasting value
Galactokinase (B)	Neonates >1 y	102 (89–121) nmol/min × gHb 28.2 (21–35) nmol/min × gHb		
Galactose-1-phosphate Uridyltransferase (B)	All ages	30.3 (24–33) µmol/h × gHb		
Galactose (S)	Neonates Older children	→ 350 µmol/l 127 (0–410) µmol/l	→ 6 mg/dl 2.3 (0–7.4) mg/dl	Postprandial
Bile acids (total) (S)	1–7 d 7–30 d 1–9 months 2 y 4 y >4 y	9.5 (1.96–17.0) µmol/l 11.8 (5.54–18.1) µmol/l 6.14 (1.2–11.1) µmol/l 2.93 (0–6.09) µmol/l 3.80 (0–8.14) µmol/l 4.25 (1.49–7.01) µmol/l	3.9 (0.8–6.9) mg/l 4.8 (2.3–7.4) mg/l 2.5 (0.5–4.5) mg/l 1.2 (0–2.5) mg/l 1.6 (0–3.3) mg/l 1.7 (0.6–2.9) mg/l	
Clotting factors (Citrate, P) Fibrinogen	1 d >1 d		245 (190–300) mg/dl 315 (255–375) mg/dl **Adult values (100%) will be attained**	
Factor II Factor V Factor VII Factor VIII Factor IX Factor X Factor XI Factor XII Factor XIII Antithrombin III Plasminogen Protein C Protein S	Neonates Neonates Neonates Neonates Neonates Neonates Neonates Neonates Neonates Neonates Neonates Neonates Neonates	45 (30–60)% 100 (60–140)% 55 (40–70)% 105 (70–140)% 30 (20–40)% 55 (40–70)% 30% 50% 100 (70–130)% 45 (30–80)% 50% 35 (20–50)% 35 (10–60)%	after 6 months at birth after 6 months at birth after 6 months from the 2nd month after 6 mohths from the 2nd month at birth after 3–6 months after 6 months after 12 months after 6 months	In premature neonates, factors II, V, VII, VIII, and XII are markedly lowered (in comparison with mature neonates)
Fibrin split products	All ages	<10 µg/ml		
Quick test (Thromboplastin time)	Neonates >14 d	80 (40–100)% 70–100%		
Partial thrombo- plastin time (PTT)	<6 months Older children	38 (30–47) s 33 (25–41) s		
Thrombin time (Plasma thrombin time)	>1 month	9–11 s		Dependent on thrombin activity

* B, blood; P. plasma; S, serum.

MEMORIX PEDIATRICS

Substance/cells (Material)* Method	Age group	Reference values ($\bar{x}$ + 2 SD) SI units	Reference values ($\bar{x}$ + 2 SD) Conventional units	Remarks and clinical values
Glucose (B)	1 d 2 d 5 d Infants Others	2.22¹–5.55 mmol/l 2.22¹–5.0 mmol/l 2.22¹–4.16 mmol/l 3.33–5.0 mmol/l 3.33–5.55 mmol/l	40¹–100 mg/dl 40¹–90 mg/dl 40¹–75 mg/dl 60–90 mg/dl 60–100 mg/dl	¹Lower limits fixed for neuro-energy grounds
Glucose-6-phosphate dehydrogenase (B)		131 (105–157) mU/10⁶ Erythrocytes		
Glucose tolerance test (B)	Schoolchildren	1 h value: ≤8.3 mmol/l Δ 150 mg/dl 2 h value: ≤7.3 mmol/l Δ 131 mg/dl		Oral: 2 g/kg oligo-saccharide
Glutamate dehydrogenase GLDH (S)	Neonates 1–6 months 7–12 months 2–3 y 3–5 y Schoolchildren		1.9 (0–6.6) U/l 1.5 (0–4.3) U/l 0.9 (0–3.5) U/l 0.9 (0–2.6) U/l → 3.2 U/l → 3.5 U/l	
Serum glutamic-oxaloacetic transaminase (S)	Neonates Infants Older children		21.9 (5.91–37.9) U/l 17.3 (7.38–27.3) U/l 13.4 (4.7–22.2) U/l	
Serum glutamic-pyruvic transaminase (S)	Neonates Infants Older children		12.4 (4.47–32.4) U/l 14.9 (6.23–35.7) U/l 9.61 (4.5–20.5) U/l	
γ-Glutamyl transpeptidase (S)	Neonates 2–3 months from 4 months		47.8 (13.9–163) U/l 13.3 (1.95–90.8) U/l 7.32 (3.1–17.3) U/l	
Hematocrit (EDTA, B)	1 d 7 d 14 d 1 month 2 months 3–6 months 0.5–2 y 2–6 y 6–12 y 12–18 y		58 (45–72)% 55 (43–67)% 50 (42–66)% 43 (31–55)% 35 (28–42)% 35 (29–41)% 36 (33–39)% 37 (34–40)% 40 (35–45)% 41 (36–46)% 43 (37–49)%	♀ ♂
Hemoglobin (total) (EDTA, B)	1 d 7 d 14 d 1 month 2 months 3–6 months 0.5–2 y 2–6 y 6–12 y 12–18 y	12.1 (9.0–14.5) mmol/l 10.9 (8.7–13.7) mmol/l 10.2 (8.1–12.4) mmol/l 8.7 (6.2–11.1) mmol/l 7.1 (5.6–8.7) mmol/l 7.1 (5.9–8.4) mmol/l 7.5 (6.5–8.4) mmol/l 7.8 (7.1–8.4) mmol/l 8.4 (7.1–9.6) mmol/l 8.7 (7.5–9.9) mmol/l 9.0 (8.1–9.9) mmol/l	19.5 (14.5–23.4) g/dl 17.5 (14.0–22.0) g/dl 16.5 (13.0–20.0) g/dl 14.0 (10.0–18.0) g/dl 11.5 (9.0–14.0) g/dl 11.5 (9.5–13.5) g/dl 12.0 (10.5–13.5) g/dl 12.5 (11.5–13.5) g/dl 13.5 (11.5–15.5) g/dl 14.0 (12.0–16.0) g/dl 14.5 (13.0–16.0) g/dl	♀ ♂
Hemoglobin A₂ (EDTA, B) Column chromatography	Neonates 1 month 2 months 3 months 5 months 6 months Older children		0.19–0.6% 0.71–1.38% 1.08–2.01% 1.44–2.08% 1.50–2.38% 1.60–2.40% 2.08–3.17	

* B, blood; P, plasma; S, serum; EDTA, ethylenediamine tetra-acetic acid.
¹ ••.

BASICS/NORMAL VALUES/DIAGNOSTIC METHODS

Substance/cells (Material)* Method	Age group	Reference values ($\bar{x} + 2$ SD) SI units	Conventional units	Remarks and clinical values
Hb A$_{1a-c}$ (glycosylated Hb) (EDTA, B)	6–12 months → 2 y → 4 y 5–12 y 13–20 y		10.0 (5.4–14.6)% 9.2 (7.0–11.4)% 7.7 (5.7–9.7)% 7.1 (5.3–8.9)% 7.1 (5.5–8.7)%	
Carboxyhemoglobin (HbCO) (B)		1.2% of total Hb		
Hemoglobin electrophoresis HB F (EDTA, B) Alkali denaturing	Neonates Adults 7 d 1 month 2 months 3 months 4 months 6 months 1 y	**Hb A$_2$** 17.3 (13.1–22.3)% 2.5% 97%	**Hb A$_2$** 0.25 (0.05–0.45)% 2.5% 60.1 (51.4–68.3)% 45.5 (30.3–58.3)% 26.6 (18.8–39.2)% 14.5 (4.5–27.1)% 9.6 (0.2–15.9)% 1.0 (0–8.4)% ≤1.3%	**Hb F** 81.7 (77.5–85.9)% 0.5%
Hb Fe^{3+} (methemoglobin) (B)	Neonates Infants Older children	0–0.37 mmol/l 0–0.19 mmol/l 0–0.2 mmol/l	0–0.58 g/dl 0–0.29 g/dl 0–0.33 g/dl	
Haptoglobin (S) Nephelometry	→ 7 d → 1 y Older children		→ 40 mg/dl → 110 mg/dl 10–140 mg/dl	
Urine – erythrocytes – leukocytes – volume/24 h	 → 6 months → 2 y → 7 y → 15 y >15 y	<5/µl <10/µl 35 ml/kg × d 200 ml/d 400 ml/d 800 ml/d → 2000 ml/d		Morning urine Morning urine
Uric acid (S) (Urine)	Neonates Infants Older children 7 d 1 y 2 y 6 y 10 y 18 y	182 (38.2–326) µmol/l 197 (68.1–325) µmol/l 232 (111–353) µmol/l **g Uric acid/g creatinine** 1.55 (0.18–2.91) 1.45 (0.62–2.27) 2.37 (0.85–2.01) 0.88 (0.59–1.26) 0.61 (0.22–1.00) 0.40 (0.16–0.69)	3.1 (0.6–5.5) mg/dl 3.3 (1.1–5.5) mg/dl 3.9 (1.9–5.9) mg/dl **mol Uric acid/ mol creatinine** 1.04 (0.12–1.96) 0.98 (0.42–1.53) 1.60 (0.57–1.35) 0.59 (0.30–0.85) 0.41 (0.15–0.67) 0.30 (0.11–0.52)	Dependent on nutritive purine load
Urea–N (S) (Urine)	Neonates Infants Older children Neonates Infants Small children Schoolchildren	3.93 (1.06–6.79) mmol/l 4.60 (2.04–7.17) mmol/l 5.06 (2.12–8.0) mmol/l	11.0 (3.0–19.0) mg/dl 12.9 (5.7–20.1) mg/dl 14.2 (6.0–22.5) mg/dl 0.15–1.0 g/d 1.0–4.0 g/d 4.0–8.0 g/d 8.0–20.0 g/d	Urea–N × 2.14 = urea
Homovanillic acid (24 h urine) HPLC	3–6 y 6–10 y 10–16 y	14.3 (7.7–23.6) µmol/l 6.1 (3.4–9.6) mmol/mol creatinine 19.8 (11.5–25.8) µmol/l 5.0 (2.7–7.1) mmol/mol creatinine 23.6 (13.2–47.7) µmol/l 3.3 (2.0–6.4) mmol/mol creatinine	2.6 (1.4–4.3) mg/d 9.9 (5.4–15.5) mg/g creatinine 3.6 (2.1–4.7) mg/d 8.0 (4.4–11.5) mg/g creatinine 4.3 (2.4–8.7) mg/d 5.3 (3.3–10.3) mg/g creatinine	

* B, blood; P, plasma; S, serum; EDTA, ethylenediamine tetra-acetic acid; Hb, hemoglobin; HPLC, high pressure liquid chromatography.

MEMORIX PEDIATRICS

Substance/cells (Material)* Method	Age group	Reference values ($\bar{x} \pm 2$ SD) SI units	Conventional units	Remarks and clinical values
Immunoglobulin (S) Nephelometry IgA	Neonates Infants 1–3 y Older children		<10 mg/dl 10–70 mg/dl 20–130 mg/dl 40–240 mg/dl	
IgG	7 d 1–12 weeks 3–12 months 1–3 y 4–7 y >8 y		700–2000 mg/dl 150–900 mg/dl 200–800 mg/dl 400–1300 mg/dl 600–1600 mg/dl 700–1800 mg/dl	
IgM	Neonates Infants 1–3 y Older children		<20 mg/dl 20–100 mg/dl 50–200 mg/dl 50–220 mg/dl	
IgE Enzyme immunoassay	Neonates Infants 1–5 y 6–9 y 10–15 y		→ 1.5 IU/ml → 15 IU/ml → 60 IU/ml → 90 IU/ml → 200 IU/ml	
Potassium (S) Flame photometry	Neonates Infants Older children	4.84 (3.56–6.11) mmol/l 4.74 (3.65–5.83) mmol/l 4.14 (3.13–5.15) mmol/l		
(Urine)	1 d 2 d 7 d	0.36 (0.08–0.5) mmol/kg × d 0.45 (0.17–0.93) mmol/kg × d 0.95 (0–2.25) mmol/kg × d 2.11 (0.51–3.71) mmol/kg × d		after breast milk after cows' milk
	1–6 months 1–2 y 4–5 y 6–10 y	2.27 (0–4.89) mmol/kg × d 4.06 (2.94–5.18) mmol/kg × d 2.33 (0.83–3.83) mmol/kg × d 22.5 (17.4–27.5) mmol/d 31.9 (27.0–36.7) mmol/d		♀ ♂
	10–14 y	38.0 (30.9–45.0) mmol/d 39.3 (34.4–44.3) mmol/d		♀ ♂
Complement (S) C1-inactivator Immune diffusion			36.9 (28–49) mg/dl	
C3-factor Nephelometry	Neonates 1–12 months 1–2 y Older children		60–220 mg/dl 60–150 mg/dl 80–170 mg/dl 80–120 mg/dl	
C4-factor Nephelometry	Neonates 1–12 months Older children		10–40 mg/dl 5–30 mg/dl 10–40 mg/dl	
CH 50 (Total hemolytic activity)			33 (20–50) U/l	
Creatinine (S) Jaffé's reaction	Neonates Infants Older children	53.5 (2.15–104) μmol/l 45.8 (9.71–81.8) μmol/l 55.7 (21.0–90.4) μmol/l	0.6 (0.02–1.2) mg/dl 0.5 (0.1–0.9) mg/dl 0.6 (0.2–1.0) mg/dl	
(24 h urine)	0–0.5 y 0.5–1 y 1–2 y 2–3 y 3–4 y 4–5 y 5–7 y 7–10 y 11–13 y >13 y	0.13–0.53 mmol/l 0.49–0.8 mmol/l 0.71–1.42 mmol/l 0.97–1.59 mmol/l 1.15–2.30 mmol/l 1.86–3.45 mmol/l 2.30–4.60 mmol/l 3.19–6.37 mmol/l 8.53 (7.01–10.1) mmol/l 71–265 μmol/kg × d	15–60 mg/d 55–90 mg/d 80–160 mg/d 110–180 mg/d 130–260 mg/d 210–390 mg/d 260–520 mg/d 360–700 mg/d 792–1140 mg/d 8–30 mg/kg × d	

* B, blood; P, plasma; S, serum.

BASICS/NORMAL VALUES/DIAGNOSTIC METHODS

Substance/cells (Material)* Method	Age group	Reference values ($\bar{x} \pm 2\,SD$) SI units	Reference values ($\bar{x} \pm 2\,SD$) Conventional units	Remarks and clinical values
Creatine clearance (S) (24 h urine)	5–7 d	50.6 (39.0–62.2) ml/min × 1.73 m²		
	1–2 months	64.6 (53.0–76.2) ml/min × 1.73 m²		
	3–4 months	85.8 (76.2–95.4) ml/min × 1.73 m²		
	5–8 months	87.7 (63.9–112) ml/min × 1.73 m²		
	9–12 months	86.9 (70.1–104) ml/min × 1.73 m²		
	3–6 y	130 (120–140) ml/min × 1.73 m²		
	7–13 y	136 (124–149) ml/min × 1.73 m²		
Creatine kinase CK (S)	Infants		47.7 (16.7–136) U/l	
	Older children		38.8 (15.6–93.8) U/l	
Creatine kinase MS	>4 months		0.5–5 U/l	
Copper (S)	0–0.5 y	3.1–11.0 µmol/l	20–70 µg/dl	
	6 y	14.1–19.8 µmol/l	90–190 µg/dl	
	Schoolchildren	10.3–21.4 µmol/l	66–136 µg/dl	
(Urine)	Schoolchildren	5.7–119 µmol/mol Creatinine	3.2–67 µg/g Creatinine	
Lactate (P)	1 h	0.9–2.7 mmol/l	8.1–24.3 mg/dl	
	5 h	0.9–2.0 mmol/l	8.1–18.0 mg/dl	
	1 d	0.8–1.2 mmol/l	7.2–10.8 mg/dl	
	7 d	0.5–1.4 mmol/l	4.5–12.6 mg/dl	
	Older children	0.9–1.8 mmol/l	8.1–16.2 mg/dl	
(CSF)		0.9–2.8 mmol/l	8–25 mg/dl	Fasting value
Lactate dehydrogenase LDH (S)	Neonates		410 (200–838) U/l	
	Infants		285 (156–521) U/l	
	Older children		213 (131–344) U/l	
Leucine aminopeptidase (S)	Neonates		15–33 U/l	
	1–6 months		13–39 U/l	
	7–12 months		15–35 U/l	
	1–2 y		13–31 U/l	
	2–3 y		12–31 U/l	
	Older children		14–36 U/l	

Leukocytes (EDTA, B)

(Count/µl, rel. %)

Age	Total count	Neutrophils	Lymphocytes	Monocytes	Eosinophils
Birth	18.1 (9.0–30.0)	11.0 (6.0–26.0) 61%	5.5 (2.0–11.0) 31%	1.1 6%	0.4 2%
12 h	22.8 (13.0–38.0)	15.5 (6.0–28.0) 68%	5.5 (2.0–11.0) 24%	1.2 5%	0.5 2%
1 d	18.9 (9.4–34.4)	11.5 (5.0–21.0) 61%	5.8 (2.0–11.5) 31%	1.1 6%	0.5 2%
7 d	12.2 (5.0–21.0)	5.5 (1.5–10.0) 45%	5.0 (2.0–17.0) 41%	1.1 9%	0.5 4%
14 d	11.4 (5.0–20.0)	4.5 (1.0–9.5) 40%	5.5 (2.0–17.0) 48%	1.0 9%	0.4 3%
1 month	10.8 (5.0–19.5)	3.8 (1.0–9.0) 35%	6.0 (2.5–16.5) 56%	0.7 7%	0.3 3%
6 months	11.9 (6.0–17.5)	3.8 (1.0–8.5) 32%	7.3 (4.0–13.5) 61%	0.5 5%	0.3 3%
1 y	11.4 (6.0–17.5)	3.5 (1.5–8.5) 31%	7.0 (4.0–10.5) 61%	0.6 5%	0.3 3%
2 y	10.6 (6.0–17.0)	3.5 (1.5–8.5) 33%	6.3 (3.0–9.5) 59%	0.5 5%	0.3 3%
4 y	9.1 (5.5–15.5)	3.8 (1.5–8.5) 42%	4.5 (2.0–8.0) 50%	0.5 5%	0.3 3%
6 y	8.5 (5.0–14.5)	4.3 (1.5–8.0) 51%	3.5 (1.5–7.0) 42%	0.4 5%	0.2 3%
8 y	8.3 (4.5–13.5)	4.4 (1.5–8.0) 53%	3.3 (1.5–6.8) 39%	0.4 4%	0.2 2%
10 y	8.1 (4.5–13.5)	4.4 (1.8–8.0) 54%	3.1 (1.5–6.5) 38%	0.4 4%	0.2 2%
16 y	7.8 (4.5–13.0)	4.4 (1.8–8.0) 57%	2.8 (1.2–5.2) 35%	0.4 5%	0.2 3%
21 y	7.4 (4.5–11.0)	4.4 (1.8–7.7) 59%	2.5 (1.0–4.8) 34%	0.3 4%	0.2 3%

Substance/cells	Age group	SI units	Conventional units	Remarks
Leukocytes (CSF)	Neonates	0–20/µl		
	Infants	0–5/µl		
	Older children	0–4/µl		
Lipase (S)	Neonates		→ 80 U/l	
	Older children		→ 115 U/l	

* B, blood; P, plasma; S, serum; EDTA, ethylenediamine tetra-acetic acid.

MEMORIX PEDIATRICS

Substance/cells (Material)* Method	Age group	Reference values ($\bar{x} \pm 2$ SD) SI units	Conventional units	Remarks and clinical values
Lipoprotein (S) Electrophoresis				
α-Lipoprotein	Schoolchildren		52.9 (34.9–68.2) rel. %	
Pre-β-lipoprotein	Schoolchildren		3.5 (0–12.9) rel. %	
β-Lipoprotein	Schoolchildren		42.5 (28.8–59.5) rel. %	
Magnesium (P) Absorption spectrometry	7 d	0.79 (0.58–0.99) mmol/l	1.91 (1.41–2.41) mg/dl	
	6–14 y	0.89 (0.73–1.05) mmol/l	2.15 (1.37–2.93) mg/dl	
Sodium (S)	Neonates	140 (132–147) mmol/l		
	Infants	136 (129–143) mmol/l		
	Older children	139 (132–145) mmol/l		
(CSF)	Schoolchildren	141 (131–159) mmol/l		
(Urine)	1 d	0.25 (0.11–0.39) mmol/kg × d		
	2 d	0.22 (0–0.56) mmol/kg × d		
	7 d	1.78 (0–4.36) mmol/kg × d		
		2.68 (1.62–3.74) mmol/kg × d		Breast milk
	1–6 months	0.79 (0–1.63) mmol/kg × d		Cows' milk
	1–2 y	3.36 (1.40–5.32) mmol/kg × d		
	4–5 y	3.12 (1.20–5.04) mmol/kg × d		
	6–10 y	44.6 (35.9–53.3) mmol/d		♀
		78.1 (66.4–89.9) mmol/d		♂
	10–14 y	108 (86.8–130) mmol/d		♀
		120 (103–136) mmol/d		♂
(Sweat)	Neonates	35–50 mmol/l		
	Infants	3–40 mmol/l		
	1–4 y	4–48 mmol/l		
	5–9 y	6–44 mmol/l		
	10–14 y	0–54 mmol/l		
Osmolality (S)		294 (285–303) mosm/l		
(CSF)		286 (280–292) mosm/l		
(Urine)		200–1300 mosm/kg		
Phosphate (inorganic phosphorus) (S)	Neonates	2.32 (1.56–3.08) mmol/l	7.2 (4.8–5.9) mg/dl	
	Infants	2.06 (1.58–2.54) mmol/l	6.4 (4.9–7.9) mg/dl	
	Older children	1.54 (1.09–2.00) mmol/l	4.8 (3.4–6.2) mg/dl	
(CSF)	7–10 y	0.41 (0.2–0.57) mmol/l	1.3 (0.6–1.8) mg/dl	GFR = glomerular filtration rate
(Urine)	Schoolchildren	1.8 (1.1–2.7) mmol/dl GFR	5.7 (3.3–8.2) mg/dl GFR	
Alkaline phosphatase (S)	1–7 d		150–300 U/l	
	8–14 d		190–450 U/l	
	15–21 d		180–430 U/l	
	22–28 d		180–450 U/l	
	2–6 months		245–470 U/l	
	7–12 months		274–460 U/l	
	13–24 months		220–450 U/l	
	3–6 y		233–380 U/l	
	7–11 y		250–358 U/l	
	12–15 y		250–340 U/l	
Acid phosphatase (S)	Neonates		10–57 U/l	
	1–6 months		10–45 U/l	
	7–12 months		10–35 U/l	
	2–9 y		10–29 U/l	
	10–14 y		10–27 U/l	
	15 y		10–22 U/l	
Phospholipids (S)	Neonates	1.94 (1.06–2.82) mmol/l	150 (82–218) mg/dl	
Pyruvate		45–91 μmol/l	0.4–0.8 mg/dl	Fasting value

* B, blood; P, plasma; S, serum.

BASICS/NORMAL VALUES/DIAGNOSTIC METHODS

Substance/cells (Material)* Method	Age group	Reference values ($\bar{x} \pm 2$ SD) SI units	Reference values ($\bar{x} \pm 2$ SD) Conventional units	Remarks and clinical values
Renin (EDTA, P)		2.15 (1.72–2.59) µg/l × h		Higher values in infants
Reticulocytes (EDTA, B)	1 d 7 d 14 d		20–60‰ 3–10‰ 0–10‰	
Platelets (B) automatic count		150–500 × 10³/µl		
Transferrin (S)	14 d 0.5–6 months 0.5–1 y 1–16 y >16 y		158–268 mg/dl 202–302 mg/dl 261–353 mg/dl 240–360 mg/dl 200–340 mg/dl	
Triglycerides (S)	Neonates Infants Small children 6–9 y 10–12 y Older children	0.66 (0.12–2.60) mmol/l 1.29 (0.50–2.32) mmol/l 1.04 (0.42–2.09) mmol/l 0.72 (0.32–1.39) mmol/l 0.74 (0.26–1.80) mmol/l 0.77 (0.33–1.70) mmol/l	58 (11–230) mg/dl 114 (44–205) mg/dl 92 (37–185) mg/dl 64 (28–123) mg/dl 65 (23–159) mg/dl 68 (29–150) mg/dl	
Vanillylmandelic acid (24 h urine)	Neonates 1–6 months 0.2–2 y 2–4 y 6–8 y 8–10 y 10–12 y 12–15 y	1.8 (0.6–3.0) µmol/d 3.2 (0.3–6.1) µmol/d 5.4 (3.0–7.8) µmol/d 8.1 (4.3–11.9) µmol/d 9.7 (6.3–13.1) µmol/d 11.7 (7.9–15.5) µmol/d 14.7 (9.1–20.3) µmol/d 18.8 (8.6–28.9) µmol/d	0.35 (0.11–0.59) mg/d 0.64 (0.06–1.22) mg/d 1.08 (0.60–1.56) mg/d 1.61 (0.85–2.37) mg/d 1.93 (1.25–2.61) mg/d 2.33 (1.57–3.09) mg/d 2.93 (1.81–4.05) mg/d 3.73 (1.71–5.75) mg/d	
Zinc (S) (Urine)	Neonates Schoolchildren Schoolchildren	11.6 (7.9–15.3) µmol/l 11.2 (7.6–13.3) µmol/l 12.6 (9.8–16.8) µmol/l 595 (155–1470) µmol/mol Creatinine	75.7 (51.7–99.7) µg/dl 73.5 (49.5–87) µg/dl 82.5 (63.8–110) µg/dl	♀ ♂

* B, blood; P, plasma; S, serum; EDTA, ethylenediamine tetra-acetic acid.

MEMORIX PEDIATRICS

Catheter sizes
French catheter scale (Charrière scale) 1 French (Fr) = 1 Charrière (Charr) = 1/3 mm

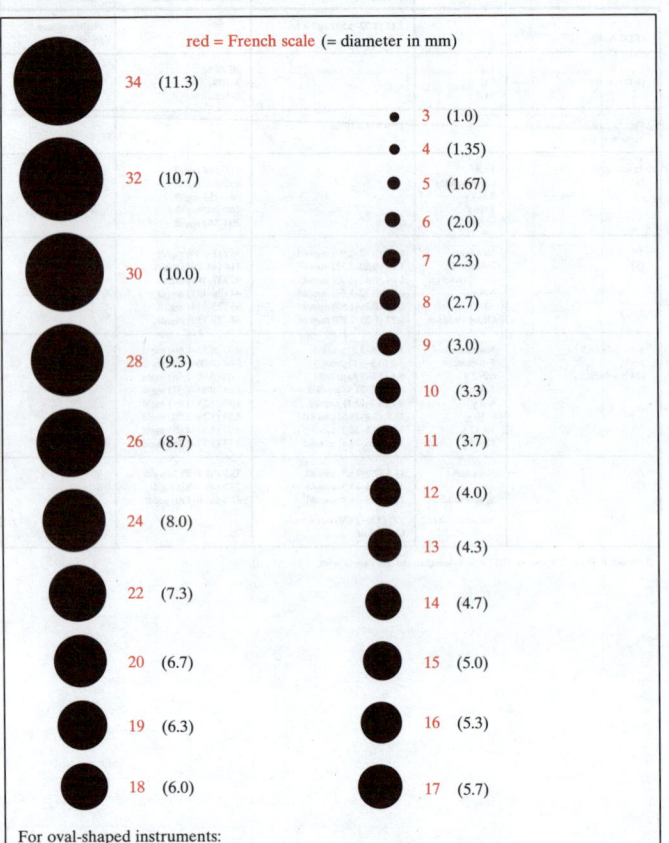

red = French scale (= diameter in mm)

French	(mm)
34	(11.3)
32	(10.7)
30	(10.0)
28	(9.3)
26	(8.7)
24	(8.0)
22	(7.3)
20	(6.7)
19	(6.3)
18	(6.0)

French	(mm)
3	(1.0)
4	(1.35)
5	(1.67)
6	(2.0)
7	(2.3)
8	(2.7)
9	(3.0)
10	(3.3)
11	(3.7)
12	(4.0)
13	(4.3)
14	(4.7)
15	(5.0)
16	(5.3)
17	(5.7)

For oval-shaped instruments:
lay a strip of lined paper around the circumference, and read off the value on the scale on the left.

0 5 10 15 20 25 30 35 40

BASICS/NORMAL VALUES/DIAGNOSTIC METHODS

Calculation of drip speed for infusions
(Approximate value for water solutions: 20 drops = 1 ml)

$$\text{Drops/min} = \frac{\text{infusion amount (ml)}}{\text{Infusion time (h)} \times 3}$$

Infusion-amount (ml)	½	1	2	3	4	5	6	7	8	9	10	11	12	14	16	18	20	22	24
							Drip count per min												
100	67	33	17	11	8	7	6	5	4										
200	133	67	33	22	17	13	11	10	8	7	7	6	5						
250	167	83	42	28	21	17	14	12	10	9	8	8	7	6	5		4	4	3
300	200	100	50	33	25	20	17	14	13	11	10	9	8	7	6	5	5	5	4
400	267	133	67	44	33	27	22	19	17	15	13	12	11	10	8	7	7	6	6
500	333	167	83	56	42	33	28	24	21	19	17	15	14	12	10	9	8	8	7
1000		333	167	111	83	67	56	48	42	37	33	30	28	24	21	19	17	15	14
1100		367	183	122	92	73	61	52	46	41	37	33	31	26	23	20	18	17	15
1200			200	133	100	80	67	57	50	44	40	36	33	29	25	22	20	18	17
1300			217	144	108	87	72	62	54	48	43	39	36	31	27	24	22	20	18
1400			233	156	117	93	78	67	58	52	47	42	39	33	29	26	23	21	19
1500			250	167	125	100	83	71	63	56	50	45	42	36	31	28	25	23	21
2000			333	222	167	133	111	95	83	74	67	61	56	48	42	37	33	30	28
2500				278	208	167	139	119	104	93	83	76	69	60	52	46	42	38	35
3000				333	250	200	167	143	125	111	100	91	83	71	63	56	50	45	42
4000					333	267	222	190	167	148	133	121	111	95	83	74	67	61	56

Prefixes for mutiplication and division of decimal units

Prefix	Symbol	Order of magnitude	Description
Exa	E	10^{18}	Million million million times
Peta	P	10^{15}	Thousand million million times
Tera	T	10^{12}	Million million times
Giga	G	10^{9}	Thousand million times
Mega	M	10^{6}	Million times
Kilo	k	10^{3}	Thousand times
Hecto	h	10^{2}	Hundred times
Deka	da	10^{1}	Ten times
Deci	d	10^{-1}	Tenth
Centi	c	10^{-2}	Hundredth
Milli	m	10^{-3}	Thousandth
Micro	µ	10^{-6}	Millionth
Nano	n	10^{-9}	Thousand millionth
Pico	p	10^{-12}	Million millionth
Femto	f	10^{-15}	Thousand million millionth
Atto	a	10^{-18}	Million million millionth

Conversion of Anglo-American units to the metric system and SI units

(Abbreviations in brackets)

Length
mile (mi) × 1.6093 = km
yard (yd) × 0.91440 = m
foot (ft) × 0.3048 = m
inch (in) × 2.54 = cm

Area
square inch (in^2) × 6.4516 = cm^2

Volume
cubic inch (in^3) × 16.387 = cm^3
fluid ounce (floz) × 28.413 = cm^3 (UK)
fluid ounce (floz) × 29.574 = cm^3 (USA)

Weight
pound (lb) × 453.59 = g

Strength
pound-force (lbf) × 4.4482 = N

Pressure
pound-force/square inch (psi) × 6894.76 = Pa

Work/Energy
foot-pound-force (ft lbf) × 1.35582 = J

Temperature
(Fahrenheit [°F] – 32) × 0.5555 = °C = $\dfrac{°F - 32}{1.8} = \dfrac{5}{9}(°F - 32)$

BASICS/NORMAL VALUES/DIAGNOSTIC METHODS

Diagnostic principle of ELISA
(enzyme-linked immunosorbent assay)

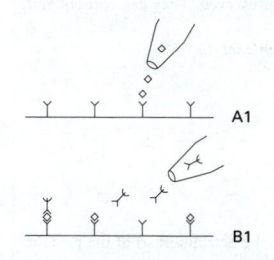

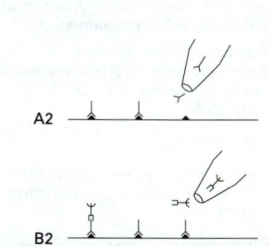

- Y Antibody (fixed)
- ▲ Antigen (fixed)
- ◇ Antigen (sample)
- λ Y Antibody (sample)
- Ψ Ψ Conjugated antibody enzyme
- °₀° Substrate/color complex

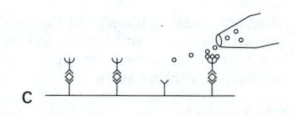

MEMORIX PEDIATRICS

DNA, RNA and protein analysis by the blot technique

Definition
Blotting is the delivery of DNA or proteins from a solution or a gel into a containing material (e.g. nitrocellulose sheet) in which they are preserved. They can consequently be used for qualified substantiation.

DNA analysis (Southern blot)
The technique used for RNA analysis is essentially the same and is called Northern blot.)

Protein analysis

① DNA isolation.

② Cutting into fragments (more than 1000 base pairs) using a restriction endonuclease.

③ Electrophoretic separation of the mixed fragments in a gel. The differing migration of the fragments depends on their length. Fragment length isolation.

③ Gel electrophoresis of the protein mix.

④ Southern transfer: transfer of the banded DNA pattern from the gel on to a nitrocellulose sheet through capillary or vacuum suction.

④ Southern transfer. In Western transfer the proteins migrate electrophoretically from the gel into the nitrocellulose sheet.

⑤ Southern blot.

⑤ Southern blot or Western blot.

⑥ Denaturing of the double strand DNA to single strand DNA.

⑥ Blocking of more free-binding fragments in the sheet with a known protein solution.

⑦ Hybridization with a gene probe. Gene probes are specific. Use DNA single strand fragment marked with a ^{32}P isotope.

⑦ Showing the required protein band by enzyme-immunoassay (binding on enzyme-labeled specific antibody + color reaction) or binding the proteins on antibodies (immunoblotting), excluding the complexes by enzyme immunoassay. Metallic colloids (gold, silver).

Ⓐ Wash out the noncomplement-bound DNA.

⑧ Demonstration of the required DNA base sequence by autoradiography.

⑧ Or with radioisotope-labeled anti-IgG-antibody.

BASICS/NORMAL VALUES/DIAGNOSTIC METHODS

DNA/RNA analysis   **Protein analysis**

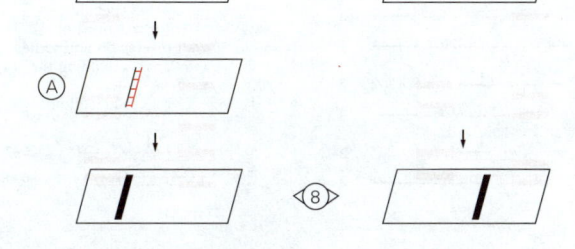

MEMORIX PEDIATRICS

Principle of the polymerase chain reaction (PCR)

PCR is the enzymatic increase (polymerase) of specific DNA segments of defined length (so-called target DNA). Before the PCR, RNA must be transcribed by the reverse transcriptase to DNA.

Reaction components: Heat-stable polymerase, two non-identical primers, deoxynucleotide (dATP, dGTP, dCTP, dTIP) for the polymerization and the target DNA as the matrix.

Technique: Cyclical repetition of three reaction steps:

A) Separation of the double-stranded DNA into complementary single strands by heating to 90–98°C.

B) Placing the primer on the target DNA matrix by cooling to 40–50°C. The primers are short DNA single strands of 20–25 bases (oligonucleotides). They place themselves in complementary fashion at definite positions on the target DNA sequence.

C) A DNA polymerase is used which, through basal pairing with the matrix DNA (target DNA), adds new nucleotides extending the primers in opposite directions.

With the third cycle, exponential increase in the target sequences commences. This technique can be used for all diagnostic methods in molecular biology.

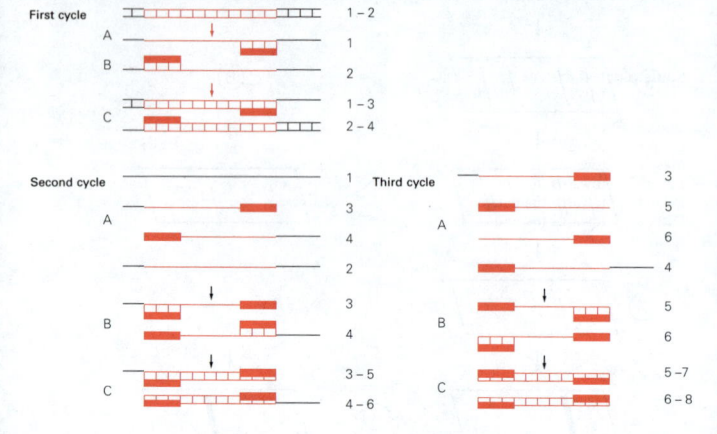

BASICS/NORMAL VALUES/DIAGNOSTIC METHODS

International double-digit dental chart
(After the Fédération Dentaire Internationale (1970).)
Encircled number = first digit; second digit = numbering of the teeth from the incisor to the molar. It is the patient's side that is referred to in each case.

Permanent teeth

① Top right   Top left ②

18	17	16	15	14	13	12	11	21	22	23	24	25	26	27	28
48	47	46	45	44	43	42	41	31	32	33	34	35	36	37	38

④ Bottom right   Bottom left ③

Primary (milk) teeth

⑤ Top right   Top left ⑥

55	54	53	52	51	61	62	63	64	65
85	84	83	82	81	71	72	73	74	75

⑧ Bottom right   Bottom left ⑦

Somatological sites for localization

	Direction			Direction
Buccal	towards the cheek		Apical	towards the root apex
Lingual	towards the tongue		Cervical	towards the tooth neck
Mesial	towards the midline of the mouth		Incisal	towards the cutting edge
Labial	towards the lips		Occlusal	towards/on the chewing area
Palatal	towards the palate		Proximal	the surface of a tooth in relation to its neighbor
Distal	towards the end of the row			

MEMORIX PEDIATRICS

Sequence of dentition (unilateral chart)

First dentition			Second dentition
Primary teeth		*Permanent teeth*	
Average and range (months)	5 4 3 2 1	1 2 3 4 5 6 7 8	Average and range (years)
8.6		○ ○ ○ ○ ○ ●	6.6
6–11.5	○	● ○ ○ ○ ○ ●	5–11
10.4	○	● ○ ○ ○ ○ ●	7.5
7.3–13.5	○	● ○ ○ ○ ○ ●	5.5–11.5
12.3	○ ○	● ● ○ ○ ○ ●	8.1
9–15.6	○	● ○ ○ ○ ○ ●	6–12
14.2	○ ○	● ● ○ ● ○ ●	10.2
10.9–17.5	○ ○	● ● ○ ○ ○ ●	6.5–14.5
15.5	○ ○ ○	● ● ○ ● ○ ●	10.8
12.2–18.81	○ ○	● ● ○ ● ○ ●	7–15
16.4	○ ○ ○	● ● ○ ● ● ●	11.2
13.2–19.2	○ ○ ○	● ● ● ● ○ ●	6.5–15
19.5	○ ○ ○ ○	● ● ● ● ● ●	11.8
15.9–23.1	○ ○ ○	● ● ● ● ● ●	7–15
19.9	○ ○ ○ ○	● ● ● ● ● ●	12.0
16.4–23.4	○ ○ ○ ○	● ● ● ● ● ●	8–15
25.0	○ ○ ○ ○ ○	● ● ● ● ● ●	12.6
22.1–27.5	○ ○ ○ ○ ○	● ● ● ● ● ●	9–15
		● ● ● ● ● ● ●	Variable
		● ● ● ● ● ● ●	>14

BASICS/NORMAL VALUES/DIAGNOSTIC METHODS

Epidemiological definitions

Morbidity: number of cases of a defined disease in a population within a defined period (weeks, months, years, or the end of an epidemic) = absolute M.
Relative M = disease cases/10 000 inhabitants of a defined population.
Mortality: number of deaths in a population resulting from a defined disease during a defined period = absolute M.
Relative M = number of deaths/10 000 inhabitants in a population.
Lethality: number of deaths (%) per 100 patients in a given period.
Prevalence: statistical measure of the number of individuals with a definite characteristic of a disease or the disease itself.

$$P = \frac{\text{Number of individuals with the characteristic of a disease or the disease itself}}{\text{Number of all individuals in a defined population}}$$

Incidence: dynamic measure for the frequency of a sign or an event occurring (or developing) during a defined period.

$$I = \frac{\text{Number of individuals in a defined population in a defined period who develop a sign or meet with an event}}{\text{Number of individuals in the same population within the same defined period who show the sign or are affected by the event}}$$

Examples of annual incidences

$$\text{Perinatal mortality} = \frac{\text{Number of deaths before, during and seven days after birth}}{1000 \text{ total births (dead and live)}}$$

$$\text{Neonatal mortality} = \frac{\text{Number of dead neonates (up to four weeks old)}}{1000 \text{ live births}}$$

$$\text{Infant deaths} = \frac{\text{Number who die in their first year}}{1000 \text{ live births}}$$

Note: In chronic diseases (e.g. TB) the prevalance is much higher than the incidence. Obversely, acute diseases (e.g. varicella) have a high incidence and a lower prevalence.

MEMORIX PEDIATRICS

Assessment of diagnostic tests

Characteristics of the validity of a test are its sensitivity and specificity.
Sensitivity: the percentage of patients with a true-positive diagnostic test (test result = A).
Specificity: the percentage of healthy people with a true-negative (test result = D).

Test result	Patients	Healthy
positive	A = true-positive	C = false-positive
negative	B = false-negative	D = true-negative

$$\text{Sensitivity}(\%) = \frac{A}{A+B} \times 100$$

$$\text{Specificity}(\%) = \frac{D}{D+C} \times 100$$

Positive predictive value: percentage of subjects with a positive test who are actually ill.

$$\text{Positive predictive value}(\%) = \frac{A}{A+C} \times 100$$

Negative predictive value: percentage of subjects with a negative test who are later found to be healthy.

$$\text{Negative predicitive value}(\%) = \frac{D}{D+B} \times 100$$

Predictive efficiency: proportion of test results that are correct (positive + negative) out of all test results.

$$\text{Predictive efficiency}(\%) = \frac{A+D}{A+B+C+D} \times 100$$

Statistical symbols

N	Test extent	s_r	Relative standard deviation
$\bar{x}$	Mean value	r	Correlation coefficient
s, SD	Standard deviation	V	Coefficient of variation
$s_{\bar{x}}$	Standard deviation of the mean		

BASICS/NORMAL VALUES/DIAGNOSTIC METHODS

Morphological terminology of developmental disorders

(From Spranger *et al.* (1982).)

Single morphological defects

Agenesis	Organ anlage absent.
Aplasia	Organ anlage present but no organ development.
Hypo-/hyperplasia	Under-/overdevelopment of a tissue, organ or organism through diminished or increased cell-count.
Dysplasia	Abnormal development of an individual tissue (dyshistogenesis) through variation in quantity relation (e.g. phacomatoses) or a functional defect of a single component (e.g. osteogenesis imperfecta).
Neoplasia	Clonal increase in certain cells.
Hypo-/hypertrophy	Decrease/increase in the size of cells, tissues and organs.
Atrophy	Decrease in a normally developed tissue or organ through reduction in cell size and cell count.
Malformation	Malformation is a genetically conditioned disorder in part of an organ, the whole organ or a body region.
Disruption	A morphological defect due to exogenous injury of a normal and until then normally developing organ or part.
	Causal agents: ischemia, infection, teratogenic substances, ionizing radiation.
Deformation	Variation in shape through mechanical forces in a primarily normally-sited and developing part of the body. After these forces have ceased, a return to normal shape is possible, e.g. in foot deformities.

Patterns of morphological defect

Polytopic area defect	Widely distributed morphological defects through disorder of a single blastogenetic or embryogenetic developmental factor through primary (malformation) or secondary (disruptive) malformation.
Sequence	Serial mutiple morphological developmental disorders as a consequence of a single malformation, disruption or deformation. Examples: Potter's syndrome, arthrogryposis.
Syndrome	Pattern of multiple anomalies considered to be pathogenetically connected but which cannot be classified as sequential or polytopic area defects. The term disease is used instead of syndrome if the cause of the anomalies is identifiable. Syndrome is dropped in favor of sequence if a uniform pathogenesis is known, and the term polytopic defect is employed if a special embryogenetic classification is possible.
Association	Non-accidental appearance of multiple anomalies which, because the cause(s) and/or pathogenesis is unknown, cannot be classified among any of the morphological patterns described above, e.g. VACTERL association.

MEMORIX PEDIATRICS

Symbols for the documentation of a family tree

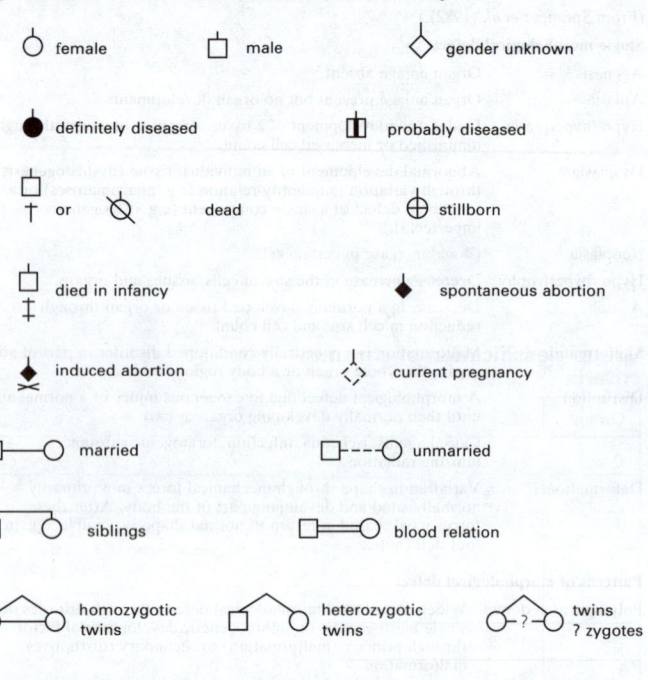

○ female   □ male   ◇ gender unknown

● definitely diseased   ◐ probably diseased

□† or ⦰ dead   ⊕ stillborn

□‡ died in infancy   ◆ spontaneous abortion

◆ induced abortion   ◇ current pregnancy

□—○ married   □---○ unmarried

□—○ siblings   □═○ blood relation

homozygotic twins   heterozygotic twins   twins ? zygotes

↗ referred patient

30

BASICS/NORMAL VALUES/DIAGNOSTIC METHODS

Indications for chromosome analysis in children

1. Prenatal analysis
   - Age of mother ⩾35 years
   - Previous birth of a sibling with a chromosomal aberration
   - Known structural (inversion, translocation) or numeric (mosaic) chromosomal aberration in a parent
   - Sonographically dysplastic child
   - Liability for one or both parents to chemical or radiobiological chromosomal disorder.

2. Postnatal analysis
   - Phenotypical suspicion of a chromosome aberration (pathogenetically unclear malformation, somatic and statomotor retardation + dysplasias, symptoms of a known syndrome)
   - Intersexual external genitalia
   - Non-development of secondary sex characteristics
   - Primary amenorrhea
   - For typing leukemia.

Group classification of chromosomes on morphological criteria

Group	Chromosome number	Remarks
A	1–3	
B	4–5	
C	6–12	X-chromosome corresponds to this group
D	13–15	
E	16–18	
F	19–20	
G	21–22	Y-chromosome resembles this group

MEMORIX PEDIATRICS

X-chromosomal inherited diseases

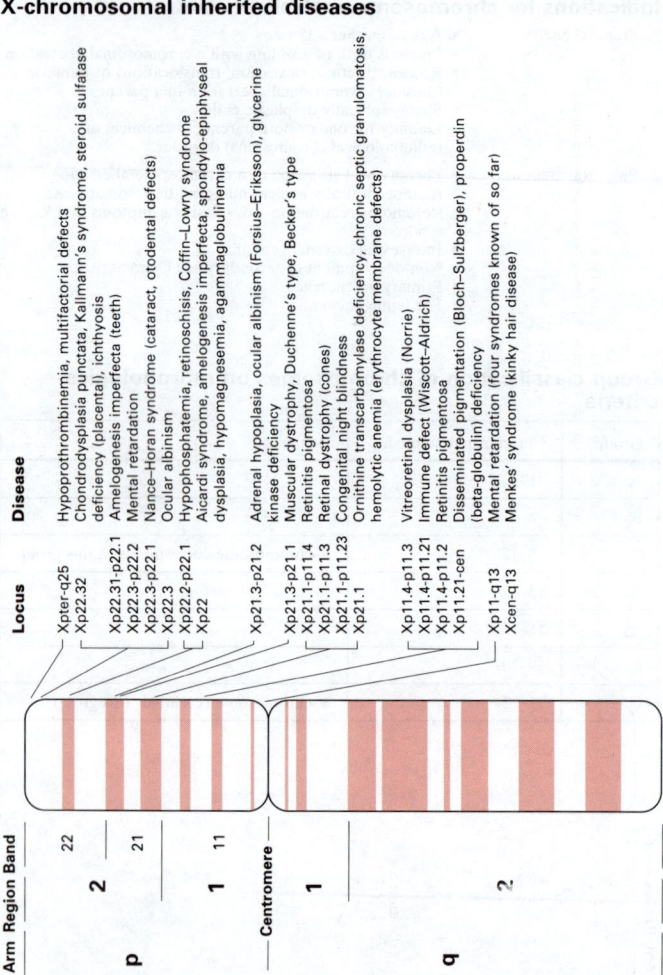

Locus	Disease
Xpter-q25	Hypoprothrombinemia, multifactorial defects
Xp22.32	Chondrodysplasia punctata, Kallmann's syndrome, steroid sulfatase deficiency (placental), ichthyosis
Xp22.31-p22.1	Amelogenesis imperfecta (teeth)
Xp22.3-p22.2	Mental retardation
Xp22.3-p22.1	Nance–Horan syndrome (cataract, otodental defects)
Xp22.3	Ocular albinism
Xp22.2-p22.1	Hypophosphatemia, retinoschisis, Coffin–Lowry syndrome
Xp22	Aicardi syndrome, amelogenesis imperfecta, spondylo-epiphyseal dysplasia, hypomagnesemia, agammaglobulinemia
Xp21.3-p21.2	Adrenal hypoplasia, ocular albinism (Forsius–Eriksson), glycerine kinase deficiency
Xp21.3-p21.1	Muscular dystrophy, Duchenne's type, Becker's type
Xp21.1-p11.4	Retinitis pigmentosa
Xp21.1-p11.3	Retinal dystrophy (cones)
Xp21.1-p11.23	Congenital night blindness
Xp21.1	Ornithine transcarbamylase deficiency, chronic septic granulomatosis, hemolytic anemia (erythrocyte membrane defects)
Xp11.4-p11.3	Vitreoretinal dysplasia (Norrie)
Xp11.4-p11.21	Immune defect (Wiscott–Aldrich)
Xp11.4-p11.2	Retinitis pigmentosa
Xp11.21-cen	Disseminated pigmentation (Bloch–Sulzberger), properdin (beta-globulin) deficiency
Xp11-q13	Mental retardation (four syndromes known of so far)
Xcen-q13	Menkes' syndrome (kinky hair disease)

BASICS/NORMAL VALUES/DIAGNOSTIC METHODS

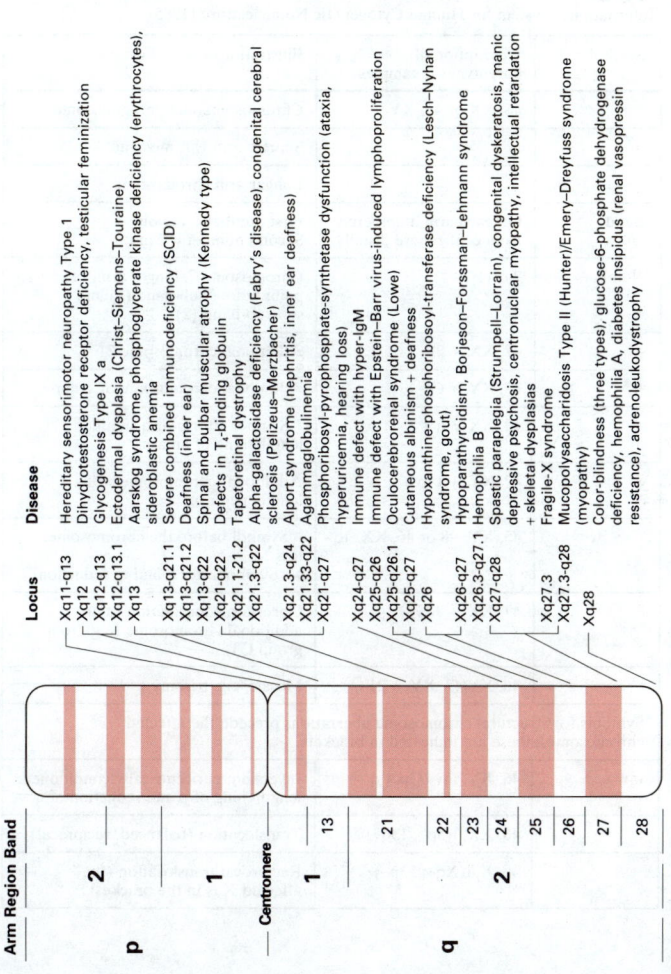

Locus	Disease
Xq11-q13	Hereditary sensorimotor neuropathy Type 1
Xq12	Dihydrotestosterone receptor deficiency, testicular feminization
Xq12-q13	Glycogenesis Type IX a
Xq12-q13.1	Ectodermal dysplasia (Christ–Siemens–Touraine)
Xq13	Aarskog syndrome, phosphoglycerate kinase deficiency (erythrocytes), sideroblastic anemia
Xq13-q21.1	Severe combined immunodeficiency (SCID)
Xq13-q21.2	Deafness (inner ear)
Xq13-q22	Spinal and bulbar muscular atrophy (Kennedy type)
Xq21-q22	Defects in T$_3$-binding globulin
Xq21.1-21.2	Tapetoretinal dystrophy
Xq21.3-q22	Alpha-galactosidase deficiency (Fabry's disease), congenital cerebral sclerosis (Pelizeus–Merzbacher)
Xq21.3-q24	Alport syndrome (nephritis, inner ear deafness)
Xq21.33-q22	Agammaglobulinemia
Xq21-q27	Phosphoribosyl-pyrophosphate-synthetase dysfunction (ataxia, hyperuricemia, hearing loss)
Xq24-q27	Immune defect with hyper-IgM
Xq25-q26	Immune defect with Epstein-Barr virus-induced lymphoproliferation
Xq25-q26.1	Oculocerebrorenal syndrome (Lowe)
Xq25-q27	Cutaneous albinism + deafness
Xq26	Hypoxanthine-phosphoribosyl-transferase deficiency (Lesch-Nyhan syndrome, gout)
Xq26-q27	Hypoparathyroidism, Borjeson-Forssman–Lehmann syndrome
Xq26.3-q27.1	Hemophilia B
Xq27-q28	Spastic paraplegia (Strumpell–Lorrain), congenital dyskeratosis, manic depressive psychosis, centronuclear myopathy, intellectual retardation + skeletal dysplasias
Xq27.3	Fragile-X syndrome
Xq27.3-q28	Mucopolysaccharidosis Type II (Hunter)/Emery-Dreyfuss syndrome (myopathy)
Xq28	Color-blindness (three types), glucose-6-phosphate dehydrogenase deficiency, hemophilia A, diabetes insipidus (renal vasopressin resistance), adrenoleukodystrophy

Cytogenetic nomenclature
(International System for Human Cytogenetic Nomenclature (1985).)

Symbol	Description of karyotypes (examples)	Illustrations
	46, XX or 46, XY	Chromosome number, gonosomes
p		Shorter arm chromosome
q		Longer arm chromosome
Band index	On each arm, numbered from centromere distally	First number = region Second number = band
Numbers 1–8	7 q 11.22	Chromosome 7, longer arm, region 1, point before sub-band (2) and sub-sub-band (2)
+	47, XX, + 21	Additional chromosome 21
+	47, XY, + G	Additional chromosome of group G
+	46, XX, 3 q +	+ Symbol after p or q signifies lengthening of an arm
+	47, XY, + 14p +	Additional chromosome with lengthened arm
–	45, XY, –8 or 46, XX. 1q–	– Symbol before the chromosome: loss – Symbol after p and q: reduction
?	47, XX, + ? G	Uncertain coordination of an additional chromosome (e.g. from group G)
/	46, XY/47, XY, + 21	Mosaic, e.g. trisomy

Symbols for structural chromosome aberrations precede the affected chromosomes; these are indicated in brackets

inv	46, XY, inv (Gp + q –)	Inversion, pericentrically conditioned: lengthening of p and reduction of q
t	46, XX, t(5p–; 13q+)	Translocation (balanced, reciprocal)
	46, X, t(Xq+; 13p–)	Reciprocal translocation (the affected X is in the bracket)

BASICS/NORMAL VALUES/DIAGNOSTIC METHODS

Symbol	Description of karyotypes (examples)	Illustrations
t	45, XX, –D, –G, +t(DqGq)	Formation of a translocation chromosome by centric fusion of Dq and Gq
mat	46, XX, t(4q–; 11p+) mat	Maternal origin of translocation
pat	46, XY, t(11p–; 13q+) pat	Paternal origin of a karyotype
r	46, XY, r(14)	Ring chromosome (e.g. number 14)
i	46, X, i (Xq)	Normal X chromosome and an isochromosome from two long arms of X
dic	46, X dic (Y)	X chromosome and a dicentric Y chromosome
mar	+2 mar 13	Marker chromosome (number before mar gives the number of structurally abnormal chromosomes, the number after mar indicates the marker chromosome)
h	46, XX, 14qh +	h = secondary constriction; +/– = lengthening or shortening
s	46, XY, 20 s +	s = satellite; + = enlarged; – = reduced
ss	46, XY, 21 psqs	Duplication of chromosomal structures are represented by the double symbol
fra	fra (8) (q21)	Fragile position (in 8q21)
var	46, XX, var (6) (cen, C24)	var = variable chromosome regions (e.g. centromere region of number 6) C24 = code for band position

Fracture of a chromosome is shown by the band in which it is situated. If it is between two bands, the distal one of the two is named, counting from the centromere outwards. Fractures at the border of two bands are described by naming the band plus the word 'or', e.g. 1q22 or 23. Localization of a band is done by giving the distance from the proximal margin, e.g.
2q 1204 = 4/10 bandwidth from the proximal border to band 2q 12

Symbol	Description of karyotypes (examples)	Illustrations
System for the recognition of structural aberrations 1. Definition of the altered chromosome by specifying the fracture sites. Sequence: type of rearrangement, chromosome in brackets, bands in brackets, fractures on p are named before those on q. With three fractures, the one named first is the one where the chromosomal segment is repositioned. The segmental designation follows the fracture site.		
ins	inv (3) (p12 q21)	Pericentric inversion of chromosome 3
	inv ins (3) (q12 p22 p11)	Inverse insertion segment of p11–p22 at q12 of chromosome 3
If more chromosomes participate, they are separated by a semicolon		
rcp	rcp (5; 8) (q21; q32)	Reciprocal translocation of the long arms on the fracture sites 5q21 and 8q32
2. Extended system for describing chromosomal structural variations. Sequence: chromosome count, gonosomes, symbol of the variation type, changed chromosome(s) are in brackets denoting the band variations, beginning with the end of p, to the end of q. A colon indicates the chromosomal fracture, two colons (::) signify the fracture and reunion of the fragments.		
del	46, XY, del (5) (pter → q31:) 46, XY, del(5) (q31)	Deletion (del), pter: (terminals) distal ends of the short arms, chromosome fracture at q31. The altered chromosome extends from the end of the short arms to band 31 of the long arms. Arrow: from to. Shorthand description after 1.
	46, XY, del(3) (pter → q11::q22 → qter): interstitial deletion of the segment from q11 to q22	
inv	46, XX, inv (1) (pter → p32::p12 → p32::p12 → qter): paracentric inversion of segment p32 → p12 in chromosome 1	
	46, XX, inv (8) (pter → p13::q21 → p13::q21 → qter): pericentric inversion of segment p13 → q21 in chromosome 8	
r	46, XY, r (3) (p22 → q13) 46, XY, r (3) (p22q13)	Ring chromosome after fracture at p22 and q13, as well as deletion of the distal segment. Description after 1.

BASICS/NORMAL VALUES/DIAGNOSTIC METHODS

Symbol	Desription of karyotypes (examples)	Illustration
dup	46, XY, inv dup (1) (pter → p31::p12 → p31::p31 → qter):	Duplication of segment p31 → p12, which is inserted at p31 into chromosome 1.
	46, XY, inv.dup (1) (p31 → p12)	Shorthand description after 1.
dir	46, XY, dir dup (1) (pter → p31::Lp31 → p12::p31 → qter): Direct duplication of segment p31 → p12	
dic	46, X, dic (Y) (pter → p12::p12 → pter): dicentric Y chromosome	
	46, X, dic (Y) (q12)	Shorthand description after 1.
t	46, XX, t(5; 13) (5pter → 5q31::13q22 → 13qter; 13qter → 13q22::5q31 → 5qter)	Reciprocal translocation (the terminal segments of the long arms are reciprocally appended to 5q31 and 13q22)
t	45, XY, t(14; 21) (14qter → 14p11::21q11 → 21qter):	Robertson translocation
	45, XY, t(14;21) (p11; q11)	Shorthand description after 1.
t	46, XX, t(1; 2) (1pter → cen → 2qter; 1qter → cen → 2pter):	Translocation of an entire arm.
	46, XX, t(1; 2) (1p2q; 1q2p)	Shorthand description after 1.
cen		Centromere, e.g. cen 1 or cen 2 indicates the origin of the centromere from chromosome 1 or 2
der		derivative chromosomes (e.g. 1p2q; 1q2p)
dir ins	46, XX, dir ins (3) (pter → p12::q31 → q21::p12 → p21::q31 → qter)	Direct insertion of segments q21 → q31 in the short arm of p12
	46, XX, dir ins (3) (p12q21q31)	Shorthand description after 1.
dir ins	46, XY, dir ins (7; 3) (7pter → 7p14::3q12 → 3q28::7p14 → 7qter; 3pter → 3q12::3q28 → 3qter)	Direct insertion between two chromosomes (e.g. segment 3q12q28 is included in 7p14). The recipient chromosome is named first.
	46, XY, dir ins (7; 3) (p14; q12q28)	Shorthand description after 1.

MEMORIX PEDIATRICS

Symbol	Description of karyotypes (examples)	Illustrations
inv ins	46, XX, inv ins (3) (pter → p12::q21 → q31::p12 → q21::q31 → qter)	Inverse insertion of segments q21 → q31 in the short arm of chromosome 3
	46, XX, inv ins (3) (p12q31q21)	Shorthand description after 1.
inv ins	46, XY, inv ins (7; 3) (7 pter → 7p14::3q28 → 3q12::7p14 → 7qter; 3pter → 3q12::3q28 → 3qter)	Inverse insertion between two chromosomes
	46, XY, inv ins (7; 3) (p14; q28q12)	Shorthand description after 1.
t	46, XY, t(3; 5; 7) (p12; q12; q31)	Complex translocation (shorthand description after 1). The chromosomes are numbered in series. This is followed by the bands which are separated and rejoined. Sequence: the segment distal 3p12 was joined at 5q12, segment distal 5q12 at 7q31, segment distal 7q31 at 3p12.
ter rea	45, XX, ter rea (12; 13) (12qter → cen → 12p13::13p13 → 13qter)	Terminal rearrangement (end-to-end junction of two chromosomes). Only the active centromere is numbered, e.g. here in chromosome 12.
psu dic	47, XY, psu dic (10) t (10; 8) (10pter → cen → 10q12::8q12 → 8pter)	Pseudodicentric chromosome (e.g. after translocation between number 8 and number 10). The chromosome with the active centromere is named first.
	47, XY, psu dic (10) t (10; 8) (q12; q12)	Shorthand description after 1.
Acquired chromosomal aberrations		
ct		Chromatid aberration (only one chromatid of one chromosome)
ctg	ctg (6) (q21)	Chromatin gap (achromatic region q21 of a chromatid from number 6)
ctb	ctb (6) (q21)	Chromatid fracture (e.g. at q21) in chromosome number 6

BASICS/NORMAL VALUES/DIAGNOSTIC METHODS

Symbol	Description of karyotypes (examples)	Illustrations
cte	cte (6; 11) (q21; q12)	Chromatid exchange (e.g. 6q21 and 11q12)
ct del	ct del (6) (q12q26)	Chromatid deletion of segments 6q12 → 5q26
ct inv	ct inv (6) (q12q26)	Chromatid inversion of segments 6q12 → 6q25
sce	sce (3) (q22q28)	Sister chromatid exchange (e.g. on bands 3q22 and 3q28)
cs		Aberration of both chromatids of a chromosome at the same locus
	csg csb cse	Analogous to ct (see above) both chromatids are changed
pvz	pvz (2)	Pulverization (multiple breaks in one chromatid or chromosome (e.g. number 2)
f		Fragment
ace		Acentric fragment

MEMORIX PEDIATRICS

DNA diagnosis: restriction fragment length polymorphism (RFLP)

Definition
Variations in the DNA sequence are ascertained by the changed localization of specific cuts by a restriction enzyme (gene scissors). (Indirect method of DNA diagnosis.) Each restriction enzyme has its own sequence in the DNA. In its region, or within a defined distance of it, the specific restriction enzyme cuts the double-stranded DNA into fragments. If the sequences in the DNA are displaced or individual sequences deleted, the points of cutting are changed and with it the DNA segments (fragments) between them.

Technique
Enzymatic cutting of the DNA → gel electrophoresis. The fragments migrate in the electrical field to a varying extent, according to their negative charge or length. The distance traveled corresponds to the logarithm of the length of the fragments.
→ Southern blot → hybridization with marked complementary DNA probe.

Application
1. Restriction mapping of DNA.
2. Coupling analysis. This serves as a marker if the polymorphism in the DNA is inherited together with the searched-for gene. An example follows.

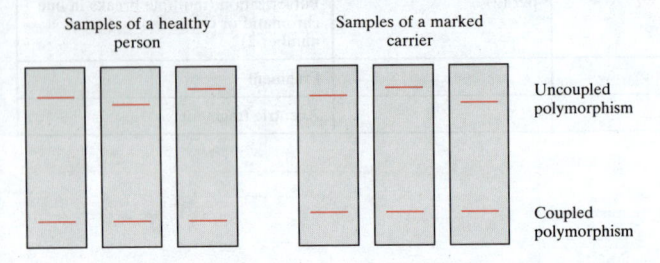

Samples of a healthy person   Samples of a marked carrier

Uncoupled polymorphism

Coupled polymorphism

BASICS/NORMAL VALUES/DIAGNOSTIC METHODS

Organ development: sensitive periods

The critical periods in organ development comprise the early organ anlagen (embryopathies). During the fetal period small morphologic anomalies and/or functional defects may occur.
(Time specifications after Hinrichsen (1990).)

Weeks after conception	Embryonic period 3–8	Fetal period 9–40
Central nervous system	██████████████	██████████████
Spinal cord	███	
Ear, labyrinth	████████████	████████
Heart, vessels	████████	
Hips	██	
Eye	██████████	██████
Upper limbs	████	
Lower limbs	█████	
Respiratory tract	██ ← Esophagotracheal fistula ████	████████
Vertebral column	████████████	██
Face, jaws	████ ←Lips, jaws, clefts ██████	← Cleft palate
Diaphragm	████	
Intestines	██████	████████
Kidney, ureter	██████	████████
Gonads	█████	██████████
Genitalia	██████	████████
	Embryopathies	Fetopathies

MEMORIX PEDIATRICS

Early prenatal development

Gestational age in weeks: 15–42 days.
(After Moore and Lütjen-Drecoll (1990).)

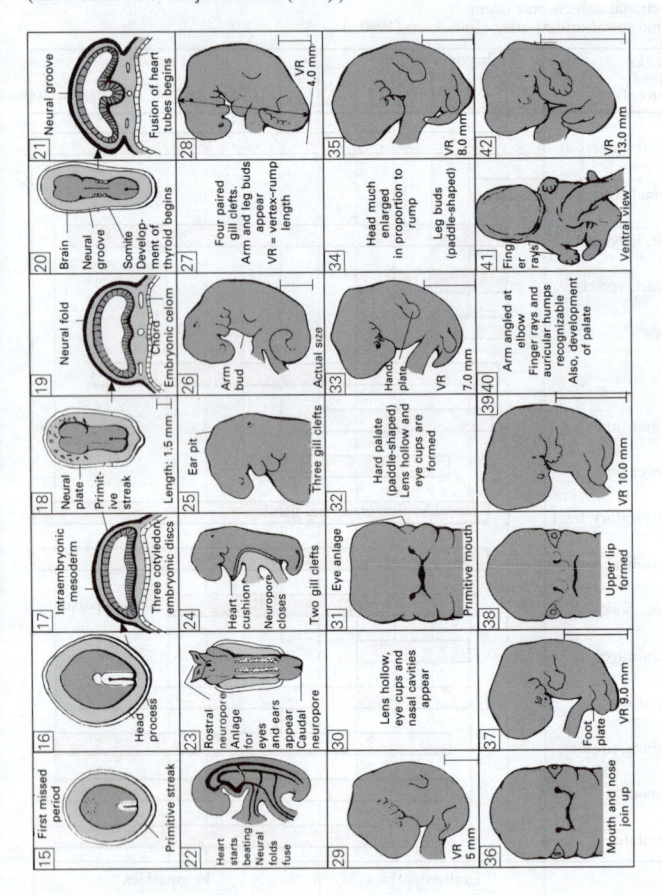

BASICS/NORMAL VALUES/DIAGNOSTIC METHODS

Gestional age in weeks: 43–70 days.
(After Moore and Lütjen-Drecoll (1990).)

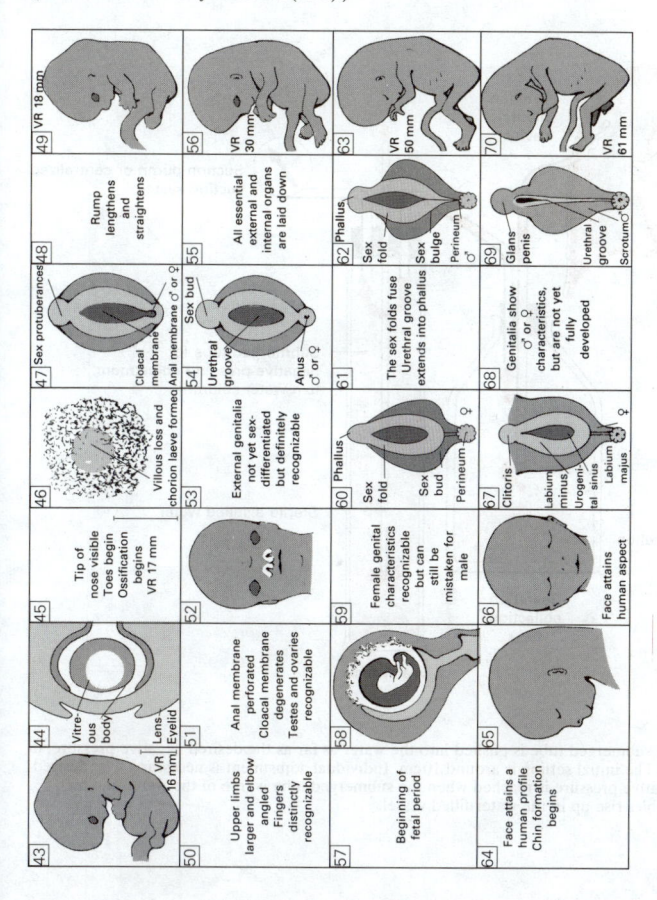

49 VR 18 mm	56 VR 30 mm	63 VR 50 mm	70 VR 61 mm
48 Sex protuberances ♂ or ♀	55 Rump lengthens and straightens	62 Phallus / Sex fold / Sex bulge / Perineum ♂	69 Glans penis / Urethral groove / Scrotum ♂
47 Sex protuberances / Cloacal membrane / Anal membrane ♂ or ♀	54 Sex bud / Urethral groove / Anus ♂ or ♀	61 All essential external and internal organs are laid down	68 Genitalia show ♂ or ♀ characteristics, but are not yet fully developed
46 Villous loss and chorion laeve formed	53 External genitalia not yet sex-differentiated but definitely recognizable	60 The sex folds fuse Urethral groove extends into phallus	67 Phallus / Sex fold / Sex bud / Perineum ♀
45 Tip of nose visible Toes begin Ossification begins VR 17 mm	52	59 Female genital characteristics recognizable but can still be mistaken for male	66 Clitoris / Labium minus / Urogenital sinus / Labium majus ♀
44 Vitreous body / Lens / Eyelid	51 Anal membrane perforated Cloacal membrane degenerates Testes and ovaries recognizable	58 Beginning of fetal period	65 Face attains human aspect
43 VR 16 mm	50 Upper limbs larger and elbow angled Fingers distinctly recognizable	57	64 Face attains a human profile Chin formation begins

43

MEMORIX PEDIATRICS

Thoracic suction drainage

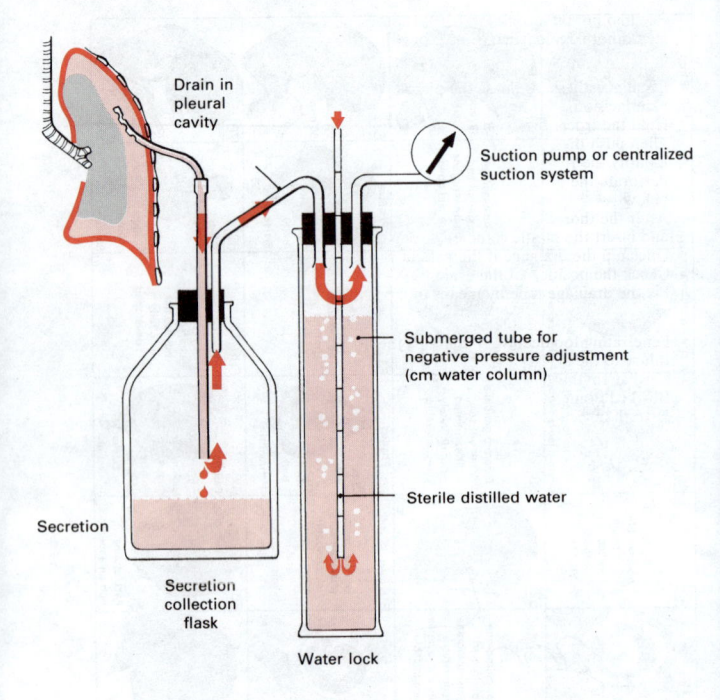

The submerged tube is pushed into the water as far as the desired negative pressure, in cm. The initial setting is around 10 cm. Individual adjustment is necessary. The desired negative pressure is reached when the submerged tube is free of the water and air bubbles rise up in the water-filled vessel.

BASICS/NORMAL VALUES/DIAGNOSTIC METHODS

Thoracic puncture

Needle puncture sites
– Pneumothorax: second intercostal space anteriorly in the midclavicular line
– Hemothorax: midaxillary line, not below the nipple.

Procedure
– Local anesthesia as far as the pleura
– Skin incision
– Hold the trocar firmly so as to avoid penetrating too deeply
– Then push the trocar at right angles through the thoracic wall
– Identify the ribs with the trochar point
– Perforate the thoracic wall with a short firm stab at the upper border of the rib below
– After the thoracic cavity has been entered, guide the point in the desired direction and insert the plastic catheter through the metal rod
– Unclamp the drainage if the patient is breathing spontaneously
– Check the position of the drain by X-ray
– Fix the drainage tube by means of a purse-string suture.

Complications and problems
– Penetrating too deeply → injury to the diaphragm or intra-abdominal organs
– Injury to the surface of the lung
– Cardiac rhythm disorder from drain touching heart
– Blocked drainage
– Extrathoracic (subcutaneous) malposition.

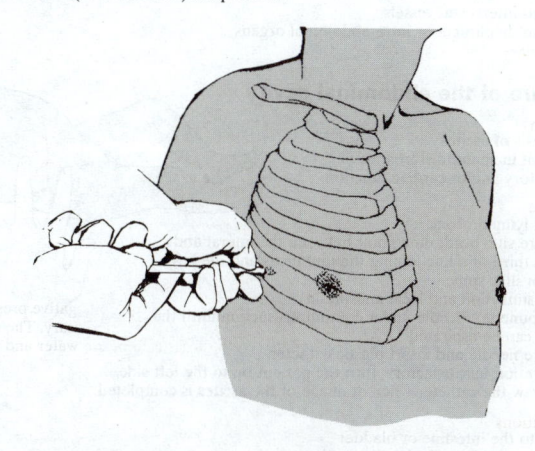

MEMORIX PEDIATRICS

Pleural puncture

Indications
- Evidence of pockets of intrapleural fluid
- Relief of pneumothorax, pleural effusion or empyema.

Procedure
- Needle puncture with the patient sitting or with trunk elevated; arm on the affected side raised above the head
- Puncture site in the middle or posterior axillary line in fourth/fifth intercostal space if patient lying down, or fifth/sixth intercostal space if sitting; (best to establish the extent of the effusion sonographically beforehand)
- Skin disinfection and local anesthesia as far as the parietal pleura
- Needle puncture at right angles to the skin at the upper margin of the rib below
- Push in the cannula under continuous suction until the effusion can be aspirated
- Withdraw the puncture needle and insert the plastic cannula
- Aspirate the effusion; coughing is stimulated when the cavity is nearly emptied.

Complications
- Pneumothorax, hemothorax
- Injury to intercostal vessels
- Injury to diaphragm or intra-abdominal organs
- Infection.

Puncture of the abdominal cavity

Indications
- Diagnosis of ascites
- Relief of incipient disturbance of respiratory and/or cardiac function.

Procedure
- Patient lying on back
- Puncture site: borderline point between the lateral and middle third of a line joining the umbilicus and the left anterior iliac spine
- Skin disinfection and local anesthesia
- Insert puncture needle under continuous suction until the ascites can be aspirated
- Remove needle and insert plastic catheter
- If aspiration unsatisfactory, turn the patient on to the left side
- Withdraw the catheter when drainage of the ascites is completed.

Complications
- Injury to the intestine or bladder
- Injury to the abdominal wall vessels
- Electrolyte and protein loss
- Circulatory collapse due to too rapid evacuation of the ascitic fluid.

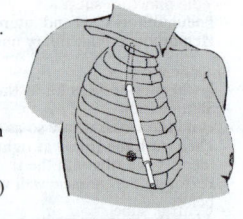

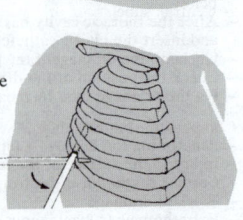

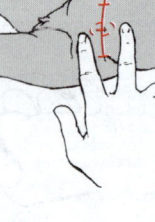

BASICS/NORMAL VALUES/DIAGNOSTIC METHODS

Venepuncture: central venous catheter

Indications
– Circulatory shock
– Total parenteral nutrition
– Administration of high molecular solutions or vessel-irritating intravenous medication
– Central venous pressure measurement
– Insertion of temporary pacemaker.

Contraindication
– Coagulation disorder.

Site
– Peripheral: cephalic vein, basilar vein
– Central: subclavian, internal and external jugular, external femoral veins

Complications

General	Special
Infection	Pneumothorax
Thrombosis	Intrathoracic infusion
Arterial puncture	Hemothorax
Nerve injury	Air embolism
Vascular perforation	Pericardial tamponade
Malposition	

Errors in caval catheter placement
– Bilateral attempts at puncture near clavicle without previous exclusion of a pneumothorax
– Withdrawal of catheter through sharp puncture needle
– Forcible insertion of the catheter or guidewire against resistance
– Omitting to check the position of the catheter before starting the infusion.

Positioning of patient
– If puncture is near the clavicle or at the throat, head-down position (upper body lowered by about 20°).

① **Puncture of subclavian vein**

Puncture site: below the clavicle at the crossing point of first rib and clavicle (approximately in the midclavicular line).

Procedure
– Push the puncture needle forward under the clavicle
– Insert it further horizontally between the clavicle and first rib behind the clavicle in the direction of the sternoclavicular joint
– The subclavian vein runs immediately behind the clavicle and in front of the subclavian artery.

② **Puncture of the internal jugular vein**

Puncture site: about 0.5–1 cm lateral to the palpable common carotid artery, immediately below the crossing of the external jugular vein over the sternocleidomastoid muscle.

Procedure
– Palpation of the common carotid artery with the finger of the free hand
– Insertion of the needle at an angle of 35–40° to the skin surface
– Direction of insertion towards the median border of the sternocleidomastoid muscle at its clavicular insertion
– The right internal jugular vein is preferred because of its straight course.

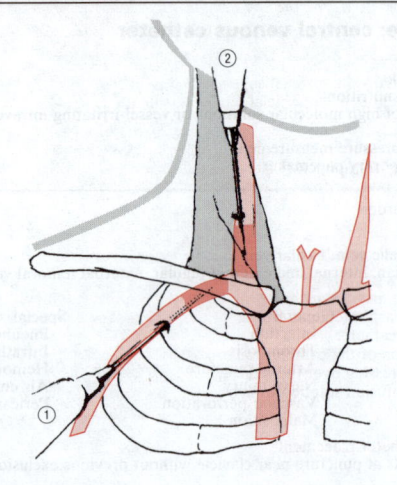

Puncture of the external jugular vein

Puncture site: at about the middle of the sternocleidomastoid muscle.

Procedure

- Head turned to the opposite side and in slight dorsiflexion
- Compression of the vessel directly above the clavicle
- Puncture in the direction of the recognizable venous track.

Puncture of the femoral vein

Procedure

- Patient lying on back, thighs slightly abducted and externally rotated
- Skin sterilization
- Palpation of femoral artery
- Position of femoral vein: 0.5–1 cm (according to age) medial to the artery, approximately in the middle of the groin
- Puncture at about 45° to the skin surface in the direction of the centre of the inguinal ligament; advance the needle under suction.
  (Mnemonic for the position of the vessels in the groin: IVAN – internal vein, then artery, then nerve.)

Complications

- Thrombosis, thrombophlebitis
- Hematoma
- Injury to femoral nerve
- Infection of hip joint
- Creation of an arteriovenous fistula.

BASICS/NORMAL VALUES/DIAGNOSTIC METHODS

Venepuncture: epicutaneous catheter
(Modified from Chávez la lama, Lentze and Versmoldt (1980).)

Puncture sites: cubital vein, internal saphenous vein at the inner ankle; see: external jugular vein, superficial temporal veins.

Procedure
- Skin sterilization
- Measure distance from puncture site to right atrium
- Wash the talcum powder from gloves (thrombophlebitis)
- Dress the puncture site with sterile towels
- Fill the catheter with 5% glucose (heparin)
- Puncture vein with a butterfly needle with the tube end cut off
- When blood flows out, push the catheter with forceps into the needle and advance it into the vein for a previously measured length
- The length of the inserted catheter can be read from the markings on it
- If blood is easily aspirated, pull out the butterfly needle and remove it over the distal end of the catheter
- Check the position of the catheter radiologically, correcting it if necessary
- Apply a sterile dressing over the puncture site
- Heparinize the infusion solution to avoid clotting in the catheter.

MEMORIX PEDIATRICS

Arterial puncture and catheterization

Radial artery puncture (for taking blood)
Procedure
- Wrist joint overextended and fixed in this position
- Palpate the radial artery
- Allen test (check for sufficient collateral circulation via the ulnar artery): in this test the radial and ulnar arteries are compressed until the hand becomes blue. The ulnar artery compression is then released. If the hand regains its normal color, there is an adequate supply via the ulnar artery
- Skin sterilization
- Puncture site is directly proximal to the first skin crease of the wrist
- Puncture needle (23–25 G) with 1 ml heparinized syringe inserted at an angle of 30–45° to the skin
- Aspirate blood
- After removal of the cannula compress the puncture site firmly for five min. (N.B. hematoma formation.)

Catheterization of the radial artery
- Preparations as for arterial puncture
- Insertion of indwelling catheter (22–24 G) at an angle of 30–45° to the skin into the artery
- If pulsating blood appears, push the indwelling catheter flat into the vessel
- Removal of the puncture needle (pulsating blood must be seen flowing from the indwelling catheter)
- Connect the catheter to drip or tubing as needed (e.g. for pressure recording)
- The indwelling catheter must be continuously flushed with heparinized NaCl solution (1–3 ml/h).

Arterial puncture of the femoral artery (for taking blood)
Procedure
- Preparation as for femoral vein puncture
- Palpation of femoral artery with two fingers of the free hand
- With fingers slightly spread, insert the puncture needle with syringe at an angle of 30–45° through the skin
- Needle advanced until blood appears
- After removal of needle, firm compression of puncture site for at least five min.

Complications
- As for femoral vein puncture
- Subsequent gangrene of the lower limb from thrombosis at the puncture site.

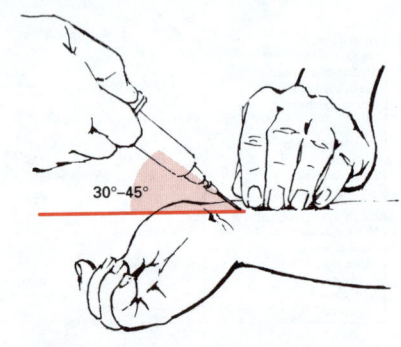

BASICS/NORMAL VALUES/DIAGNOSTIC METHODS

Establishment of brain death

Definition: brain death is the death of the human being. It is a condition of irreversible extinction of the total functions of the cerebrum, cerebellum and brain stem, while cardiovascular functions may still be maintained and gas exchange continued by artificial ventilation.

Assumptions
- Primary brain damage (supra-, infra-tentorial
- Examples: severest brain injury, intracranial hemorrhage, cerebral infarct, malignant tumor, acute obstructive hydrocephalus
- Secondary brain damage result of hypoxia, cardiovascular conditioned circulatory arrest, shock

Exclude:
- Intoxication (association with cerebral circulatory arrest is proven)
- Neuromuscular block
- Hypothermia
- Circulatory shock
- Endocrine coma
- Metabolic coma

Symptoms/findings (two independent examiners, not associated with a transplantation team)
- Unconsciousness
- Dilated pupils (slight, medium)
- Eliminate mydriatic drug cause
- No oculocephalic reflex obtainable (doll's eye phenomenom)
- No corneal reflex obtainable
- No reaction to painful stimulus in the trigeminal area (e.g. nasal septum)
- No pharyngeal reflex obtainable (e.g. by aspiration)
- No spontaneous respiration (negative apnoea test, 60 mmHg obligatory)

Supplementary investigations
- EEG, isoelectric (0-line) over 30 min in adults
- Brainstem auditory evoked responses
- Median SEP: no reaction above neck line
- Doppler sonography
- Bilateral angiography
- Aortic arch DSA
- Demonstration of cerebral circulatory arrest
- Nuclear medicine: brain flow study

Observation time
- Adults with 10 degree brain damage: 12 h
- Adults with 20 degree brain damage: 72 h
- Children with 10 degree brain damage: 24 h
- Early newborn with 10 degree brain damage: 72 h

Time of death – time of establishment of final diagnosis

International brain death criteria
(Modified from Frowein *et al.* (1985).)

	Germany, 1991	USA, 1981	GB, 1976	Switzerland, 1983
Preconditions				
Diagnosis	+	+	+	+
No intoxication	+	+	+	+
No hypothermia	+	+	+	+
No hypovolemia	+	+	+	+
Clinical findings				
Coma	+	+	+	+
Apnea test	+	+	+	+
(pCO_2 mmHg)	>60	>60	>50	>50
Mydriasis dilation	+	+	+	+
Brain stem reflex	+	+	+	+
No. of signatures	2	1	2	1
Observation time (h)				
In primary brain damage	12	12	6	6
In secondary brain damage	72	24	12	48
Additional investigations				
EEG, no response	30 min	6 h/30 min	–	2 in 24 h
AEP absent	+	–	–	–
Circulatory arrest	Angiography	Nuclear medicine	–	Angiography
ICP above systolic RR	–	Brain flow study	–	+

X-ray investigations

General X-ray diagnosis (terminology)
(From Droste and v. Planta (1989).)

Position of patient – **supine**, lying face upwards
 – **prone**, lying face downwards
 – **erect**, standing or sitting upright

Projection defines the direction taken by the X-rays through the patient (from the X-ray tube to the X-ray film).

Antero-posterior (AP)
back of body
lying on film

Postero-anterior (PA)
front of body
lying on film

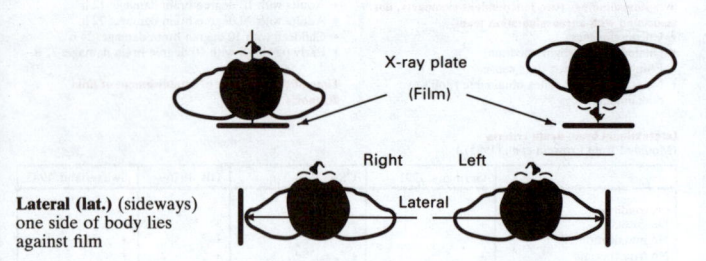

Lateral (lat.) (sideways)
one side of body lies
against film

Oblique all positions between AP, PA and lateral. For special imaging, e.g. coronary angiography, the angle is usually specified.

Right anterior oblique (RAO)
Oblique diameter I: Right
shoulder in front

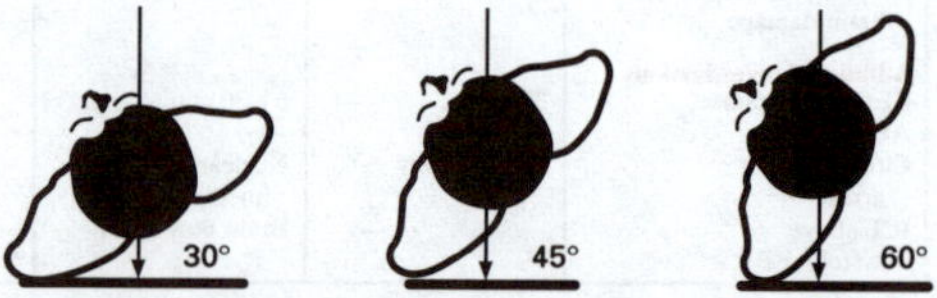

BASICS/NORMAL VALUES/DIAGNOSTIC METHODS

Left anterior oblique (LAO)
Oblique diameter II: left shoulder in front

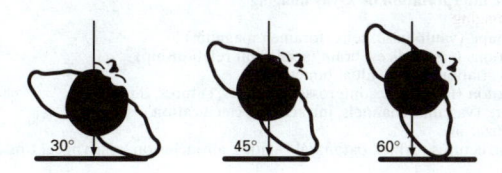

30°   45°   60°

Left lateral oblique   **Right lateral oblique**

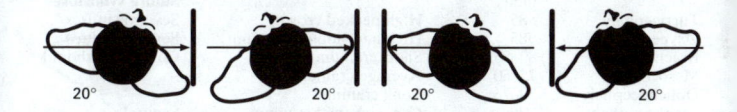

20°   20°   20°   20°

MEMORIX PEDIATRICS

X-ray diagnosis

Systematic interpretation of X-ray imaging
Cranial imaging
- Skull shape (vault, base, sella, foramen magnum)
- Proportions (size indices, brain/facial skull relationship)
- Shape variation in individual bones
- Ossification (fontanelles, interosseous bones, sutures, diploë)
- Structure (vascular channels, intracranial calcification, osteolysis)
- Mineralization
- Facial structures (orbits, paranasal cavities, air inclusion, pharyngeal tonsils (lateral view)
- Cervical vertebral column
- Extracranial artefacts (biplane imaging).

Typical cranial dysplasias

	Length–breadth index		Suture synostoses
Turricephaly	>85	High peaked crown	Several sutures
Oxycephaly	>85	High and sloping cranium	Several sutures
Brachycephaly	80–85	Short cranium	Coronal/lambdoid
Mesocephaly	75–60	Average cranium	–
Dolichocephaly	70–75	Long cranium	–
Scaphocaphaly	<70	Canoe-shaped cranium	Sagittal
Plagiocephaly	–	Asymmetrical cranium	Coronal/lambdoid Unilateral
Trigonocephalus	–	Triangular cranium	Frontal

$$\text{Length–width index} = \frac{\text{maximum cranial width}}{\text{maximum cranial length}} \times 100$$

Commonest origins of intracranial calcification
Asymptomatic – Pineal body
 – Choroid plexus
 – Dura mater (falx, tentorium)
 – Sella (interclinoid, petroclinoidal ligaments).

Pathological – Prenatal infection – Hypocalcemia
 – Tumors – Hypoparathyroidism
 – Phakomatoses – Generalized elastorrhexis
 – Angiodysplasias – Cockayne's syndrome (progressive dystrophy)
 – Hemorrhage – Gorlin–Goltze syndrome (calcification of falx cerebri)
 – Cerebral infarction – Fahr's disease (intracerebral calcification)
 – Urbach–Wiete's disease (paraseller calcification).

Artifacts: ointments, EEG paste, dressings, hairclips, etc.

BASICS/NORMAL VALUES/DIAGNOSTIC METHODS

Thickness and/or density of the cranial bones in X-ray imaging

Increased

Generalized
Mucopolysaccharidoses
Hyperphosphatasia
Osteopetrosis
Craniometaphyseal dysplasias
Pyknodysostosis
Cortical hyperostosis (van Buchem)
Metaphyseal dysplasia (Pyle)
Craniodiaphysial dysplasia
Tubular stenosis + hypocalcemia (Kenny–Caffey)
Otopalatodigital syndrome
Chronic anemia
Fluorosis
Myelosclerosis
Phenytoin
Hypervitaminosis D
Microcephaly
Hydrocephalus
Radiation

Circumscribed
Cephalohematoma
Chronic osteomyelitis
Tumors

Cranial osteolysis
Meningo-encephalocele
Osteomyelitis
Fracture
Aneurysmal bone cyst
Fibrous dysplasia
Postoperative or radiation necrosis

Decreased

Generalized
Cranial ossification defects
Intracranial pressure increase
Osteogenesis imperfecta
Rickets
Hypophosphatasia
Hypothyroidism
Hyperparathyroidism
Prematurity
Premature aging (progeria)
Osteodysplasia (Melnick–Needles)

Circumscribed
Arachnoid cyst
Porencephaly
Hygroma

Tumors: Histiocytosis
Hemangioma
Dermoid, epidermoid
Sarcoma
Lymphoma
Metastases

Skeletal imaging
- Total skeleton (aplasia, absent secondary ossification in epi- and apophyses)
- Shape (symmetry, axis-true posture, deformities, hypo- and hyperplasia)
- Structure (diaphyses, metaphyses, epiphyses, trabeculation of the spongiosa, thickness and density of the cortex, periosteal thickness and thinning)
- Mineralization (thickness of cortex and spongiosa, particularly metaphyseal)
- Skeletal age
- Joint contours, joint spaces
- Associated soft tissues (ligaments, muscles, subcutaneous).

MEMORIX PEDIATRICS

Base-of-skull angle δ
Angle construction: draw a line from the inner intersection of the frontal bone and the base of the skull to the basolateral synchondrosis of the occipital bone (base-of-skull tangent). The second tangent is drawn from the top of the first upper jaw incisor to the occipital bone.
Angle measurement: δ = 33° ± 3° in neonates, average growth = 0.5%/y.

Clivus angle η
Angle construction: base of skull tangent and tangent of the dorsum sellae
Angle measurement: neonatal η = 37 ± 7°, η in children = 35 ± 5°.

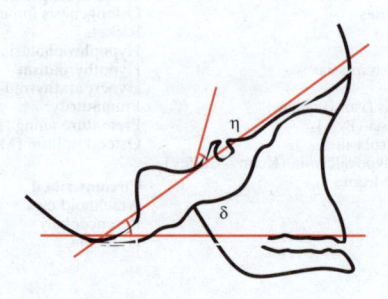

Development of the paranasal sinuses
(unilateral diagram)

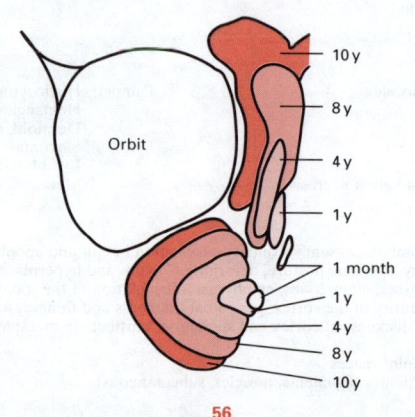

BASICS/NORMAL VALUES/DIAGNOSTIC METHODS

Thoracic imaging

- Technique
  Symmetry of the image, phase of breathing, position of diaphragm. In normal inspiration the domes of the diaphragm are between the fifth and eighth anterior ribs, above that in expiration, below it in deeper inspiration. The exposure is correct if the intervertebral spaces are recognizable through the cardiac silhouette. Sharpness of contour can be judged from the vascular shadows and the diaphragm.
- Lungs
  Transparency, pulmonary structure, air bronchogram, vascular markings.
- Hilus
  Size
  Borders
  – sharp, indistinct, position in mediastinum
  Structure
  – homogeneous, inhomogeneous, streaked, dense, coarsely or finely patchy.
- Mediastinum
  How centred in picture, its width, wall contours, mediastinal lines, thymus shadow, air tracheogram and bronchogram, position of an endotracheal tube, the great vessels, shape of the heart, its size and position, position of ventriculo-atrial shunt.
- Pleura
  Space, recesses, effusion, pneumothorax including pneumomediastinum.
- Thoracic skeleton
  Symmetry, shape, rib count and shape, clavicles, vertebral column.
- Cervical and upper abdominal regions; extrathoracic tissues (may be included in the film) (breast shadow).

General abdominal imaging

- Technique
  Plain film, contrast imaging, patient position (erect), head position (inverted position).
- Form
- Structure
  Air distribution pattern, free air, fluid levels, calcification and other radio-opaque shadows, concretions in the region of the gallbladder, bile duct, urinary tract.
- Viscera
  Size, internal structures
- Tumor shadows
- Associated bony structures
  Thorax, vertebral column, pelvis.

MEMORIX PEDIATRICS

Computed tomography (CT): window technique

CT-imaging assessment
Radiological densities (Hounsfield units (HU)) of tissues and body fluids

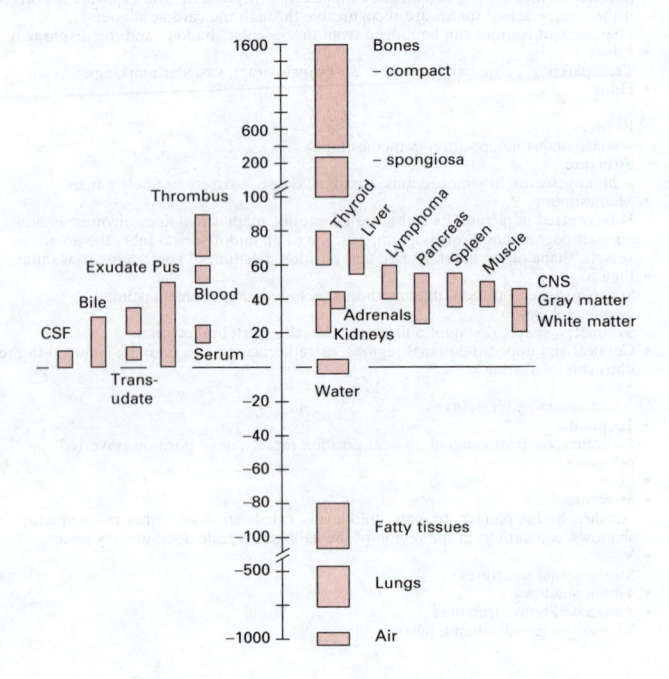

CT Window technique: the density scale of –1000 to +2000 Hounsfield units comprises 3000 gray steps although these cannot be differentiated visually. Depending on the radiological densities of the tissues under investigation, limited regions of the scale become visible as a window with a series of gray steps between black and white.

BASICS/NORMAL VALUES/DIAGNOSTIC METHODS

CT characteristics

Bleeding, effusion, abscess, necrosis

Bleeding: Absorption of X-rays proportional to the amount of hemoglobin
(compare extravasated with intravascular blood)
Initial	isodense
After hours	isodense → hyperdense
During absorption	hyperdense → isodense → hypodense
Connective tissue organization	isodense → hyperdense → slightly hyperdense
calcification	isodense → asymmetrically hyperdense

Effusion: (compare with venous blood)
Transudate, cyst contents	hypodense
Exudate	hypodense → isodense

Abscess: (compare with surrounding tissues)
Pus	as for solid tissues
Fatty degeneration	isodense → hypodense
Caseation	strongly hypodense
Wall consolidation	isodense → hyperdense
Hypodense areas	smooth/irregular, sharp/ill-defined border, possibly with fluid level, septa, vesicles

Necrosis: (compare with vital tissues) hypodense

MEMORIX PEDIATRICS

CT imaging topography

Arteries
1. Aorta
2. Pulmonary trunk
3. Pulmonary aorta
4. Brachiocephalic trunk
5. Common carotid artery
6. Left subclavian artery
7. Celiac trunk
8. Hepatic artery
9. Splenic artery
10. Superior mesenteric artery
11. Femoral artery

Veins
12. Superior vena cava
13. Brachiocephalic vein
14. Azygos vein
15. Inferior vena cava
16. Superior mesenteric vein
17. Femoral vein
18. Renal vein
19. Pulmonary vessels

Organs
20. Heart, left ventricle
21. Heart, right ventricle
22. Heart, left atrium
23. Heart, right atrium
24. Trachea
25. Main bronchus
26. Lungs
27. Thymus
28. Esophagus
29. Diaphragm
30. Liver
31. Gallbladder
32. Stomach
33. Spleen
34. Pancreas
35. Duodenum
36. Jejunum
37. Colon
38. Rectum
39. Adrenals
40. Kidneys
41. Renal pelvis
42. Ureter
43. Bladder
44. Uterus
45. Prostate
46. Lymph nodes

Bones
47. Ribs
48. Sternum
49. Vertebrae
50. Symphysis
51. Sacrum
52. Coccyx
53. Psoas muscle

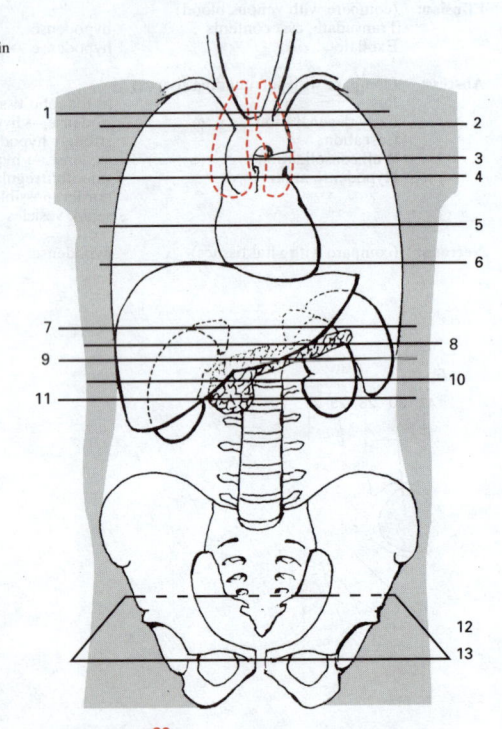

BASICS/NORMAL VALUES/DIAGNOSTIC METHODS

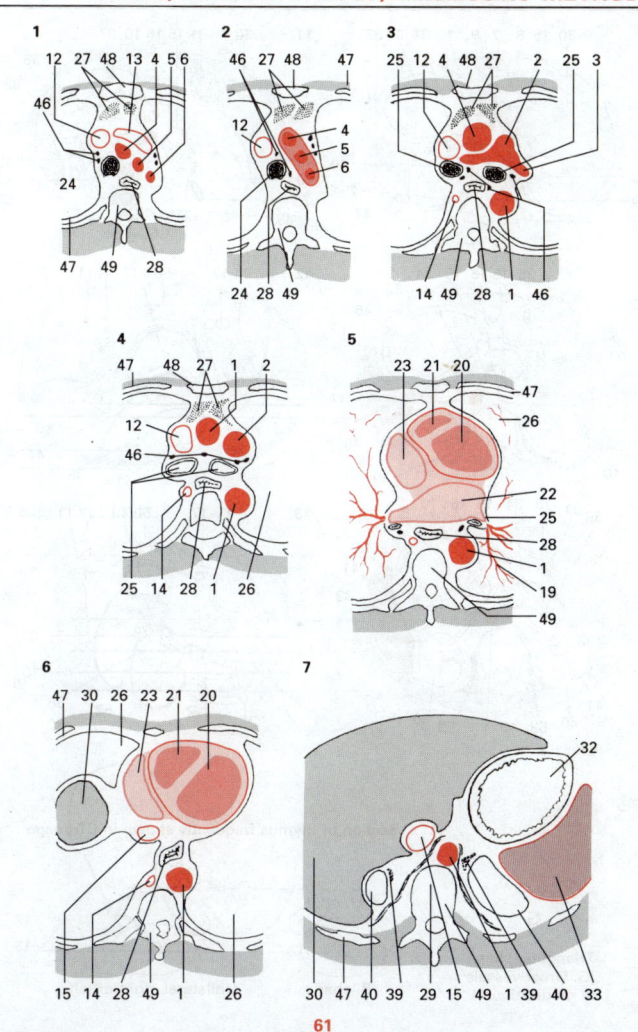

MEMORIX PEDIATRICS

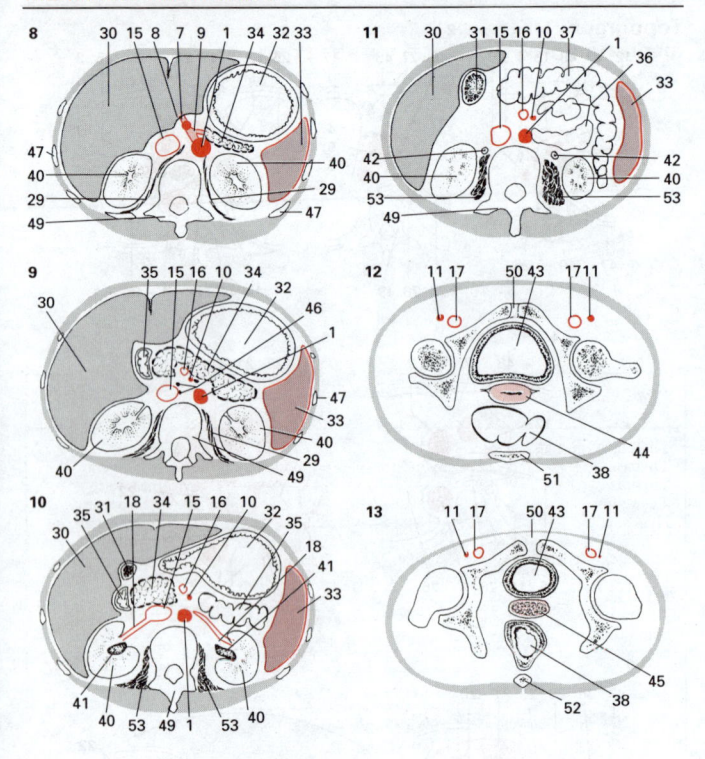

Section of thymus frequently shown in CT image

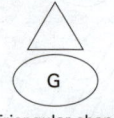

Triangular shape (G: Great vessels in mediastinum)

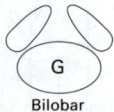

Bilobar

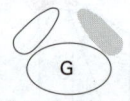

Unilateral, right or left

62

BASICS/NORMAL VALUES/DIAGNOSTIC METHODS

Topography of space-occupying structures in the mediastinum in X-ray and CT imaging

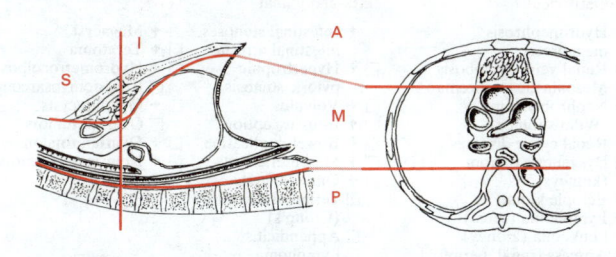

Anterior mediastinum (A)	Mid-mediastinum (M)	Posterior mediastinum (P)
Thymus hyperplasia Thymoma Thymus cyst Thymolipoma Hygroma Lymphadenitis Mediastinitis, abscess Hodgkin's lymphoma Non-Hodgkin's lymphoma Teratoma Seminoma Morgagni's hernia (liver)	**Superior mediastinum (S)** Paratracheal cyst Cystic esophageal duplication Esophageal diverticulum Lymphadenitis Lymphoma Histiocytosis X Metastases Aneurysms (aorta, etc.) **Inferior mediastinum (I)** Bronchogenic cyst Lymphadenitis Lymphoma Pericardial effusion Coronary aneurysm Achalasia Hiatus hernia	Neuroblastoma Ganglioneuroma Neurofibroma Pheochromocytoma Vertebrogenic tumors Aortic aneurysm Neurenteric cyst Bochdalek's hernia

MEMORIX PEDIATRICS

Space-occupying structures in the abdomen
+ Mostly in neonates ☐ In infants and older children

Retroperitoneal
- ☐ + Hydronephrosis megaureter
- + Renal vein thrombosis
- + Mesoblastic nephroma
- ☐ + Nephroblastoma (Wilm's tumor)
- ☐ + Renal cystic diseases
- ☐ Dysgenetic tumors (kidneys)
- ☐ + Ectopic kidney
- + Lymphoma (renal)
- ☐ Leukemia (kidney)
- ☐ Abscess (renal, perirenal)
- ☐ + Urachal diverticulum, urachal cyst
- ☐ + Splenic cyst
- ☐ Inflammatory splenomegaly
- ☐ Splenomegaly (storage diseases)
- ☐ Mesenchymal splenic tumors – benign, malignant
- ☐ + Accessory spleens
- ☐ + Splenic vein thrombosis
- ☐ Spleen sequestration (sickle cell anemia)
- ☐ Splenic torsion
- ☐ Mobile spleen
- + Adrenal hemorrhage
- ☐ Adrenal adenoma, adrenal carcinoma
- ☐ + Neuroblastoma
- ☐ Pheochromocytoma
- ☐ + Hygroma
- ☐ + Teratoma
- ☐ Lymphoma
- ☐ + Sarcoma
- ☐ Neurofibroma
- ☐ + Hematoma
- ☐ Aortic aneurysm
- + Ventral meningocele

Intra-abdominal
- + Intestinal stenoses, intestinal atresias
- ☐ + Hypertrophic pyloric stenosis
- ☐ + Volvulus
- ☐ + Intussusception
- ☐ + Bowel duplication
- ☐ + Mesenteric cysts
- ☐ + Omental cysts
- ☐ + Terminal ileitis (Crohn's)
- ☐ Appendicitis
- ☐ Lymphoma
- + Segmental bowel dilatation
- + Roser's cyst (residual yolk-duct)
- + Yolk-duct cyst
- ☐ + Gallbladder hydrops
- ☐ Torsion of gallbladder
- ☐ + Bile duct cyst
- + Tumors of gallbladder
- ☐ + Annular pancreas
- ☐ Pancreatic pseudocyst
- ☐ Hepatomegaly (storage)
- ☐ Liver cysts
- ☐ Parasitic liver cysts
- ☐ Liver abscess
- ☐ Liver metastases
- ☐ Hemangio-endothelioma
- ☐ Hepatoblastoma
- ☐ Hepatocellular carcinoma

Pelvic
- + Megacyst
- ☐ + Teratoma
- ☐ + Hydrometrocolpos
- ☐ Rhabdomyosarcoma
- ☐ + Ovarian cysts
- ☐ Ovarian tumors
- ☐ + Ovarian torsion
- ☐ + Neurogenic tumors

BASICS/NORMAL VALUES/DIAGNOSTIC METHODS

Nuclear medicine diagnosis

Problem	Method	Radiopharmaceuticals	Remarks
CSF fistula	Scintigraphy in two planes after 2 and 3 h. Comparing the two sides, measuring activity in the nasal or ear tampon	^{111}In-DTPA; ^{111}indium-diethylenetriamine pentaacetic acid (pentetic acid)	
Suspected osteomyelitis	Three-phase scintigraphy Ⓐ → 60 s perfusion phase (sequential scintigraphy) Ⓑ → 10 min extravasation phase (early static scintigraphy) Ⓒ → 2 h mineral phase (late static scintigraphy)	^{99m}Tc-methylenediphosphonate	Confirmation: Ⓐ Hyperemia Ⓑ Edema Ⓒ Reactive bone formation at the edge of the inflammation
Suspected multilocular bone tumor	Static scintigraphy (bones)	^{99m}Tc-phosphonate	
	Scintigraphy mostly positive in: 1. Benign tumors: osteoblastoma, osteoid osteoma, chondroma (extraosseous), osteoclastoma 2. Tumor-like bone processes: fibrous dysplasia of bone (Jaffe–Lichtenstein disease), eosinophilic granuloma 3. Primary malignant bone tumors: osteosarcoma, Ewing's sarcoma, undifferentiated chondrosarcoma, reticular cell sarcoma **Scintigraphy generally negative in:** 1. Benign tumors: osteoma, osteochondroma, chondroblastoma, non-ossifying bone fibroma, cartilagenous exostoses, enchondroma, hemangioma, neuroma 2. Primary malignant tumors: malignant fibrosing histiocytoma, malignant bone lymphoma, fibrosarcoma		
Metastases identification	Static whole-body scintigraphy	^{99m}Tc-methylenediphosphonate (^{99m}Tc-MDP) ^{99m}Tc-hydroxymethylene-diphosphonate (HMDP)	Metastases from: neuroblastoma, lymphoma, rhabdomyosarcoma, hepatoblastoma, retinoblastoma, thyroid carcinoma
Sonographically absent kidney	Static scintigraphy	^{99m}Tc-dimercaptobernstein acid (DMSA, dimercapto-succinic acid)	Demonstration of parenchyma, 100% tubular secretion
Urodynamic significance of a urinary tract obstruction	Functional scintigraphy with furosemide (frusemide)	^{123}I-orthoiodohippuric acid (I-hippuran) ^{99m}Tc-mercaptoacetyltri-glycerine (MAG$_3$)	^{123}I-hippuran filtration is 20% glomerular and 80% tubular. Only after furosemide is given can obstruction be distinguished from dilatation
Extent of chronic renal insufficiency	Functional scintigraphy	MAG$_3$	Perfusion trial with ^{99m}Tc-DTPA (filtered through glomeruli only)
Search for a source of bleeding, eg Meckel's diverticulum or a polyp	Static scintigraphy	^{99m}Tc-diethylenetriamine pentaacetic acid (DTPA, pentetic acid)	Marking of erythrocytes *in vivo* or *in vitro* with ^{99m}Tc
Intestinal protein loss	Activity measurement in feces after 5–6 days	^{51}Cr-serum protein or ^{51}CrCl$_3$	Normal excretion <1%
Megaloblastic anemia, vitamin B$_{12}$ deficiency	Schilling test: whole-body measurement	^{57}Co-vitamin B$_{12}$ orally	Pathologically reduced absorption = retention <45%, excretion in urine <4%

MEMORIX PEDIATRICS

Problem	Method	Radiopharmaceuticals	Comments
Autoimmune hemolytic anemia: splenectomy?	Spleen scintigraphy, liver scintigraphy	^{51}Chromate marked erythrocytes	Specific activity spleen: liver > 1.5 (= argument for splenectomy)
Search for accessory spleens	Spleen scintigraphy	^{51}Cr- or ^{99m}Tc-marked patient's erythrocytes	
Hypothyroidism: athyroidism? Ectopy?	Static thyroid scintigraphy	^{123}I Na (= sodium iodide)	^{123}I, ^{99m}Tc-scintigram to be considered
Function in multinodular goiter, search for thyroid carcinoma metastases Check after ^{131}I-treatment	Functional scintigraphy Static scintigraphy Static scintigraphy	^{123}I Na (= sodium iodide) ^{123}I Na (= sodium iodide) ^{123}I Na (= sodium iodide)	No X-ray contrast media to be used beforehand
Hypertension: suspected pheochromocytoma	Static scintigraphy		Accumulation in chromaffin tissues

Changes in radioiodine uptake
(After Winkel (1990).)

Reduced by:		Duration
X-ray contrast media	Excretion urography Micturition cystography Angiography	6 weeks
	Lymphography	<2 years
Iodine-containing drugs	Antiseptics Antidiarrhetics Anti-asthmatics Organic iodide	<2 weeks
	Dermatotherapeutics	<2 weeks
Thyrotropic drugs	Thyroxine	4 weeks
	Triiodothyronine	2 weeks
	Iodide	⩾2 weeks
	Perchlorate Thiouracil Mercaptoimidazole	⩾2 weeks
Other drugs	Corticoids Sulfonamide Androgens	<1 week
	Isoniazid, PAS	⩾2 weeks

Raised by:		
	Alimentary iodine deficiency	Pregnancy
	Failure of iodine organification	Rebound after thyrostatic agents

BASICS/NORMAL VALUES/DIAGNOSTIC METHODS

Magnetic resonance imaging (MRI)

A spectroscopic technique used in the investigation of the chemical composition of tissue.

In clinical magnetic resonance imaging (MRI), the patient is placed in a magnetic field with field strength between 0.3 and 1.5 Tesla. The precessing hydrogen nuclei ultimately allow the production of radiofrequency signals whose frequency is dependent upon the intensity of the magnetic field. A good deal of local measurable information can be extracted and reconstructed for visual record. In the resultant image, the signal intensity of the different tissues is dependent upon: (1) the two relaxation time constants (T_1- and T_2-times); (2) the repetition time (T_R); (3) the echo time (T_E); and (4) the stimulating angle.

Multiple techniques (pulse sequences) are used in MRI to produce optimal images. These may be divided into two main groups: (1) conventional spin-echo sequences; and (2) rapid pulse sequences (generally gradient echo sequences). In clinical applications, T_1- or T_2-weighted images can be acquired using both conventional and rapid techniques. The degree of weighting depends upon the choice of T_E/T_R. In 'T_1-weighted' images, most pathologic processes (inflammation, edema, fluid) are represented by decreased signal intensity with respect to the surrounding healthy tissues. T_2-weighted images are more sensitive in detecting pathology; however, resolution of the images is usually reduced with respect to T_1-weighted images, which reveal greater anatomic detail.

MRI: signal intensity of tissues and fluids

(After Bohnhof (1991).)

0 = no signal, + = poor signal, ++ = intermediate, +++ = strong signal.

Tissues, fluids	Weighting T_1	T_2
Bones, tendons, scars, cartilage	0	0
Free fluid, edema, CSF, cysts, intervertebral discs, synovia, necroses	+	+++
Abscess	+/++	+++
Hyaline cartilage	++	++
Liver, kidney, muscle	++	+/++
Fat tissue, bone marrow	+++	++

T_1 time is generally shorter than T_2.
T_R = repetition time (of the electromagnetic 90° stimulation impulse).
T_E = echo time (time difference between stimulation impulse and appearance of corresponding resonance signal).

Weight for T_1: T_R short, T_E short
T_2: T_R long, T_E long
Spin density: T_R long, T_E short.

MRI: interpretation/indications

Table for signal intensity in MRI of head and vertebral column (spin echo technique) (After Barnes and Mulkern (1992).)

| Weighting |||| Signal intensity |
T_1	T_2	Spin density	
Fat tissue	Meniscus	Fat tissue		+++
CNS – white matter	Cerebrospinal fluid	CNS gray matter		
CNS – gray matter	CNS – gray matter	Meniscus		
Meniscus	CNS – white matter	CNS – white matter		↓
Musculature	Fat tissue	Musculature		
Cerebrospinal fluid	Musculature	Cerebrospinal fluid		
Bones, dura, ligaments	Bones, dura, ligaments	Bones, dura, ligaments		
Blood vessels	Blood vessels	Blood vessels		+

Principal variations in signal intensity in MRI during postnatal myelogenesis

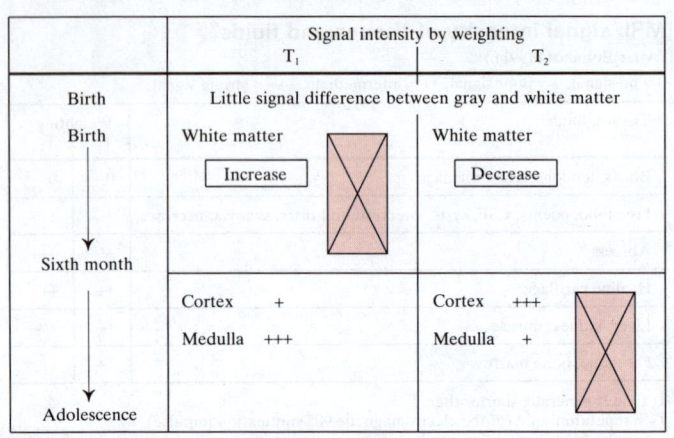

| | Signal intensity by weighting ||
	T_1	T_2
Birth	Little signal difference between gray and white matter	
Birth ↓ Sixth month	White matter [Increase]	White matter [Decrease]
↓ Adolescence	Cortex + Medulla +++	Cortex +++ Medulla +

⊠ = Investigatory method according to age.

BASICS/NORMAL VALUES/DIAGNOSTIC METHODS

Intracranial MRI

Signal intensity of MRI in physiological and pathological intracranial processes

Intensity: (+) = very little, + = little, ++ = intensity of normal brain tissue, +++ = raised.

Physiology/pathology	Signal intensity by weighting	
	T_1	T_2
– Normal intravascular flow	++	++
– Increased flow	+	+
• Stenosis, arteriovenous fistula		
• Turbulent flow (poststenotic, aneurysm)		
– Pulsating cerebrospinal fluid (arterial pulse) in area of foramen of Munro, aqueduct, foraminae of Luschka	(+)	(+)
– Reduced blood flow, stasis	+/++	++/+++
– Thrombus		
• fresh (Hb-Fe^{++})	+/++	(+)/+
• old (meth-Hb)	+++	+++
– Fibrin plug	(+)	(+)
– Bleeding (age)		
• <1 d	+	+++
• Hemolysis	+++	+++
• ~2–14 d	+/++	+
• >2–4 weeks	+++	+
• Hemosiderin	+/++	(+)
– Cerebrospinal fluid	+	+++
– Edema	+	+++
– Cyst content	++/+++	+++
– Abscess	++/+++	+++
– Calcification	+/++/+++	+/++
– Tumors (cellular)	+/++/+++	+
– Gd-DTPA*	+++	+++

* Gadolinium-diethylenetriamine penta-acetic acid.

MEMORIX PEDIATRICS

Ultrasound diagnosis

General guide to image documentation

(After Peters, Deeg and Weitzel (1987).)

Section	Image side (as seen by the viewer)	
	Left	Right
Longitudinal	Cranial	Caudal
Transverse Patient on back Patient on front	Right side of body Left side of body	Left side of body Right side of body
Sagittal (skull) Coronal (skull)	Frontal Right side	Occipital Left side
Note: Echocardiography, thoracic sonography: cranial = right of image. Transverse sections as with other structures (see above).		

- Define non-standard section terms precisely.
- Mark measurements on the picture.

General guide on description of findings
- Topographic localization
- Measure distances
- Assess surfaces/volumes arithmetically
- Shape
- Contour smooth/irregular, well/badly defined
- Structural components: echo-free (cysts), echogenic (eg: calcification), tubular (vessels), bands, lines (septa)
- Basic texture: homogeneous/inhomogeneous, fine/coarse
- Echogenicity: low/high
- Movement phenomena
- Variation in findings due to changes in transducer placement pressure.

Quality criteria for ultrasound images
- Evenly clear picture
- Good surface demarcation and many gray gradations
- Echo-free demonstration of border-free areas (cavity of urinary bladder and gallbladder, plexus-free CSF spaces).

Sonographic volume measurement using the ellipsoid formula:

Volume of organ (cm³) = length × width × $\dfrac{T_1 + T_2}{2}$ × 0.523

T_1 = depth of organ in longitudinal section
T_2 = depth of organ in transverse section

Applicable for spleen, kidneys, bladder, uterus, ovaries, testes

---

Rule for parenchymatous organs: echogenicity ↓ in acute inflammations
echogenicity ↑ in chronic inflammations

BASICS/NORMAL VALUES/DIAGNOSTIC METHODS

Ultrasound diagnosis: organs

Organ	Section	Demonstrable structures	Critical criteria, normal values pathological examples
Skull/brain, CNS	Sagittal, parasagittal	Cingular gyrus, corpus callosum ventricular system, choroid plexus, brain stem. From medial to lateral: thalamus striate body (caudate nucleus, pallidum, putamen). Basal cisterns, cerebellum	No echo: CSF, cavity, aneurysms Moderately echogenic: brain parenchyma More echogenic: plexus, vessels, fissures, sulci Highly echogenic: cerebral and cerebellar falx, cerebellar tentorium, base of skull
	Coronal	Cerebral falx, interhemispheric cleft, corpus callosum, cavity of septum lucidum, lateral ventricles, third ventricle, plexus, basal ganglia, internal capsule, Sylvian fissure, hypothalamus, cerebellum, basal cisterns, base of skull	Marking of the gyri: ↓ in brain edema, pressure hydrocephalus; ↑ brain atrophy pattern distorted by lissencephalia Ventricle width: ↑ in hydrocephalus; ↓ in edema, tumor, bleeding Ventricular shape: round; smooth border in pressure hydrocephalus; irregular in atrophy, malformation
Neck organs	Transverse, longitudinal	Thyroid (medial to the common carotid artery and jugular vein)	Echo texture fine, homogeneous Echogenicity moderate Volume: 7–8 ml in 10-year-olds 14–15 ml in adults Texture non-homogeneous in thyroiditis Echogenicity ↓ in hypothyroidism
		Parotid gland	As thyroid
		Lymph nodes	Echogenicity not homogeneous, texture coarser in lymphadenitis Echogenicity ↓ in abscess Hygroma echo-free, possibly septal Branchiogenic cysts echo-free
Mediastinum	Longitudinal, transverse First to fourth intercostal space parasternal, suprasternal, transsternal (young infants)	Thymus Lymphnodes Great vessels, heart	Moderately echogenic, finely homogeneous echotexture Echogenicity ↓ + inhomogeneous texture: thymoma, lymphoma Echo-free: hygroma, thymus cyst, bronchogenic cyst
Pleura	Subxiphoid	Enlarged pleural split Liver	Echo-free: serous effusion Internal echos: purulent serofibrinous exudate Septa
Diaphragm	Subxiphoid	Diaphragm Liver	Highly echogenic, movements registered by M-mode

71

MEMORIX PEDIATRICS

Organ	Section	Demonstrable structures	Critical criteria, normal values pathological examples
Heart	Standard planes: long axis = longitudinal heart axis (L); short axis vertical to long axis (K); four-chamber plane vertical to the long and short axes (four-chamber view) (V)		RA/LA = right/left atrium; RV/LV = right/left ventricle; AS = atrial septum, VS = ventricular septum; TV = tricuspid valve; MV = mitral valve; PV/AV = pulmonary/aortic valve; PT = pulmonary trunk; AO = aorta; PV = pulmonary vein; PA = pulmonary arteries The para- or suprasternal thymus is demonstrable depending on age. Subcostally the liver serves as an acoustic window
	Acoustic window		Comparison of the size and shape of the chambers
	1 Parasternal second to fourth left intercostal spaces		Septal defects: ECG-triggered visualization of endodiastolic loss of echo, size and shape of defect, defect margin echo-dense
	– long axis:	LA, LV, AO, AV, MV, coronary venous sinus, RV, TV, VS, PT	
	– short axis:	LA, MV, LV, AV, RA, TV, RV, PT, VS, left coronary arteries	
	2 Apical		
	– long axis:	Left heart, VS, AO, RV	
	– four-chamber view:	All chambers, MV, TV, AS, VS Pulmonary venous connection	Valve movements Valvar stenosis: • Valve margins echo-dense • Valve position in emptying phase • Limited jerky valvar action • Planimetrically reduced valve opening area • Prestenotic muscle hypertrophy • Poststenotic vessel dilatation
	3 Subcostal		
	– long axis:	RA, TV, RV, PT, PV, AS, VS, LA, MV, LV, AV, AO	
	– short axis:	LA, RA, AS, LV, RV, PT, inferior and superior vena cava	
	– four-chamber view:	LA, MV, LV, AV, AO, RA, AS, TV, PT	
	4 Suprasternal		
	– Long axis:	Ascending AO, aortic arch with vessel origins, LA, right pulmonary artery, vein innominata	
	– short, axis:	LA, ascending AO, right pulmonary artery, brachiocephalic vein, innominate vein superior vena cava	

BASICS/NORMAL VALUES/DIAGNOSTIC METHODS

Organ	Section	Demonstrable structures	Critical criteria, normal values, pathological examples
Liver	1 Sternal	Liver, aorta, celiac trunk, superior mesenteric artery, esophagus, pancreas, inferior vena cava, portal vein, splenic vein, small omentum	Shape, contour Moderate echogenicity, but less away from transducer head Texture fine, homogeneous Hepatic veins echo-free without wall echoes Portal branches echo-free with wall echoes Hepatic arteries, bile ducts seen as tubular structures, gallbladder 2–10 cm long, echo-free Echogenicity ↓ in acute hepatitis, acute obstruction, lymphoma, hemangiomatosis, metastases, hematomas Echogenicity ↑ (often with both inhomogeneous and rough texture) in chronic hepatitis, portal hypertension, storage diseases, hepatoblastoma, metastases
	2 Midclavicular right	Liver, right kidney	
	3 Flank (anterior axillary line right)	Liver, right kidney, adrenals, diaphragm	
	4 Subcostal right	Liver, hepatic veins, inferior vena cava, portal vein, gallbladder, bile duct	
Pancreas	Subxiphoid transverse	Liver, pancreas longitudinal, aorta	Shape, size (Ø = 0.7–2.5 cm) Echoes as with the liver Echogenicity ↓ in acute pancreatitis, pancreatic carcinoma Echogenicity ↑ (+ inhomogeneous texture) in chronic pancreatitis Pseudocysts echo-poor or echo-free with echo-dense wall
	Subcostal left	Stomach, pancreas (body, tail)	
	Dorsal right	Right kidney, pancreas (head)	
	Dorsal left	Left kidney, pancreas (tail)	
Spleen	1 Subcostal parallel to 10th rib (longitudinal) 2 Vertical to this (transverse)	Spleen (length, depth) Splenic artery and vein in hilus, left kidney, adrenals (neonates), stomach, colon Spleen (width, depth)	Volume Echogenicity: low to moderate Texture: fine, homogeneous Echogenicity ↓ in sepsis, obstruction Echogenicity ↑ in storage diseases, lymphomas and metastases Echo-free: splenic cysts

MEMORIX PEDIATRICS

Upper abdominal region
Sites of upper abdominal organs

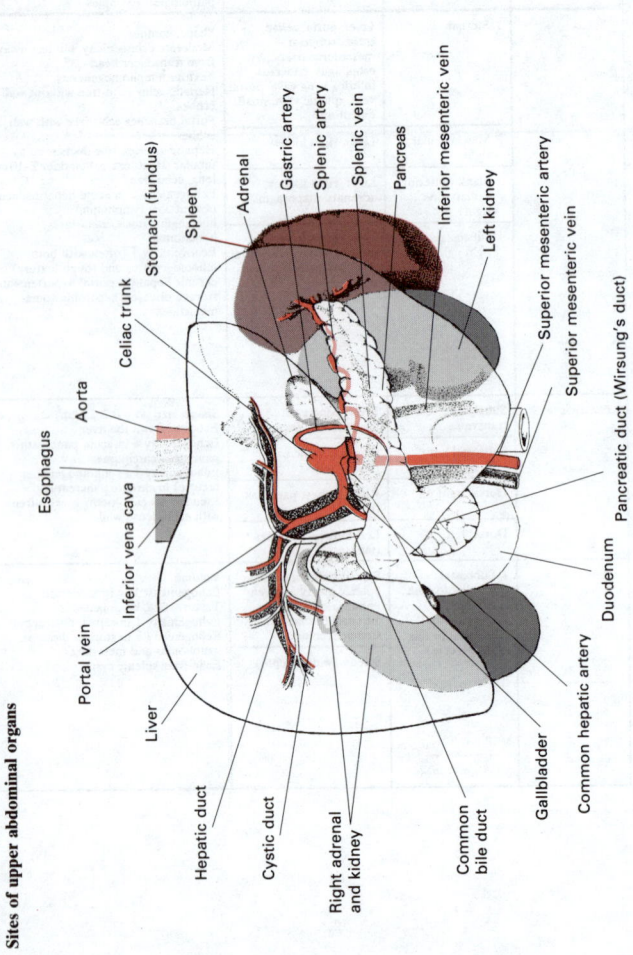

BASICS/NORMAL VALUES/DIAGNOSTIC METHODS

Organ	Section	Demonstrable structures	Critical criteria, normal values, pathological examples
Kidneys	Lateral longitudinal longitudinal loin section	Right liver, left spleen, renal parenchyma, calyces, pelvis, ureteric exit	Parenchymal edge: echogenicity moderate, echotexture fine, homogeneous Central echo (vessels, pelvis, fatty tissue): high-grade echoes, inhomogeneous Double kidneys → doubled moderate echo (in longitudinal) Pathology: divergent renal contour Parenchymal edge wide/narrow, moderate echo, less defined Echogenicity ↓: acute nephritis Echogenicity ↑: chronic nephritis Nephronophthisis, spongy renal medulla, hemolytic uremic syndrome, uric acid nephropathy, chronic transplant rejection Wilms' tumor: mostly clear contour, moderate echogenicity, moderate to coarse, inhomogeneous echo texture Echo-free: cysts
	Dorsal longitudinal, transverse	Back muscles, kidneys	
Urinary tract	Longitudinal loin section, longitudinal and transverse suprapubic	Abdominal wall, bladder, mouth of ureter	Ureter demonstrable only in reflux grade 3–5 Urinary bladder echo-free Bladder wall: 2–3 mm thick, moderate echogenic, texture fine, homogeneous Establish urinary retention: ellipsoid formula
Adrenals	Right: longitudinal in anteroaxillary line, or loin, subcostal	Liver, kidney, adrenals (cortex, medulla), inferior vena cava	Shape, size Echgoenicity: moderate Echo texture: fine, homogeneous Bleeding: echo-poor–echo-free Waterhouse–Friderichsen syndrome: echo texture inhomogeneous Neuroblastoma: mostly strongly echogenic, echo texture inhomogeneous
	Left: loin, 1st/12th intercostal space	Kidney, adrenal, spleen and vessels, tail of pancreas, stomach	

Kidney size and volume

MEMORIX PEDIATRICS

Organ	Section	Demonstrable structures	Critical criteria, normal values pathological examples
Gastrointestinal tract	Variable	Stomach wall: thickness 1–4 mm Pylorus: Ø < 15 mm – muscle: 2–3 mm thick – length < 16 mm Bowel wall: 1–2 mm thick	Wall thickness, width of lumen Ø of intestinal loops Stomach contents: tea, juices, echo-poor; milk, meals (solids), echo-rich Intestinal contents: feces high-grade echogenic, moderate echo texture Intestinal wall Echogenic: inner and outer surfaces, submucosa Echo-poor: mucosa, muscularis Peristalsis Intra-abdominal fluid (demonstrable from 10–20 ml upwards) Intra-abdominal gas Stenosis: prestenotic dilatation → piano key phenomenon (= prominent Kerkring folds), peristalsis ↑ Intussusception: target sign = concentric rings, in longitudinal/oblique sections = pseudokidney sign

Uterus, ovaries, vagina	Suprapubic, transverse, longitudinal	Abdominal wall, bladder, uterus vagina, ovaries, rectum	Uterus:
			• prepubertal: length 2–3.5 cm
			  depth 0.5–1.0 cm
			  volume 1.0 cm³
			• postpubertal: length 5–8 cm
			  depth 1.5–3 cm
			  volume 50 cm³
			Echogenicity: low-grade
			Echo texture: fine, homogeneous
			Ovaries: volume
			• prepubertal: 0.1–1.0 cm³
			• postpubertal: 2–6 cm³
			Echogenicity: moderate to high grade
			Echo texture: rough, inhomogeneous
			Vagina: tubular form, echo-rich lumen, echo-poor wall

Prostate	Suprapubic, transverse longitudinal	Abdominal wall, bladder, prostate	Echogenicity low grade Echo texture homogeneous, rough
Testes	Scrotal	Testis, epididymis	Testes: echogenicity moderate grade Echotexture fine, homogeneous Epididymis: echogenicity like testis, texture less homogeneous than testis Inhomogeneous texture in testicular torsion, orchitis, epididymitis Echogenicity ↓ in leukemia echo-free in hydrocele and spermatocele
Vessels of the abdomen	Substernal longitudinal Substernal transverse Liver hilus longitudinal = vertical to subcostal section	2 Aorta 1 Inferior vena cava Aorta, inferior vena cava 3 Portal vein longitudinal, inferior vena cava	Echo-free to echo-poor lumen Pulsation synchronous with heart beat Ø 4–5 mm (body size > 55 cm) Ø 11–14 mm (body size > 150 cm) Echo-poor lumen Aorta round, vena cava oval, diameter of inferior vena cava on inspiration ↓, on expiration ↑ Wall echogenic, lumen echo-free Ø 3–4.5 mm (body size > 55 cm) Ø 7–10 mm (body size > 150 cm)

BASICS/NORMAL VALUES/DIAGNOSTIC METHODS

Ultrasound, normal values: spleen

Sonographic normal values for spleen volume (calculated by the ellipsoid formula, 95% confidence limits in red, regression line).
(Modified from Dittrich *et al.* (1983).)

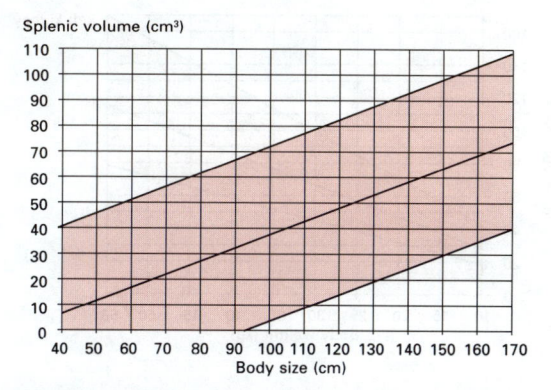

Sonographic normal values for mean kidney volume in infancy (calculated using the ellipsoid formula, 95% confidence limits in red).
(Modified from Peters *et al.* (1986).)

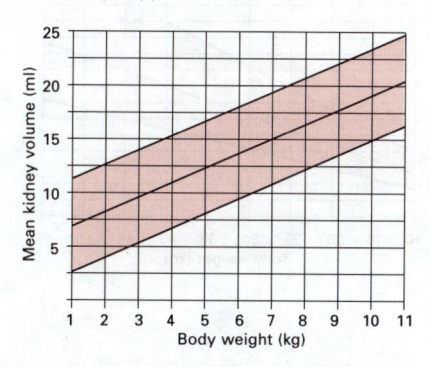

Ultrasound, normal values: kidneys

Sonographic normal values for renal volume (calculated using the ellipsoid formula, median values, R = regression line, 95% confidence limits in red).
(Modified from Dinkel *et al.* (1985).)

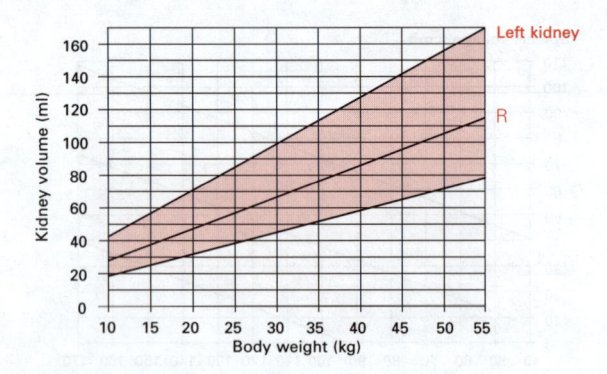

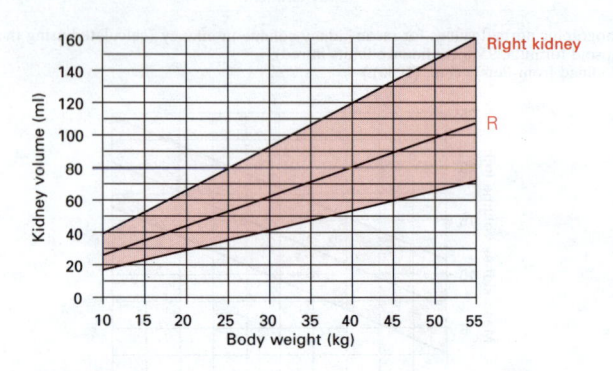

BASICS/NORMAL VALUES/DIAGNOSTIC METHODS

Intracranial hemorrhage

Grades of subependymal and intraventricular hemorrhage

Grad	Bleeding – unilateral or bilateral	Section view		
		Transverse (computed tomogram)	Parasagittal (ultrasonogram)	Coronal (ultrasonogram)
I	Small subependymal hemorrhage, no dilatation of the ventricular system			
II	Subependymal and small intraventricular hemorrhage with or without hemorrhage in the plexus. No ventricular dilatation			
III	As II, but massive bleeding in the lateral ventricles. Ventricle dilated, most often irreversibly so			
IV	As III, with added parenchymal bleeding. Later hydrocephalus and porencephalus			

Note: in the differential diagnosis of grade III, there is rarely a homogeneous echo-rich plexus reaction with the ventricle enlarged a little or moderately (? plexus hemorrhage). No progression, good prognosis.

Color-coded Doppler ultrasonography
Pulsed Doppler method

Flow features	Color code	
Direction	Towards transducer	Red
	Away from transducer	Blue
Velocity	Bright color in several steps by admixture of white (the faster, the brighter)	
Variance (simultaneous measurement of flow in different direction, e.g.: turbulence)	Mixing of green to red and blue	

Measurements in Doppler ultrasonography

Stenotic pressure gradient (kPa, mmHg) = $4 \times (\text{maximal velocity [V]})^2$

(simplified Bernoulli equation)

Stenotic pressure gradient (kPa, mmHg) = $4 \times (V^2 \text{ distal} - V^2 \text{ proximal})$

Maximal systolic velocity $\qquad V_S$ (m/s)

End-systolic velocity $\qquad V_{ES}$ (m/s)

End-diastolic velocity $\qquad V_{ED}$ (m/s)

Mean flow velocity (time average velocity) TAV = mean of all speeds in measured volumes per cardiac cycle

Pulsatility index $PI = \dfrac{V_S - V_{ED}}{TAV}$

Resistance index $RI = \dfrac{V_S - V_{ED}}{V_S}$

Flow (cm³/s) = cross-section of vessel (cm²) $\times \dfrac{\text{velocity (cm/s)}}{\cos(\Theta)}$

(Θ) = Angle between ultrasound direction and flow direction, omitted if directions identical.

CARDIOLOGY

Principle of Doppler ultrasonography

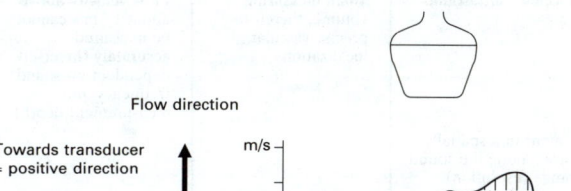

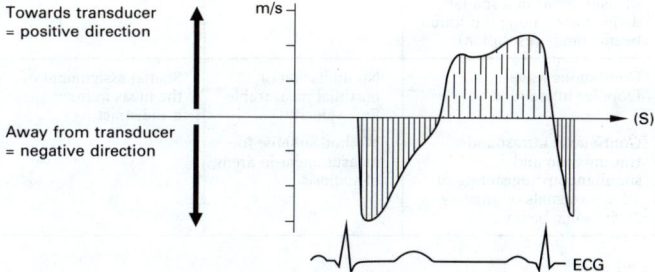

Transducer

Flow direction

Towards transducer
= positive direction

Away from transducer
= negative direction

ECG

Registration example: Continuous wave (CW) Doppler ultrasonogram of the pulmonary trunk of a neonate. Transducer position left parasternal. Below the baseline, systolic forward flow away from the transducer. Above the baseline, oppositely directed diastolic flow via the persistent ductus arteriosus.

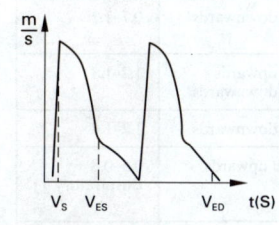

Measurement of the flow velocity

V_S maximum systolic flow velocity
V_{ES} end systolic flow velocity
V_{ED} end diastolic flow velocity

MEMORIX PEDIATRICS

Doppler ultrasound

Procedure	Advantages	Disadvantages
Pulsed Doppler ultrasound Measurement in a spatially defined area along the sound beam (range resolution)	Small measuring volume, therefore precise vascular localization	Flow velocity above about 1.5 m/s cannot be measured accurately (inversely dependent on sound frequency and measurement depth)
Continuous wave Doppler ultrasound Continuous ultrasound transmission and simultaneous registering of all echo signals originating in the sonic beam	No limitation of maximal measurable flow velocity Method suitable for measurement in areas of stenosis	Spatial assignment of the measurement sites is indistinct

Ultrasound measurement of normal flow velocities in the heart and great vessels

Transducer position	Measurement site flow	Presentation in image (leading outward)	Flow velocity (m/s)
Apical	Mitral flow, distal at mitral valve edge	Diastolic upwards two peaks	0.8–1.3
Apical	Left ventricular outflow tract	Systolic downwards	0.7–1.2
Suprasternal Apical	Ascending aorta Ascending aorta	Systolic upwards Systolic downwards	1.2–1.8
Suprasternal	Descending aorta	Systolic downwards	1.2–1.8
Apical, parasternal short axis	Tricuspid flow, distal at valve edge	Diastolic upwards	0.5–0.8 (inspiratory ↑)
Parasternal short axis	Pulmonary trunk	Systolic downwards	0.7–1.1

BASICS/NORMAL VALUES/DIAGNOSTIC METHODS

AZ = ejection time of the left ventricle

M-mode echocardiography
Example of recording principle: aortic valves

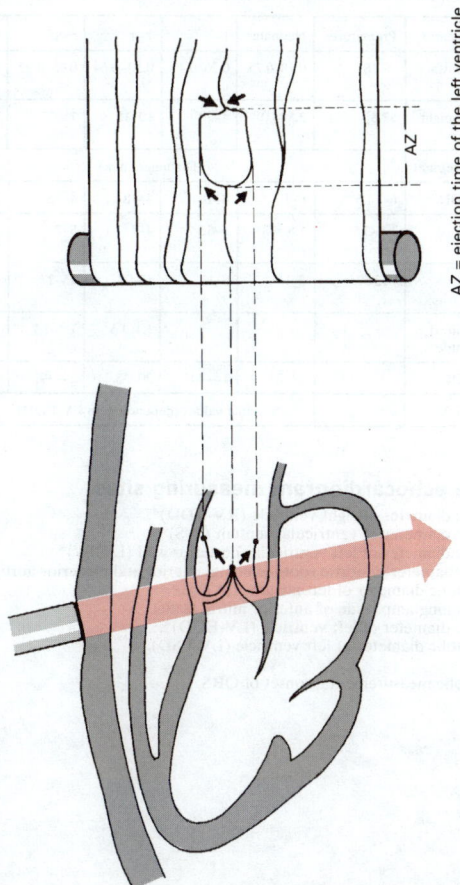

Measurements with M-mode echocardiogram
(After Peters, Deeg and Weitzel (1987); Keutel (1979).)

	Age (years)	Prematures	Neonates	1	1–4	5–8	9–14	>14
	Body surface (m^2)	<0.18	0.18–0.25	0.26–0.49	0.50–0.64	0.65–0.95	1.0–1.5	>1.5
	Body weight (kg)	>2.5	2.5–4.0	4–10	10–15	15–25	25–40	>40
N	Measurement	\multicolumn{7}{c}{Diameter (mm)}						
a	RV-EDD	6–14.5	6–17	4–18	4–18	4–18	7–18	8–30
b	IVS	1.5–3.5	1.8–4.3	3–6.5	4–7	5–7	5–8	5–13
c	LVPW							
d	Ao	–12.5	5–13	8–17	13–24	15–27	15–35	15–40
e	LA							
f	D-E mitral amplitude				1.1–1.5	1.4–1.7	1.9–2.3	>2.0
g	LV-EDD		12–25	14–30	20–33	24–39	30–48	37–55
h	LV-ESD	\multicolumn{7}{c}{variable values (depending on LV-EDD)}						

M-mode echocardiogram measuring sites
a diastolic diameter of right ventricle (RV-EDD)*.
b diastolic diameter of ventricular septum (IVS)*.
c diastolic diameter of left ventricular posterior wall (LVPW)*.
d systolic diameter of aortic root including anterior and posterior aortic wall (Ao).
e end-systolic diameter of left atrium (LA).
f D-E opening amplitude of anterior mitral leaflet.
g diastolic diameter of left ventricle (LV-EDD)*.
h end-systolic diameter of left ventricle (LV-ESD).

* end-diastolic measurement at onset of QRS.

CARDIOLOGY

One-dimensional (M-mode) echocardiography

Measurements of left ventricle

Volumes

Calculation using simplified ellipsoid formula: length × width × depth
Assumption: width = depth [= transverse diameter] (measuring on M-mode record)
Length is measured in two-dimensional sections.

S = end-systolic; D = end-diastolic; HR = heart rate; EDD = diastolic diameter;
ESD = systolic diameter; EDV = end diastolic volume; ESV = end-systolic volume;
ADD = atrial diastolic diameter.

V_S = (transverse diameter)^2 × longitudinal diameter (cm^3)
V_D = (transverse diameter)^2 × longitudinal diameter (cm^3)

Stroke volume (SV): $\quad SV = V_D - V_S$ (cm^3)

Cardiac output: $\quad CO$ (l/min) $= SV \times HR \times 10^{-3}$

Shortening fraction of left ventricle (SF)

$$SF = \frac{EDD - ESD}{EDD} \times 100(\%) \quad \text{Normal range: 26–42\%}$$

Ejection fraction of left ventricle (EF)

$$EF = \frac{EDV - ESV}{EDV} \quad \text{Normal range: right ventricle: 0.58–0.68}$$
$$\text{left ventricle: 0.65–0.77}$$

Mean velocity of circumferential fiber shortening (Vcf)

$$Vcf \text{ (circumference/s)} = \frac{EDD - ESD}{EDD \times AT} \quad (AT = \text{left ventricular ejection time} = \text{aortic valve opening time})$$

Vcf normal values: Neonates   1.51 ± 0.04
                      Infants   1.74
                      Children >1 y   1.33 ± 0.19

MEMORIX PEDIATRICS

Cardiac cycle

Calculation of the circulation values from invasive measurement of pressure and O₂ saturation

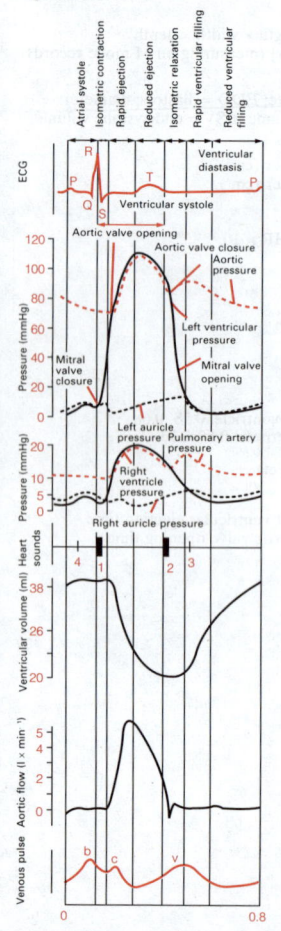

Cardiac output (CO)

$$= \frac{O_2 \text{ consumption } (cm^3/min)}{\text{arteriovenous } O_2 \text{ diff.} (cm^3/100\,cm^3) \times 10 \times BS} (l/min \times m^2)$$

O_2 consumption data are obtained from tables of normal values for age and sex
BS = body surface (m²)
Arteriovenous O_2 differences (cm³O_2/100 cm³ blood (%))
* systemic circulation O_2 saturation aorta (arteries) – mean O_2 saturation venae cavae (%)
* pulmonary circulation O_2 saturation pulmonary veins – mean O_2 saturation venae cavae (%)

Mean vena cava saturation

$$= \frac{2 \times O_2(\%) \text{ superior vena cava} + O_2(\%) \text{ inferior vena cava}}{3} (\%)$$

Mean arterial pressure

$$= \frac{p_{syst} + 2 \times p_{diast}}{3} (mmHg \times 0.1333 = kPa)$$

$$= p_{diast.} + \frac{p_{syst.} - p_{diast.}}{3}$$

Mean atrial pressures (p_{mRA}, p_{mLA})

$$= \frac{a + x + v + y}{4} (mmHg, kPa)$$

a = atrial contraction wave, x = end of ventricular systolic pressure fall
v = AV-valve opening wave, y = early systolic minimum pressure

Vascular resistance (Rs, Rp)
CO_s in systemic circulation
CO_p in pulmonary circulation
p_m = mean pressure

Peripheral total resistance $R_R = \frac{p_{mAo} - p_{mRA}}{CO_s} (U \times m^2)$

Pulmonary vessels resistance $R_p = \frac{p_{mPA} - p_{mLA}}{CO_p} (U \times m^2)$

Shunt volumes
LRS = left-right shunt   RLS = right-left shunt

Normal: $\frac{CO_p}{CO_s} = 1$ LRS: $\frac{CO_p}{CO_s} > 1$ RLS: $\frac{CO_p}{CO_s} < 1$

$$LRS = \frac{O_2(\%) \text{ pulmonary artery} - O_2(\%) \text{ caval veins}}{O_2(\%) \text{ pulmonary vein} - O_2(\%) \text{ caval veins}} \times 100$$

$$(= \text{shunt in \% of } CO_p)$$

$$RLS = \frac{O_2(\%) \text{ pulmonary vein} - O_2(\%) \text{ Ao}}{O_2(\%) \text{ pulmonary vein} - O_2(\%) \text{ caval veins}} \times 100$$

$$(= \text{shunt in \% of } CO_s)$$

CARDIOLOGY

Normal values for cardiovascular pressures and O$_2$ saturation

Vessels/cavities	Pressure (mmHg (kPa)) Systolic	Diastolic (end diastolic)	Mean pressure	O$_2$ saturation (%)
Superior vena cava	–	–	–	70
Inferior vena cava	–	–	–	76
Right atrium	a wave: 5 (0.66)	v wave: 3 (0.4)	4 (0.52)	72
Pulmonary veins	–	–	–	97
Left atrium	a wave: 7 (0.93)	v wave: 10 (1.33)	6 (0.8)	95
Right ventricle	20–35 (2.7–4.7)	0 (5 [0.66])	12 (1.6)	72
Pulmonary trunk	20–35 (2.7–4.7)	7–20 (0.9–2.7)	12 (1.6)	72
Left ventricle	80–120 (10.7–16)	0 (6 [0.8])	40 (5.3)	95
Ascending aorta	80–120 (10.7–16)	50–65 (6.6–9.0)	70 (9.3)	95

Pulmonary vascular resistance: normal range 1–4 U/m^2

Ratio of total resistance in the systemic (R_s) and pulmonary (R_p) circulation:
R_p/R_s = 0.2   normal
      = 0.6   limiting value for operability in transposition of the great arteries
      = 0.8   limiting value for operability in cardiac anomalies with left–right shunt.

Arterial pulse types – diagnostic significance

Quality	Physiological significance	Diagnostic points
Rapid	Heart rate ↑	Emotion, work, fever, myocarditis, anemia, hypoxia, hypovolemia, pericardial effusion, endocardial fibrosis, infection, hyperthyroidism, poisoning (atropine, digitalis, carbon monoxide), pheochromocytoma, cardiac failure, tachycardias, cerebral seizures
Slow	Heart rate ↓	Sleep, vagotonia, ↑ intracranial pressure, anorexia, athlete's heart, carotid sinus syndrome, acute myocarditis, abnormal intracardiac impulse conduction, hepatitis
Irregular	Rhythm	Extrasystoles, mitral valve prolapse
Fast and bounding	Rising velocity ↑ (*Windkessel* function)	Aortic valve regurgitation, aortopulmonary septal defect, persistent ductus arteriosus, aortic coarctation (proximal)
Poor (narrow)	Amplitude ↓	'low output' shock, aortic valve stenosis, aortic (coarctation) (distal), pericardial effusion, constrictive pericarditis, infusion thorax (extravascular infusion)
Alternans	Amplitude ~	Cardiomyopathy, cardiac failure
Hard	Blood pressure ↑	Hypertension
Soft	Blood pressure ↓	Hypotension, cardiac failure
Paradoxical	Inspiratory filling deficit	Pericarditis, left–right shunt ↑, status asthmaticus

Normal values for heart rate
(After Garson (1987).)

Age	Mean values	Extreme range
1 d	123	88–168
1–2 d	123	57–170
3–6 d	129	87–166
1–3 weeks	148	96–188
1–2 months	149	114–204
3–5 months	141	101–188
6–11 months	134	100–176
1–2 y	119	68–165
3–4 y	108	68–145
5–7 y	100	60–139
8–11 y	91	51–145
12–15 y	85	51–133

CARDIOLOGY

Heart murmurs – grades of intensity

Grade 1/6: Very faint murmur, audible during apnea or after concentrated auscultation in quiet surroundings

Grade 2/6: Soft murmur, audible without intensive auscultation

Grade 3/6: Medium intensity murmur without a thrill

Grade 4/6: Loud murmur with added soft thrill

Grade 5/6: Very loud murmur with marked thrill

Grade 6/6: Murmur so loud that it is audible with the stethoscope up to 1 cm away from the thoracic wall

Auscultation points (maximum murmurs) in congenital heart defects

S systolic, D diastolic, SD systolic–diastolic sound, 1–5 intercostal spaces (ICS), → sound direction.

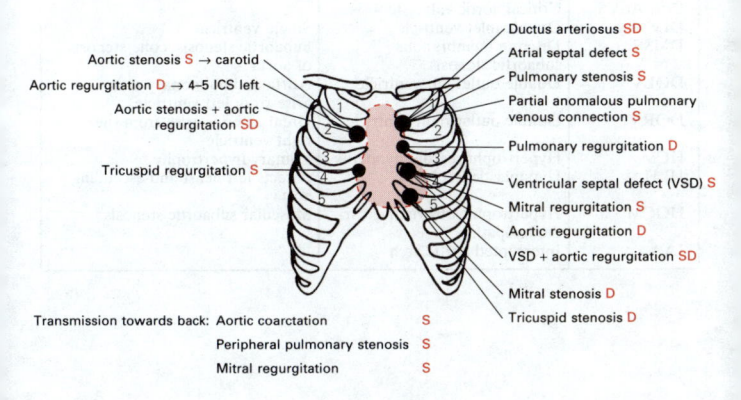

Aortic stenosis S → carotid
Aortic regurgitation D → 4–5 ICS left
Aortic stenosis + aortic regurgitation SD
Tricuspid regurgitation S

Ductus arteriosus SD
Atrial septal defect S
Pulmonary stenosis S
Partial anomalous pulmonary venous connection S
Pulmonary regurgitation D
Ventricular septal defect (VSD) S
Mitral regurgitation S
Aortic regurgitation D
VSD + aortic regurgitation SD
Mitral stenosis D
Tricuspid stenosis D

Transmission towards back: Aortic coarctation S
Peripheral pulmonary stenosis S
Mitral regurgitation S

Congenital defects: glossary (heart and great vessels)
(See Schumacher and Bühlmeyer (1989).)

Abbreviation	Description	Synonyms/supplementation
AI	Aortic regurgitation	Aortic valve insufficiency
AoA	Aortic atresia	
AoVA	Aortic valve atresia	
AoVS	Aortic valve stenosis	Valvar aortic stenosis
APSD	Aortopulmonary septal defect	
APW	Aortopulmonary window	
AS	Aortic stenosis	Valvar, supra-, or subvalvar
ASD	Atrial septal defect	
ASD I	ASD primary type	Primary ostium defect
ASD II	ASD secondary type	Secondary ostium defect
ASH	Asymmetrical septum hypertrophy	Muscular subaortic stenosis
AVSD	Atrioventricular septal defect	Defect of the atrioventricular canal, endocardial cushion defect
CA	Coarctation of the aorta	Pre-, juxta-, postductal
CAT	Common arterial trunk	
CAVSD	Complete AVSD	Complete AV canal
CCT	Congenitally corrected transposition of the great arteries	Aorta runs leftward in front of the pulmonary trunk
Crit. AoVS	Critical aortic valve stenosis	
DIV	Double inlet ventricle	Single ventricle
DMSS	Discrete membranous subaortic stenosis	Subaortic stenosis, cone stenosis of aorta
DOLV	Double outlet left ventricle	Aorta and pulmonary artery arise from left ventricle
DORV	Double outlet right ventricle	Great arteries arise from the right ventricle
HCM	Hypertrophic cardiomyopathy	Primary hypertrophy
HLH	Hypoplastic left heart	Affects left heart and ascending aorta
HOCM	Hypertrophic obstructive cardiomyopathy	Muscular subaortic stenosis
IAA	Interrupted aortic arch	

CARDIOLOGY

Congenital defects: glossary (continued)

Abbreviation	Description	Synonyms/supplementation
IHSS	Idiopathic hypertrophic subaortic stenosis	Asymmetrical septal hypertrophy
Inf. PS	Infundibular pulmonary stenosis	Infundibular stenosis
MR	Mitral (valve) regurgitation	Mitral insufficiency
MS	Mitral stenosis	Valvar mitral stenosis, supra- or subvalvar
MvA	Mitral valve atresia	See HLH
MvP	Mitral valve prolapse	
NOCM	Non-obstructive cardiomyopathy	Primary NOCM: endocardial fibroelastosis, secondary NOCM = symptomatic
PA	Pulmonary atresia	
PAPVC	Partial anomalous pulmonary venous connection	Pulmonary venous transposition
PaVA	Pulmonary valve atresia	
PaVS	Pulmonary valve stenosis	
PAVSD	Partial atrioventricular septal defect	Partial AV canal, primum ostium defect, endocardial cushion defect
PDA	Patent (persistent) ductus arteriosus	
PFO	Patent foramen ovale	Persistent foramen ovale
PS	Pulmonary stenosis	Valvar, supra-, subvalvar, central/peripheral supravalvar PS
SAS	Subaortic stenosis	Subaortic stenosis, cone stenosis of aorta
SV	Single ventricle	See DIV, biatrial univentricular heart
SVAS	Supravalvar aortic stenosis	
TA	Tricuspid atresia	
TAC	Truncus arteriosus communis	
TAPVC	Total anomalous pulmonary venous connection	Pulmonary venous transposition
TGA	Transposition of the great arteries	Transposition of the great vessels
TOF	Tetralogy of Fallot	Fallot's tetrad
VSD	Ventricular septal defect	

MEMORIX PEDIATRICS

Pressures and oxygen saturation in congenital heart defects
(Partly modified from Schumacher and Bühlmeyer (1989).)
Pressure values: systolic/diastolic or systolic/diastolic/end-diastolic, m = mean pressure, % O_2 saturation.
SVC/IVC = superior, vena cava/inferior, RA/LA = right/left atrium, RV/LV = right/left ventricle, PT = pulmonary trunk, RPA/LPA = right/left pulmonary artery, PV = pulmonary vein, AO = aorta, Aod = descending aorta, PDA = persistent ductus arteriosus, BT = brachiocephalic trunk, LCCA = left common carotid artery, LSA = left subclavian artery.

Normal pressure and saturation values

SVC: 72%
IVC: 78%
RA: 75%, m = 5
RV: 75%, 25/0/5
PT: 75%, 25/14
LA: 96%, m = 6
LV: 96%, 110/0/6
AO: 96%, 120/80

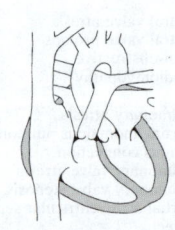

Aortic valvar stenosis

LA: m = 10
LV: 95%, 160/0/10
AO: 80/40

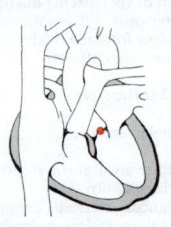

Ventricular septal defect

RV: 80%, 60/0/5
LV: 95%, 100/0/6
PT: 88% → 87%, 60/30
LA: m = 6

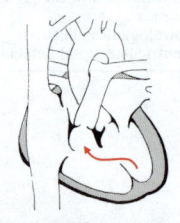

CARDIOLOGY

Persistent ductus arteriosus (see p. 92 for key)

RV:	50/0/5
PT:	78%, 50/25
RPA/LPA:	84%
LA:	m = 7
AO:	100/60

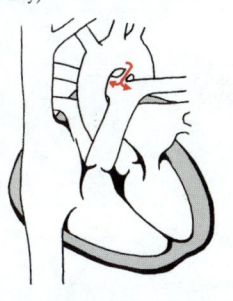

Aortic coarctation (isthmus stenosis: preductal)

SVC:	47%
IVC:	52%
RA:	62%, m = 6
RV:	65/0/5
PT:	62%, 50/30
LA:	94%, m = 11
PV:	95%
RPA:	55/35

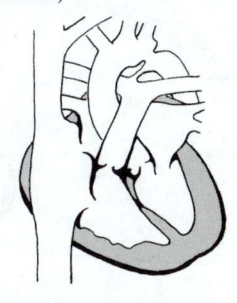

Pulmonary valve stenosis

SVC:	60%
IVC:	62%
RA:	59%, m = 7.5
RV:	58%, 215/0/10
PT:	55%, 13/9
LA:	95%

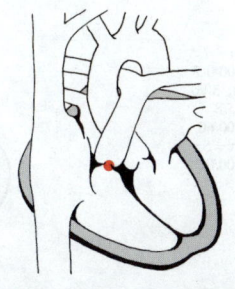

MEMORIX PEDIATRICS

Atrial septal defect (septum secundum) (see p. 92 for key)

SVC: 68%
IVC: 74%
RA: 86%, m = 3
RV: 86%, 35/0/5
PT: 86%, 24/12
LA: m = 4

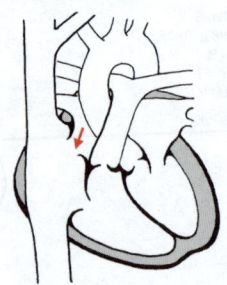

Complete AV canal

SVC: 42%
IVC: 66%
RA: 71%, m = 6
RV: 79%, 75/0/5
PT: 76%, 70/24
PV: 95%
LA: 86%, m = 7.5
LV: 89%, 75/0/4

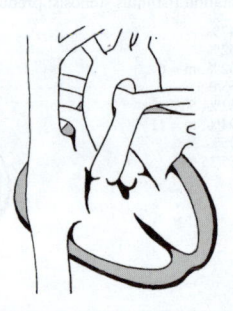

Tetralogy of Fallot

SVC: 48%
IVC: 54%
RA: 50%, m = 7
RV: 51%, 100/0/7
Infundibulum: 30/0
PT: 50%, 15/8
AO: 70%, 100/60
LA: 95%, m = 5
LV: 90%, 100/0/5

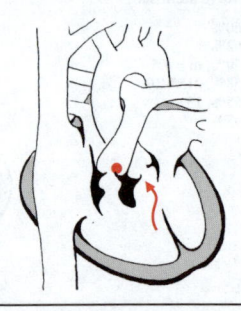

CARDIOLOGY

Transposition of the great arteries (TGA)

SVC: 24%
IVC: 31%
RA: 28%, m = 3
RV: 30%, 65/0/3
AO[a]: 30%, 55/40
LA: m = 5
LV: 95%, 55/0/2.5

[a] Ascending aorta; see p. 92 for full key.

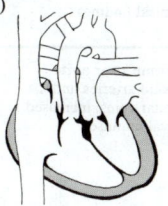

Possible recurrence risk (%) for congenital defects (heart and great vessels)
(After Nora (1989).)

I Mother or Father with congenital cardiac defect

Defect	Mother = patient	Father = patient
AV septal defect	14	1
Aortic stenosis	13–18	3
Tetralogy of Fallot	6–10	1.5
Ventricular septal defect	6	2
Pulmonary stenosis	4–6.5	2
Atrial septal defect	4–4.5	1.5
Aortic coarctation	4	2
Persistent ductus arteriosus	3.5–4	2.5

II Sibling with a congenital cardiac defect

Defect	Recurrence risk (%)
Endocardial fibroelastosis	4
Ventricular septal defect	3
Persistent ductus arteriosus	3
Atrial septal defect	2.5
Tetralogy of Fallot	2.5
Pulmonary stenosis	2
Aortic coarctation	2
Aortic stenosis	2
Atrioventricular septal defect	2
Hypoplastic left heart	2
Transposition of the great arteries	1.5
Common arterial trunk	1
Pulmonary atresia	1
Tricuspid atresia	1
Ebstein's anomaly	1

MEMORIX PEDIATRICS

Defect	Clinical findings	
Aortic stenosis	Murmur over aorta, carotid arteries and jugular veins; increased apical impulse	Gradient (Δp) = 40 mmHg
Aortic coarctation	Pulsation in neck and in jugular region; reduced pulse or pulse difference; absent femoral or pedal pulse; arterial hypertension with blood pressure gradient between upper and lower body regions	

EC = ejection click; LVH = left ventricular hypertrophy; HS = heart sound; → = valve; P = pulmonary valve.

CARDIOLOGY

Auscultation (heart sounds)	ECG	Radiography
Mild to medium grade	Often inconspicuous	Normal to slightly abnormal
First HS and second HS NAD: early systolic e.c., coarse spindle-shaped systolic murmur; maximal point. Second ICS right → carotids, jugular area, apex	P mitrale, LVH, abnormal repolarization in left precordial leads	Enlarged heart shadow, possibly dilatation of aorta
Higher grade		
No e.c., possibly third and fourth HS The more marked the stenosis, the later in systole is the murmur maximum	The height of the R wave and size of the heart in the X-ray image do not correlate well with the severity of the stenosis	
First HS normal, second HS possibly accentuated; early systolic click, midsystolic crescendo murmur with late systolic maximum amplitude; maximal murmur heard dorsally between the shoulder blades	Normal or LVH	Heart often normal size, possibly dilated ascending aorta in upper mediastinum Rib knotching usually not before school age

radiating to; ICS = intercostal space; NAD = nothing abnormal detected; A = aortic

Defect	Clinical findings	
Coarctation syndrome (CoA + VSD + PDA)	Dyspnea and tachypnea; gray–white skin color, varyingly marked cyanosis; femoral and pedal pulses weakend (but no pulse difference if a wide open PDA); left parasternal pulsation	
Aortic regurgitation	Waterhammer pulse; increased R-R amplitude	

e.c. = ejection click; LVH = left ventricular hypertrophy; HS = heart sound; electrocardiogram; PVM = pulmonary vascular markings; m.p. = maximal point; PDA markings.

CARDIOLOGY

Auscultation	ECG	Radiography
In 50% no murmur, otherwise coarse, spindle-shaped systolic murmur grade 2–3/6, m.p. second to fourth ICS left → back	Right axis deviation RVH or BVH P pulmonale, abnormal repolarization	Cardiomegaly, prominent pulmonary segment, PVM increased
First HS normal, second HS normal to accentuated; early diastolic decrescendo murmur and soft early systolic murmur third ICS left; heard particularly in sitting position		Inconspicuous in mild regurgitation; increasing heart enlargement, rounding of apex, widened aortic diameter
Higher grade regurgitation: first and second HS weakened; early to midsystolic crescendo/ decrescendo murmur, early to mid-diastolic decrescendo murmur, third and forth HS	Left axis deviation, P mitrale, LVH, abnormal left ventricular repolarization	

RVH = right ventricular hypertrophy; BVH = biventricular hypertrophy; ECG = = patent ductus arteriosus; ICS = intercostal space; PVM = pulmonary vascular

MEMORIX PEDIATRICS

Defect	Clinical findings
Mitral stenosis	Dyspnea, tachypnea, congestive cough
Pulmonary stenosis	Dyspnea and cyanosis according to severity; in slight and moderate grades of stenosis, systolic murmur over second to third, left ICS; pulsation in third to fourth left parasternal ICS

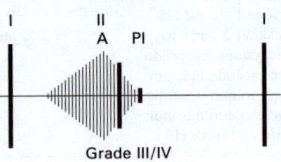

MOS = mitral opening snap; RBBB = right bundle branch block; PVM = pulmonary intercostal space; RVH = right ventricular hypertrophy.

CARDIOLOGY

Auscultation	ECG	Radiography
First HS loud, second HS normal to accentuated, mitral opening snap, rumbling mid-diastolic decrescendo murmur and late diastolic crescendo murmur over fourth left ICS and apex, particularly when lying on the left side The earlier the MOS after the second HS, the greater the stenosis	Right axis deviation, P mitrale, pulmonale or biatrial, RVH, right-sided abnormal repolarization	Enlarged left atrium with normal size of left ventricle; prominent pulmonary segment; sign of pulmonary obstruction
Slight to medium grade: First HS soft over the pulmonary region, early systolic e.c., widely split second HS; coarse, spindle-shaped mid- to high frequency systolic murmur; m.p. second to third left ICS → precordium, throat, left axilla and back Higher grade: Later onset of systolic murmur with end systolic maximum amplitude The higher grade the stenosis, the later in systole the beginning and maximum of the murmur	Mild grade: frequently inconspicuous; incomplete RBBB Moderate to high grade: right axis deviation, P pulmonale, RVH, abnormal right precordial repolarization	Mostly normal size or only slightly enlarged heart shadow; prominent pulmonary segment; PVM normal or diminished

vascular markings; e.c. = ejection click; m.p. = maximal point; HS = heart sound; ICS =

MEMORIX PEDIATRICS

Defect	Clinical findings	
Pulmonary regurgitation	Usually unremarkable; if higher grade regurgitation, possibly pulsation over the right ventricle and a systolic thrill over the second to third left ICS	I — A₂P₂ — I
Tetralogy of Fallot	Generalized cyanosis, clubbed fingers, hour-glass nails, gingival hyperplasia, increased vascular injection of mucous membranes and conjunctivae	I — A P — I

MOS = mitral opening snap; RBBB = right bundle branch block; PVM = pulmonary hypertrophy.

CARDIOLOGY

Auscultation	ECG	Radiography
First HS normal, split second HS, soft early to midsystolic crescendo/decrescendo murmur and early to mid-diastolic murmur The higher the pulmonary artery pressure, the earlier the onset of the diastolic murmur	Incomplete RBBB	Enlarged heart, accentuated pulmonary segment
First HS usually loud; possibly a systolic click, aortic valve closure sound accentuated; high frequency, coarse, spindle-shaped systolic murmur third to fourth left parasternal ICS	Right axis deviation; moderate RVH; incomplete RBBB, abnormal right precordial repolarization, P pulmonale	Normal heart size, elevated apex; definite waist; PVM usually only slightly diminished, typical boot-shaped heart

vascular markings; ICS = intercostal space; HS = heart sound; RVH = right ventricular

MEMORIX PEDIATRICS

Defect	Clinical findings	
Persistent ductus arteriosus	In large shunt: tachypnea and dyspnea in infants; waterhammer pulse; pulsation over left ventricle with apical impulse shifted toward the left	
Common arterial trunk	Severe dyspnea and tachypnea in neonates; cyanosis with reduced pulmonary flow, waterhammer pulse, heaving pulsation over the whole precordium	

e.c. = ejection click; HS = heart sound; m.p. = maximal point; ICS = intercostal space; biventricular hypertrophy; PVM = pulmonary vascular markings.

CARDIOLOGY

Auscultation	ECG	Radiography
First and second HS normal, if pulmonary hypertension second HS is accentuated; mid- to high frequency continuous systolic–diastolic crescendo–decrescendo murmur (machinery murmur), m.p. second ICS left → left shoulder and back	Usually normal findings; LVH (increased volume load); if pulmonary hypertension, RVH or BVH	In large shunts: cardiomegaly with enlarged left atrium and left ventricle, prominent pulmonary segments, increased PVM
First HS normal, early systolic e.c.; second HS mostly single and accentuated; heart murmur may be absent; uncharacteristic, rough, spindle-shaped or band-like holosystolic murmur, m.p. third to fourth ICS left → precordium, perhaps early diastolic decrescendo (truncal valve regurgitation); if increased pulmonary flow, a mid-diastolic murmur	Usually right axis deviation, P pulmonale, usually BVH, RVH or LVH	Cardiomegaly, possibly right aortic arch, PVM usually increased

LVH = left ventricular hypertrophy; RVH = right ventricular hypertrophy; BVH =

MEMORIX PEDIATRICS

Defect	Clinical findings	
Transposition of the great arteries	Dyspnea and cyanosis of varying severity, raised left parasternal pulsation	
Atrial septal defect	In large left–right shunt, dyspnea on effort; enlarged pulmonary segment; increased left parasternal pulsation	I — II (A P) — I

HS = heart sound; VSD = ventricular septal defect; PS = pulmonary stenosis; PDA = hypertrophy; LVH = left ventricular hypertrophy; PVM = pulmonary vascular space.

CARDIOLOGY

Auscultation	ECG	Radiography
First HS normal, second HS single and accentuated, heart murmurs may be absent; uncharacteristic systolic murmur associated with any accompanying defect (VSD, PS, PDA)	Right axis deviation; P pulmonale; at first, physiological RVH, then abnormal RVH with right abnormal repolarization; if additional VSD, BVH; if additional PS, LVH	At first, normal heart, often egg-shaped, then getting larger; PVM normal to slightly increased
First HS normal; second HS in large defects wide with fixed splitting; low frequency, mostly coarse, spindle-shaped early to midsystolic murmur, m.p. left parasternal second to third ICS In large defects: middle to low frequency, mid-diastolic spindle-shaped murmur in the left parasternal fourth ICS	P pulmonale, right axis deviation, incomplete, rarely complete, RBBB; RVH	Cardiomegaly, elevated and increasingly rounded cardiac apex; prominent pulmonary segment, PVM increased

patent ductus arteriosus; RVH = right ventricular hypertrophy; BVH = biventricular markings; RBBB = right bundle branch block; m.p. = maximal point; ICS = intercostal

MEMORIX PEDIATRICS

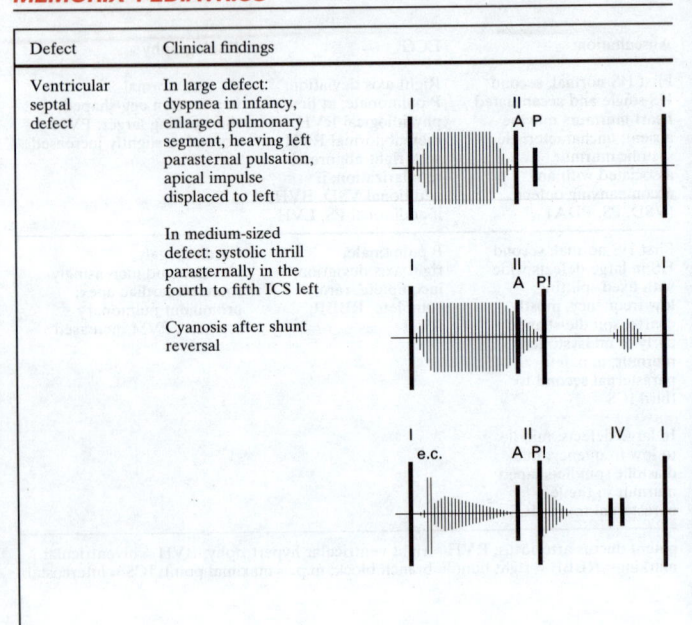

Defect	Clinical findings
Ventricular septal defect	In large defect: dyspnea in infancy, enlarged pulmonary segment, heaving left parasternal pulsation, apical impulse displaced to left
	In medium-sized defect: systolic thrill parasternally in the fourth to fifth ICS left
	Cyanosis after shunt reversal

e.c. = ejection click; m.p. = maximal point; ICS = intercostal space; LVH = left markings; HS = heart sound; RVH = right ventricular hypertrophy.

CARDIOLOGY

Auscultation	ECG	Radiography
Small defect: short, sharp, high frequency pre- to mid-diastolic murmur m.p. third to fourth left parasternal at third to fourth, grade 3–4/6	Small defects: unremarkable	Small defect: normal
Moderately large and large defects: second HS split with respiration; accentuated pulmonary valve closure; loud, high frequency, sharp, holosystolic murmur, m.p. third to fourth ICS left parasternal, grade 4–5/6; possibly low frequency spindle-shaped, mid- to late diastolic murmur over apex (mitral flow murmur)	Medium-sized and larger defects: LVH or BVH, P mitrale	Medium-sized and larger defects: heart shadow definitely enlarged to left; large prominent pulmonary artery; distinctly increased PVM
	Large defect + pulmonary hypertension: RVH or BVH	Large defects with pulmonary hypertension: decreased heart size; prominent pulmonary segments; caliber of pulmonary arteries diminished toward periphery
Large defects and pulmonary hypertension: second HS narrow, divided or single; explosive; early systolic click, fourth HS in third to fourth ICS; soft or absent systolic; soft early diastolic decrescendo m.p. second to third ICS left parasternally (pulmonary valve insufficiency)		

ventricular hypertrophy; BVH = biventricular hypertrophy; PVM = pulmonary vascular

Defect	Clinical findings
Atrioventricular septal defect	Dyspnea and tachypnea, peripheral cyanosis in infancy; central cyanosis if pulmonary hypertension; distinctly enlarged pulmonary segment; left parasternal heaving pulsation over both ventricles
Total anomalous pulmonary venous connection	Dyspnea and tachynea in neonates, increasing peripheral and central cyanosis; heaving left parasternal pulsation

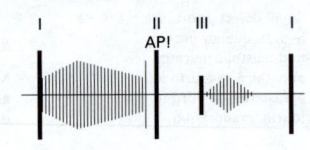

AVSD = atrioventricular septal defect; HS = heart sound; m.p. = maximal point; RBBB = right bundle branch block; RVH = right ventricular hypertrophy; BVH = hypertrophy.

CARDIOLOGY

Auscultation	ECG	Radiography
In partial AVSD: (ostium primum defect): First HS normal to slightly accentuated, second HS broad with fixed splitting, low frequency, spindle-shaped systolic murmur, m.p. second to third ICS left parasternally	Usually marked left axis deviation; AV conduction disorder, P pulmonale and/or P mitrale; incomplete, rarely complete, RBBB	Cardiomegaly, accentuated atrial bulge, elevated apex, prominent pulmonary segment; increased PVM
In complete AVSD: First HS accentuated, second HS wide with fixed, split, coarse systolic murmur, m.p. on left below the sternal border → apex and to the second to third ICS parasternally; possibly low frequency mid-diastolic murmur after third HS over fourth ICS left and at apex	RVH or BVH	
First HS accentuated; ejection click in absence of pulmonary venous obstruction; second HS wide with fixed split; heart murmur may be absent in neonates; uncharacteristic spindle-shaped systolic, possibly mid- to end-diastolic flow murmur (if no pulmonary venous obstruction)	P pulmonale in missing PVO, RVH, no LVH	Without PVO, cardiomegaly, raised apex, prominent pulmonary segment, increased PVM With PVO: normal heart size; enlarged reticular lung markings with diffuse milky pulmonary venous markings; typically figure-of-eight or 'snowman' picture in supracardiac type with connection to the left innominate vein

ICS = intercostal space; AV = atrioventricular; PVM = pulmonary vascular markings; biventricular hypertrophy; PVO = pulmonary vein obstruction; LVH = left ventricular

Hemodynamic degrees of severity of congenital heart disease

(Singer (1988).)

Hemodynamic degree of severity	Insignificant to slight	Moderate degree	Severe
CHD			
Aortic stenosis	$\Delta p \lessapprox 30(-50)$ mmHg	$\Delta p = 50 \to 80$ mmHg	$\Delta p \gtrapprox 80$ mmHg
Aortic coarctation	$\Delta p \lessapprox 20$ mmHg	$\Delta p = 20 \to 50$ mmHg	$\Delta p \gtrapprox 50$ mmHg
Pulmonary stenosis	$\Delta p \lessapprox 50$ mmHg	$\Delta p = 50 \to 80$ mmHg	$\Delta p \gtrapprox 80$ mmHg
ASD	Qp:Qs < 1.5:1	Qp:Qs 1.5 → 2:1	Qp:Qs > 2:1, mPA (↑)
VSD, PDA	Qp:Qs < 1.5:1	Qp:Qs 1.5 → 2:1, mPA (↑)	Qp:Qs ≧ 2:1, mPA (↑)
			Qp:Qs → , Rp ↑
			Qp:Qs < 1, Rp ↑↑ (>Rs)
cAVC	—	—	As for VSD
Cyanotic CHD			
– Qp ↓ Rp (↓)	—	$P_{O_2} > 35, S_{O_2} > 75$	$P_{O_2} < 35, S_{O_2} < 75$
– Qp ↓ Rp (n → (↑))	—	Qp:Qs < 2:1	Qp:Qs > 2:1
– Qp ↓ Rp ↑↑	—	—	Qp < Qs, Rp > Rs
Clinical tests			
ECG	Heart murmur, O	O → exercise tolerance ↓	Resting symptoms → CF, cyanosis
Chest X-ray	O	O → discrete overload signs	Pathological
Echo	O	O → slight changes	Pathological
Blood gas analysis	O	→ diagnosis + changes	Pathological
	O	O → pathological	Pathological

CHD = congenital heart disease; Δp = pressure gradient; ASD = atrial septal defect; VSD = ventricular septal defect; PDA = patent ductus arteriosus; Qp = pulmonary flow; Qs = systemic flow; mPA = mean pulmonary arterial pressure; Rp = pulmonary resistance; Rs = systemic resistance; cAVC = complete atrioventricular canal; P_{O_2} = arterial oxygen partial pressure; S_{O_2} = arterial oxygen saturation; O = heart murmur only, no further signs or symptoms; CF = cardiac failure.

CARDIOLOGY

Guidelines for hemodynamic assessment of operative results in congenital heart defects
(Singer (1988).)

Assessment/CHD	Very good-good	Satisfactory	Poor
Aortic stenosis	$\Delta p \geqq 30$ mmHg	$\Delta p = 31–50$ mmHg mild aortic regurgitation	$\Delta p > 50$ mmHg raised aortic regurgitation
Aortic coarctation	$\Delta p \leqq 20$ mmHg BP normal ($\uparrow$)	$\Delta p > 20$ mmHg BP $\uparrow$	$\Delta p > 30$ mmHg BP $\uparrow\uparrow$
Pulmonary stenosis	$\Delta p \leqq 20$ mmHg ($\pm$ pulmonary regurgitation)	$\Delta p = 21–50$ mmHg $\pm$ pulmonary regurgitation	$\Delta p > 50$ mmHg $\pm$ pulmonary regurgitation
ASD	Qp:Qs = 1:1 (<1.5:1)	Qp:Qs = 2:1	Qp:Qs > 2:1
VSD	Qp:Qs = 1:1 (<1.5:1) mPA, Rp normal	Qp:Qs = 2:1 mPA, Rp normal	Qp:Qs > 2:1 mPA $\uparrow$, Rp $\uparrow$ $\rightarrow$ Rp $\uparrow\uparrow$
cAVC	Qp:Qs = 1:1 (<1.5:1)	Qp:Qs = 2:1 $\pm$ little mitral regurgitation	Qp:Qs > 2:1 $\pm$ mitral regurgitation $\pm$ mitral stenosis
PDA	–	–	mPA $\uparrow$, Rp $\uparrow$ $\rightarrow$ Rp $\uparrow\uparrow$
Tetralogy of Fallot	Qp:Qs = 1:1 (<1.5:1) $\Delta p \leqq 20$ mmHg $\pm$ little pulmonary regurgitation	Qp:Qs = 1.5:1–2:1 $\Delta p = 21–50$ mmHg $\pm$ moderate pulmonary regurgitation	Qp:Qs > 2:1 (<1:1) $\Delta p > 50$ mmHg $\pm$ pulmonary regurgitation tricuspid regurgitation aortic regurgitation

CHD = congenital heart disease; Δp = pressure gradient; ASD = atrial septal defect; VSD = ventricular septal defect; PDA = patent ductus arteriosus; cAVC = complete atrioventricular canal; Qp = pulmonary flow; Qs = systemic flow; Rp = pulmonary resistance; Rs = systemic resistance; mPA pulmonary arterial pressure; BP = blood pressure.

Recommendations for participation in school sports by children with heart disease

(After Jüngst (1990).)

No participation (exempt)

Aortic stenosis
Cardiomyopathies with impaired cardiac function
Effort-induced tachyarrhythmia (long QT syndrome)
Inflammatory heart diseases
(for up to six months after the acute onset)

Non-compulsory participation (part exemption, personal decision)

Cyanotic heart defect (palliative operation)
Heart defect with Eisenmenger reaction
Third degree atrioventricular block
Pacemaker implanted

Child able to participate without sudden spurts or forced breathing (part exemption)

Left-to-right shunt with elevated pulmonary arterial pressure
Pulmonary stenosis (also after operation)
Arterial hypertension
Operated cyanotic defects, e.g. tetralogy of Fallot, transposition of the great arteries

---

Unrestricted participation

Operated atrial septal defect, ventricular septal defect, patent ductus arteriosus without complications
Heart defects with left-to-right shunt not requiring operation
Pulmonary stenosis not requiring operation

Shunt-dependent congenital heart defects
(Modified from Singer (1989).)

- Hypoplastic right heart
- Pulmonary atresia (with/without ventricular septal defect)
- Critical pulmonary stenosis
- Ebstein's anomaly/tricuspid regurgitation

→ Constriction Closure of ductus arteriosus → **Neonatal emergencies**
Cyanosis
Dyspnea
Bradycardia
P_{AO_2}, S_{O_2} ↓
Metabolic acidosis

→ Persistence of ductus arteriosus → Lung perfusion

- Hypoplastic left heart
- Critical aortic stenosis
- Coarctation syndrome

→ Constriction–closure of ductus arteriosus → Perfusion of the post-stenotic systemic circulation → **Cardiogenic shock**
Skin cold, pallid gray, moist, sweating
Recapillarization time ↑
Thready pulse
Dyspnea
Hepatomegaly
Anuria
Coagulation disorder
Respiratory + metabolic acidosis

Persistence of foramen ovale → pressure and shunt equalization at atrial level

Problem characteristic of closed ductus arteriosus: no improvement in symptoms on administration of O_2.
N.B.: Inspiratory oxygen concentration not >50%, otherwise danger of inducing ductus closure.

Treatment to keep ductus open: prostaglandin E_1, 0.01–0.1 µg/kg per min. (Begin with 0.05–0.01 µg/kg per min and adapt dose to achieve minimal maintenance dosage if P_{O_2}, S_{O_2} and diuresis ↑. Readiness to start artificial ventilation, especially during transportation.)

Side-effects of prostaglandin: cardiac rhythm disorders, hypotension, erythema, edema, fever, seizures, respiratory depression, hypoglycemia.

MEMORIX PEDIATRICS

ECG: electrode positions
Unipolar chest leads
(Wilson)

Exploring electrodes	Infants	Older children
V_1	4th ICS – sternum border	–4th ICS
V_2	4th ICS – left sternal border	–4th ICS
V_3	– midway between V_2 and V_4	
V_4	4th ICS – left midclavicular line	–5th ICS
V_5	4th ICS – left anterior axillary line	–5th ICS
V_6	4th ICS – left midaxillary line	–5th ICS
V_7	4th ICS – left posterior axillary line	–5th ICS
V_8	4th ICS – left midscapular line	–5th ICS

For particular problems (e.g. right hypertrophy, positional anomalies) additional leads V_{3a}–V_{8a} at mirror-image positions of leads V_3–V_8.
ICS = intercostal space.

Limb leads
Electrode positions and lead markings:

Right arm: red (alternatively R or one ring)
Left arm: yellow (alternatively L or two rings)
Left leg: green (alternatively F or three rings)
Right leg: black (earthing)

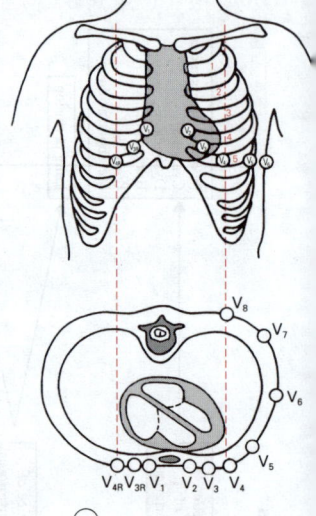

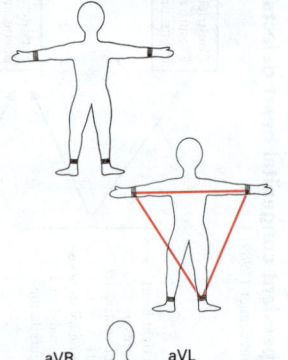

Unipolar leads
(Goldberger)
a (augmented = amplified), V (voltage)

Lead **aVR**: exploring electrode = right arm
Lead **aVL**: exploring electrode = left arm
Lead **aVF**: exploring electrode = left leg
(Indifferent electrode = connecting the two other electrodes.)

CARDIOLOGY

RS patterns of electrical axis positions/deviations
(After Gutheil (1989).)

Lead	Type ∢α	Marked right deviation +90° → +150°	Mild–moderate right deviation +60° → +90°	Normal type +30° → +60°	Left deviation +30° → -30°	Moderate left deviation +30° → -30°	Marked left deviation (inverted) -30° → -90°	Inverted right deviation -90° → -150°
Standard leads	I							
	II							
	III							
Goldberger leads	aVR							
	aVL							
	aVF							

Nomenclature of QRS wave forms
- There is no variation in the sequence Q–R–S.
- High-amplitude waves are given in capitals, lesser ones in small letters.
- Any first upward (positive) deflection: r or R.
- First downward (negative) deflection: q or Q.
- Second deflection upwards: r' or R'; it can be preceded by an s/S or followed by an s'/S'.
- Third deflection upwards: r"/R", fourth downwards: s"/S".
- If no R wave, a single negative deflection is called qs or QS.

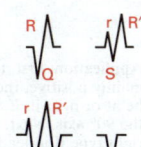

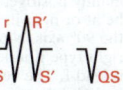

Determining positional types using the Cabrera circle
Cabrera circle: parallel move of the standard and Goldberger leads to a common intersection (midpoint of the circle). The electrical heart axis is determined by the direction of the main vector of the spread of ventricular excitation. α = angle between the main vector of the QRS complex and the horizontal line. α defines the positional type. (See next page.)

117

MEMORIX PEDIATRICS

Cabrera circle (hexaxial reference system)

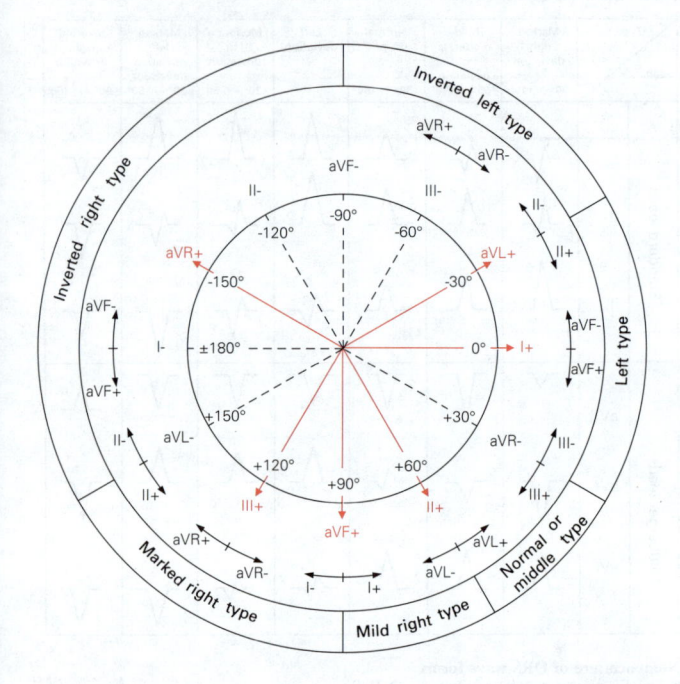

Application: first, the QRS is assessed in standard lead I. If the QRS deflections are mainly positive, the main vector will be to the right of the 90° axis, if biphasic it will be at or near it; if there is a mainly negative deflection, the vector will be to the left of the 90° axis. Next, the standard lead with the greatest positive deflection is sought: right type if in lead III, mild right type if in lead II/III, normal type if lead II, left type if lead I. The vector lies at or near the indicated axes (i.e. parallel displaced standard and Goldberger leads). Each lead is matched to its corresponding axis and the decision made whether the deflections are predominantly positive or negative (short arrows), so that they can be assigned to the appropriate electrical axis (main QRS vector).
Example: QRS negative in lead I, highly positive in III: see vector α = +120°. If QRS in aVR is more positive, α will be >120°; in the converse case, α will be <120°, but >90°.

118

CARDIOLOGY

Age-dependent normal ranges for different ECG measurements

Age	Heart rate (beats/min)	P duration in leads I–III	PR interval	QRS interval
0–2 months	100–180	0.05–0.07	0.08–0.12	0.04–0.08
2–5 months	100–180	0.06–0.07	0.08–0.12	0.04–0.08
6–12 months	100–180	0.06–0.07	0.09–0.13	0.04–0.08
2–3 years	100–180	0.05–0.07	0.09–0.15	0.04–0.08
4–6 years	60–150	0.06–0.08	0.09–0.15	0.05–0.09
7–10 years	60–130	0.06–0.08	0.10–0.18	0.05–0.09
11–16 years	50–100	0.06–0.08	0.12–0.19	0.05–0.10

Sources of normal values: Garson, Gillette and McNamara, 1980; Stoermer and Heck, 1971.

MEMORIX PEDIATRICS

ECG: relative and rate-corrected QT interval

(Both tables from Heinecker (1986).)

Ascertaining the relative QT interval from the RR interval, including the pulse rate and measured QT interval (in s).

Normal range of relative QT interval: 90% to approximately 115%.

Interval (RR or PP) (s)	Rate	Relative QT interval (%)						
		80%	90%	100%	110%	120%	130%	140%
1.50	40	0.37	0.42	0.47	0.51	0.57	–	QT interval (s)
1.32	45	0.35	0.39	0.44	0.48	0.53	0.57	
1.20	50	0.33	0.37	0.42	0.46	0.50	0.54	–
1.10	55	0.32	0.36	0.40	0.44	0.48	0.52	0.56
1.00	60	0.31	0.35	0.38	0.42	0.46	0.50	0.53
0.92	65	0.30	0.33	0.37	0.41	0.44	0.48	0.52
0.86	70	0.29	0.32	0.36	0.39	0.43	0.47	0.50
0.80	75	0.27	0.31	0.35	0.38	0.41	0.45	0.48
0.75	80	0.27	0.30	0.34	0.37	0.40	0.44	0.47
0.71	85	0.26	0.29	0.33	0.36	0.39	0.43	0.46
0.67	90	0.25	0.29	0.32	0.35	0.38	0.42	0.45
0.63	95	0.25	0.28	0.31	0.34	0.37	0.41	0.43
0.60	100	0.24	0.27	0.30	0.33	0.36	0.39	0.42
0.55	110	0.23	0.26	0.29	0.32	0.35	0.38	0.41
0.50	120	0.22	0.25	0.28	0.30	0.33	0.36	0.39
0.46	130	0.21	0.24	0.27	0.29	0.32	0.34	0.37
0.43	140	0.21	0.23	0.26	0.28	0.31	0.33	0.36
0.40	150	0.20	0.22	0.25	0.27	0.30	0.32	0.35
0.38	160	–	0.22	0.24	0.26	0.29	0.31	0.34
0.33	180	–	0.20	0.23	0.25	0.27	0.30	0.32

Ascertaining the rate-corrected QT_c interval from the RR interval, or heart rate and measured QT interval (in s).

Normal range of the QT_c: 0.35–0.43, calculated from Bazett's formula: $QT_c = QT/\sqrt{60/\text{rate}}$ or $QT/\sqrt{RR}$.

Figures within red box are those calculated by Bazett's formula (i.e. corrected for rate).

RR (s)	Rate (/min)	Measured QT interval (s)								
		0.20	0.25	0.30	0.35	0.40	0.45	0.50	0.55	0.60
1.50	40	0.16	0.20	0.25	0.29	0.33	0.37	0.41	0.45	0.49
1.32	45	0.17	0.22	0.26	0.31	0.35	0.39	0.44	0.48	0.52
1.20	50	0.18	0.23	0.27	0.32	0.37	0.41	0.46	0.50	0.55
1.10	55	0.19	0.24	0.29	0.33	0.38	0.43	0.48	0.52	0.57
1.00	60	0.20	0.25	0.30	0.35	0.40	0.45	0.50	0.55	0.60
0.92	65	0.21	0.26	0.31	0.37	0.42	0.47	0.52	0.57	0.63
0.86	70	0.22	0.27	0.32	0.38	0.43	0.49	0.54	0.59	0.65
0.80	75	0.22	0.28	0.34	0.39	0.45	0.50	0.56	0.62	0.67
0.75	80	0.23	0.29	0.35	0.40	0.46	0.52	0.58	0.64	0.69
0.71	85	0.24	0.30	0.36	0.42	0.47	0.53	0.59	0.65	0.71
0.67	90	0.24	0.31	0.37	0.43	0.49	0.55	0.61	0.67	0.73
0.63	95	0.25	0.32	0.38	0.44	0.50	0.57	0.63	0.69	0.76
0.60	100	0.26	0.32	0.39	0.45	0.52	0.58	0.65	0.71	0.78
0.55	110	0.27	0.34	0.41	0.47	0.54	0.61	0.67	0.74	0.81
0.50	120	0.28	0.35	0.42	0.50	0.57	0.64	0.71	0.78	0.85
0.46	130	0.30	0.37	0.44	0.52	0.59	0.66	0.74	0.81	0.89
0.43	140	0.31	0.38	0.46	0.53	0.61	0.69	0.76	0.84	0.92
0.40	150	0.32	0.40	0.47	0.55	0.63	0.71	0.79	0.87	0.95
0.38	160	0.32	0.41	0.49	0.57	0.65	0.73	0.81	0.89	0.97
0.33	180	0.35	0.44	0.52	0.61	0.70	0.78	0.87	0.96	1.05

CARDIOLOGY

ECG: normal values for R:S ratio and R and S amplitudes

In V_1, by age
(Both tables from Garson, Gillette and McNamara (1980).)

Age	R:S ratio	Mean	R amplitude	Mean	S amplitude	Mean
0–1 month	0.5–∞	1.5	4–25	15	0–20	10
2–3 months	0.3–10	1.5	2–20	11	1–18	7
4–12 months	0.3–4	1.2	3–20	10	1–16	8
1–3 y	0.3–1.5	0.8	1–18	9	1–27	13
4–8 y	0.1–1.5	0.7	1–18	7	1–30	14
9–11 y	0.1–1.0	0.5	1–16	6	1–26	16
12–16 y	0–1.0	0.3	1–16	5	1–23	14
>16 y	0–1.0	0.3	1–14	3	1–23	10

In V_6, by age

Age	R:S ratio	Mean	R amplitude	Mean	S amplitude	Mean
0–1 month	0.1–∞	2	1–21	6	0–12	4
2–3 months	1.5–∞	4	3–20	10	0–6	2
4–12 months	2.0–∞	6	6–20	13	0–4	2
1–3 y	3.0–∞	20	3–24	12	0–4	2
4–8 y	2.0–∞	20	4–24	13	0–4	1
9–11 y	4.0–∞	20	4–24	14	0–4	1
12–16 y	2.0–∞	9	4–22	14	0–5	1
>16 y	2.0–∞	9	4–21	10	0–6	1

MEMORIX PEDIATRICS

ECG: signs of hypertrophy

ECG criteria for right ventricular hypertrophy (RVH)

Right type/inverted right type
R′ in aVR increased
R amplitude in V_1, V_2 increased
rsR′ form in V_{4r}, V_{3r} or V_1
Time interval onset of QRS to peak of R wave (upper reversal point, URP) increased in V_1 to >0.04 s
Q wave in V_1 (qR or qRs)
S amplitude in V_6 increased
R : S ratio increased over right ventricle
Sum of $RV_1 + SV_6 > 3$ mV (Sokolow index)
Sum of $SV_1 + RV_6 < 5$ mV
Positive T wave after fifth day of life in V_{4r}, V_{3r} or V_1
Discordant negative T wave or ST depression in older patients
Indirect sign: P pulmonale

ECG criteria for left ventricular hypertrophy (LVH)

Left type/inverted left type
Sum of $R_I + S_{III} > 2.5$ mV
S amplitude in V_1, V_2 increased
R amplitude in V_5, V_6 increased
Time interval onset of QRS to peak of R wave increased in V_6 to >0.04 s in infants
>0.05 s in childhood
Wide, deep Q wave (>0.04 mV) in V_6 (in volume overload)
R in V_6 > R in V_5
R : S ratio increased over left ventricle
Displacement of the transition zone to right
Sokolow index: $RV_6 + SV_1 > 5.0$ mV
$RV_5 + SV_1 > 4.0$ mV in infants
> 6.0 mV in childhood
High peaked T wave in V_6 (in volume overload)
T wave in V_5, V_6 discordant negative with depressed ST segment (>0.1 mV), while positive T waves in V_1, V_2
Indirect sign: P mitrale

ECG criteria for biventricular hypertrophy

Definite criteria for both right ventricular hypertrophy (RVH) and left ventricular hypertrophy (LVH)

Definite criteria of RVH with some LVH criteria
Left type
R in V_5, V_6 increased
R > S in V_1 or S > R in V_6
Q in V_6 > 2 mm
URP in V_6 normal or delayed
R or S amplitude equally large in V_2–V_4 (Katz–Wachtel phenomenon)
R = S in more than half the limb leads
Transitional zone strongly displaced right
Positive criteria of LVH with some RVH criteria
Right type
Incomplete right bundle branch block and URP delayed in V_1
Difference between URP in V_6 – in V_1 = positive
Transitional zone strongly displaced to left
URP = upper reversal point (interval from onset of QRS to peak of R wave).

CARDIOLOGY

ECG: right-sided hypertrophy

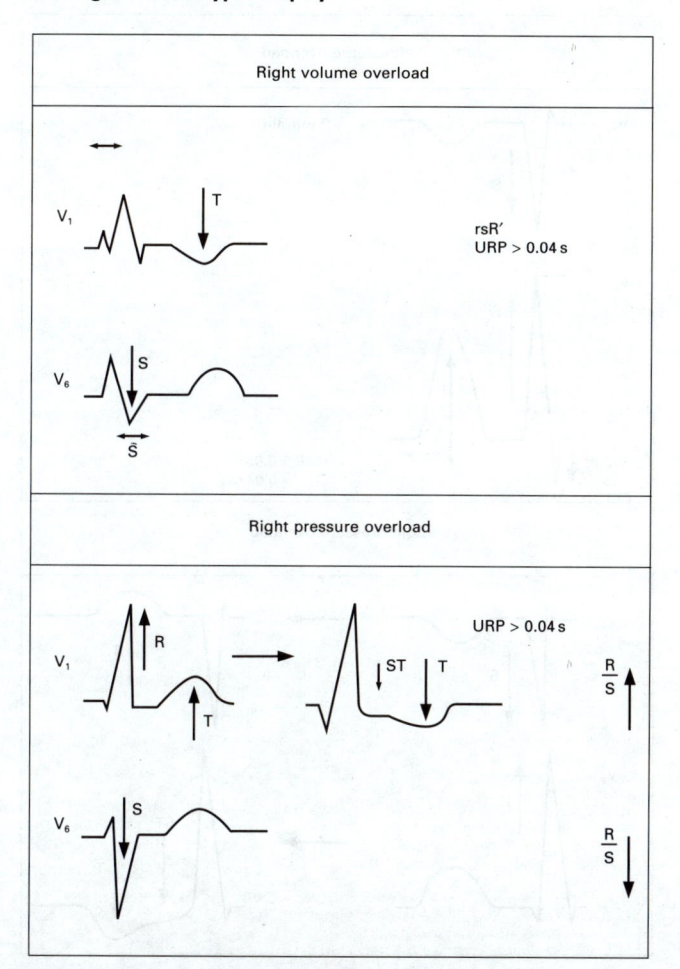

Right volume overload

V_1

rsR'
URP > 0.04 s

V_6 S, S̄

Right pressure overload

V_1 R, T → ST, T

URP > 0.04 s

$\frac{R}{S}$ ↑

V_6 S

$\frac{R}{S}$ ↓

MEMORIX PEDIATRICS

ECG: left-sided hypertrophy

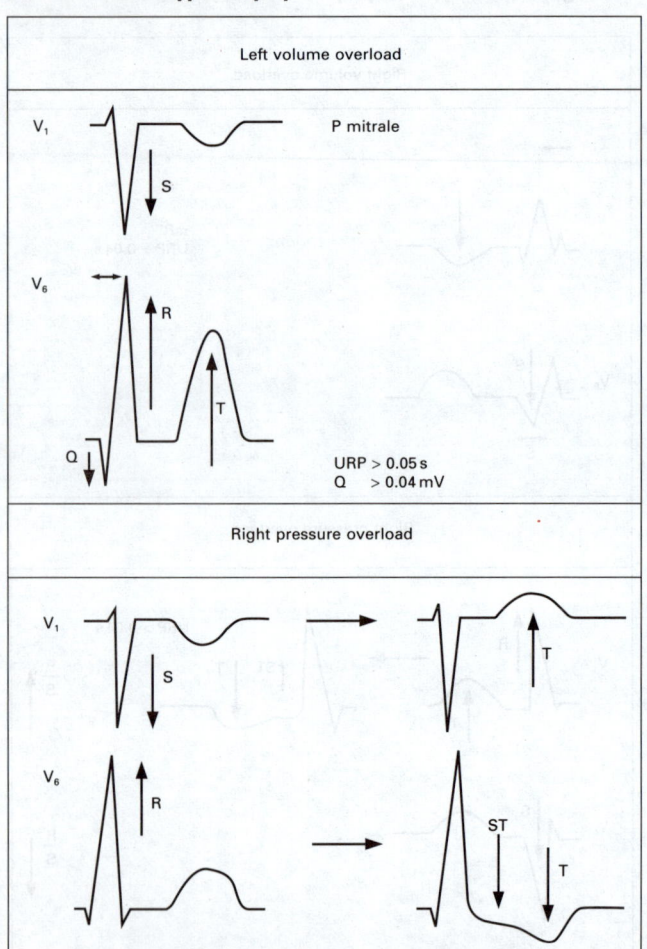

Left volume overload

V_1 — P mitrale, S

V_6 — R, T, Q

URP > 0.05 s
Q > 0.04 mV

Right pressure overload

V_1 — S → T

V_6 — R → ST, T

124

CARDIOLOGY

ECG: criteria of atrial hypertrophy

Hypertrophy of the atria shows in the ECG as a rise in amplitude and/or duration of the P wave.

RAH >3 mm

LAH >0.10

BAH

	Normal	RAH	LAH	BAH
II	RA LA	RA LA	RA LA	RA LA
V_1	RA LA	RA LA	RA LA	RA LA

	RAH	LAH	BAH
Denotation	P pulmonale	P mitrale	P biatriale
Occurrence	Tricuspid atresia, tricuspid stenosis or regurgitation Ebstein's anomaly	Mitral stenosis or regurgitation; marked hypertrophy of left ventricle; sometimes in PDA or VSD	Combined mitral defect; large ASD
P amplitude	Raised (>0.3 mV) in II, III, aVF, right accentuated in V_1, V_2	Normal Left accentuated in V_1, V_2	Raised in II, III, aVF Clearly biphasic in V_1, V_2
P duration	Normal	Prolonged (>0.1 s) in I, II, aVL, V_5, V_6	Prolonged (>0.1 s) in I, aVL, V_5, V_6
PR interval	Normal	Shortened	Shortened

RAH = right atrial hypertrophy; LAH = left atrial hypertrophy; BAH = biatrial hypertrophy; PDA = patent ductus arteriosus; VSD = ventricular septal defect; ASD = atrial septal defect.

MEMORIX PEDIATRICS

Sequence in the ECG diagnosis of cardiac arrhythmias
(After Garson, Gillette and McNamara (1980).)

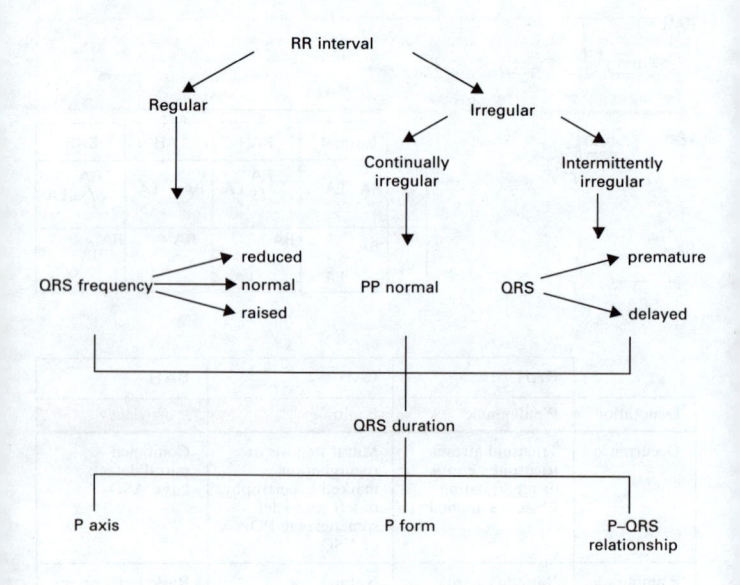

```
                            RR interval
                           /          \
                      Regular         Irregular
                         |            /        \
                         |    Continually   Intermittently
                         |     irregular      irregular
                         |         |              \
                         |         |         → premature
                    → reduced      |       QRS
QRS frequency → normal      PP normal      → delayed
                    → raised
```

	QRS duration

| P axis | P form | P-QRS relationship |

126

CARDIOLOGY

Causes of arrhythmias

Cardiac	Extracardiac
Heart defects (pre-, postoperative)	Poisoning
Infections (myocarditis)	Electrolyte disorders
Cardiomyopathies	Hypoxia/acidosis
Heart tumors	Endocrine diseases
Pre-excitation syndrome	Storage diseases
QT syndrome	Muscular dystrophies
Very frequently 'idiopathic'	

The possibility of the development of an emergency situation arising from an arrhythmia is increased by:

1. Accompanying noncardiac disease:

   Electrolyte disorders
   Acidosis
   Hypoxia
   Anemia
   Hypovolemia.

2. Cardiac disorders:

   The more severe the basic disease, the worse the cardiac function (independent of the rhythm disorder), the higher or slower the pulse rate and the longer the arrhythmia continues.

Diseases in which rhythm disturbances can potentially provoke emergency

   Valvar defects, e.g. mitral stenosis, aortic stenosis
   Obstructive and dilated cardiomyopathies
   Acute myocarditis
   Endocarditis
   Hypokalemia.

Diseases in which rhythm disorders are unlikely to provoke an emergency

   Wolff–Parkinson–White syndrome
   Hyperthyroidism
   Mitral valve prolapse.

Supraventricular tachycardia (SVT)

Symptoms: Rapid pulse; restlessness; pallor; vomiting; perhaps signs of cardiac failure and peripheral vasoconstriction; older children describe palpitations as unpleasant.

MEMORIX PEDIATRICS

ECG: Frequency 130–300/min
QRS complex usually narrow (with the exception of aberrant pathways)
P waves often not identifiable, otherwise fixed relationship with QRS complex.

Differential diagnosis: Sinus tachycardia; ventricular tachycardia; ectopic atrial tachycardia; atrial flutter.

Treatment:
- Immediate measures:
  vagal stimulation with Valsalva maneuver, iced water drinks or, in infants, ice-bags on the head (ice-water reflex)
- Hospitalization if attack not arrested after 30 minutes
- Hospital treatment
- In infants:
  – cardioversion with 2–4 (max.) W/kg (always if heart failure present)
  – rapid digitalization in 24 h
  – propafenone 0.5–1 mg/kg i.v. in 5 min, max. 3 mg/kg/24 h
- In older children:
  – verapamil 0.1–0.2 mg/kg single dose i.v., max. 5 mg (watch out for asystole)
  – resuscitation procedures ready
  – propafenone (see above)
  – no digitalization if Wolff–Parkinson–White syndrome.

Atrial flutter, fibrillation

Signs: Cardiac failure with high ventricular rate
ECG: **Flutter:** very rapid, regular, sawtooth-like change in atrial electrical activity with a rate of 240 up to >400/min; the degree of AV block determines ventricular rate.
Fibrillation: very rapid, uneven, atrial electrical activity of low amplitude with a rate of 350–700/min and irregular transmission to the ventricles. Totally irregular irregularity.

Differential diagnosis: paroxysmal atrial tachycardia with block.

Treatment:
- Cardioversion, especially if heart failure and high ventricular rate
- Digitalization
- Verapamil.

Ventricular tachycardia

Symptoms: Heart failure, palpitations, chest pain, possibly unconsciousness.

ECG: Three or more successive ventricular extrasystoles
Frequency 100–200/min
Ventricular complexes broad and deformed
P wave unrelated to the QRS complex

Differential diagnosis: Supraventricular tachycardia with aberrant AV conduction.

CARDIOLOGY

Treatment:
- If necessary, cardiac resuscitation with cardiac massage
- Cardioversion (1–2 W/kg)
- Lignocaine 1 mg/kg single dose i.v., followed by infusion at 0.5–1.5 mg/kg/h
- propafenone.

Ventricular flutter, fibrillation

Symptoms: Signs of circulatory arrest.

ECG: Completely uncoordinated electrical activity of the myocardium with rates of 250–400/min.

Treatment
- Immediate resuscitation with artificial ventilation and closed-chest heart massage
- Defibrillation
- Lignocaine with subsequent maintenance infusion.

Bradyarrhythmias

Symptoms: Low pulse rate, cardiac failure, Stokes–Adams attacks with cyanosis and unconsciousness.

ECG: Second and third degree AV block
Third degree sinoatrial block or sinus arrest
Sinus node syndrome.

Treatment:
- Resuscitation, if condition life-threatening
- Orciprenaline or atropine as temporary measure
- Temporary transvenous pacing (an absolute indication in Stokes–Adams syndrome with cardiac failure).

Critical heart rate in neonates and infants <60/min, in older children <40/min.

Sympathomimetics

	Epinephrine (WHO): adrenaline	Norepinephrine (WHO): noradrenaline	Dopamine Low dosage up to ca. 3 µg/kg/min	Dopamine Medium dosage ca. 3–7.5 µg/kg/min	Dopamine High dosage ca. over 7.5 µg/kg/min	Dobutamine	Isoprenaline (WHO): isoproterenol
Chief action on adrenergic receptors	$\alpha + \beta$ stimulator. Small doses of β, inhibit α in high doses	Mainly α stimulator	Dopaminergic	$\alpha + \beta$ stimulator — β_1	Mainly α stimulator	(Pure) β, stimulator	(Pure) $\beta_{(1+2)}$ stimulator
Cardiac β_1 — Positively inotropic (contractility ↑)	↑↑↑	↑ (↑)	+/−	↑↑	↑↑↑	↑↑↑	↑↑↑
Positively chronotropic	↑↑↑	↑	+/−	↑	↑↑	+/−	↑↑↑
Positively dromotropic (AV conduction time ↓)	↑↑↑	↑	+/−	↑	↑↑	+/−	↑↑↑
Peripheral α — Vasoconstriction (Peripheral arterioles & veins, renal, also some coronary)	High doses ↑↑↑	↑↑↑			↑↑↑	Below ca. 7.5 kg/min ↑	
β_2 — Vasodilation Bronchodilation	Small doses ↑		+/−	↑		From ca. 7.5 µg/kg/min ↑	(Muscle vessels) ↑↑↑
Dopaminergic — Vasodilation in kidneys (flow ↑, Na excretion ↑), splanchnic region	→	→	↑↑	+/−	→	+/−	+/−
Cardiac output	↑↑	+/−	+/−	↑	↑↑	↑↑↑	↑↑
Heart rate	↑↑	+/− to ↑	+/− to ↑	↑	↑ (↑)	+/− from 10 µg/kg/min upwards ↑	↑↑↑
Heterotopic excitation (rhythm disorder)	↑↑	↑	+/−	↑	↑ (↑)	+/−	↑↑↑

CARDIOLOGY

Blood pressure	Systolic	↑↑	↑↑↑	+/–	↑↑	↑↑↑	+/– to ↑	+/–
	Diastolic	low dosage ↓ high dosage ↑	↑↑	↓	↓ to +/–	↑	+/– to ↓	→
	Medium pressure	low dosage ↓ high dosage ↑	↑↑	+/–	+/–	↑↑	+/– to ↓	→
Left ventricular end-diastolic pressure		+/–	+/–	+/–	+/– to ↑	↑	→	→
Total peripheral vascular resistance		Low dosage ↓ High dosage ↑	↑↑↑ from 0.3 µg/kg/min	→	+/– to ↑	↑↑	↑ (also high dosage)	→
Total pulmonary vascular resistance		High dosage ↑	↑↑ from 0.3 µg/kg/min	→	+/– to ↑	↑↑	→	↓ (↓)
Myocardial O$_2$ consumption		↑↑		+/–	↑	↑↑	→	↑↑↑
Coronary perfusion		↑	↑	+/–	+/–	↑	↑ (↑)	↓ to +/–
Preferred use in case of:		Resuscitation, cardiac arrest, anaphylactic shock	Low output with very low blood pressure (peripheral resistance ↓)	Need to improve renal function in shock			Most cardioselective drugs have little peripheral effect, even in high doses. Drug of choice: in cardiogenic shock, perhaps with dopamine or vasodilators (sodium nitroprusside)	(Bradycardic rhythm disorder, reduced ventricular function) Bronchospasm
Recommended dose Initial dose		0.01–0.1 mg/kg (= 0.1–1.0 ml/kg of 1:10 000 solution) i.v. or endotracheally	0.05–1.0 µg/kg/min		1–30 µg/kg/min		2.5–20 µg/kg/min	
Maintenance dose		0.1–0.2 µg/kg/min	0.1–(0.2) µg/kg/min		2–5(–10) µg/kg/min		2.5–7.5(–10) µg/kg/min	0.1–2.0 µg/kg/min

Anti-arrhythmic drugs: Indications and dosages

Drug group	Example	Indications	Oral dosage	i.v. single dosage	Infusion dosage
Class I (local anesthetics)	Quinidine	Atrial flutter/fibrillation, SVT (VES, VT)	15–60 mg/kg/d in 4 doses Max 400 mg/dose	–	–
Ia (Refractory time increased)	Disopyramide	SVT, atrial flutter/fibrillation, VES, VT	1–3 mg/kg/SD (dose) every 6 h Max 200 mg/dose	0.5 mg/kg over 5 min max. 4 times (with at least 5 min between injections) Alternative: 2 mg/kg over at least 5 min	immediately (max. 30 min after main dose) 1 mg/kg/h, after 3 h reduce to 0.4 mg/kg/h
Ib (Refractory time decreased)	Lignocaine	VES, VT	–	1 mg/kg over 5 min	20–50 µg/kg/min, halve dose after 24 h
	Mexiletine	VES, VT	2.9–5 mg/kg/SD every 8 h	3 mg/kg over 15 min	0.5 mg/kg/h, max. 12 h
	Phenytoin	VES, VT Digitalis poisoning	First day 16 mg/kg/d in 4 doses, then 5–6 mg/kg/d in 2 doses	15 mg/kg over 1 h (1/12th the dose every 5 min)	10–12 mg/kg over 12–24 h
Ic (Refractory time unchanged)	Flecainide	VES, VT, tachycardia in WPW, AV nodal tachycardia, ectopic atrial tachycardia	2 mg/kg/dose (max 100 mg) 12 h	1 mg/kg over 30 min, perhaps after 20 min 0.5 mg/kg 1–2 mg/kg every 8–12 h over 30 min	4 mg/kg/d
	Propafenone	Tachycardia in WPW, VES, VT, AV nodal tachycardia	15–18 mg/kg/d for 3 d, then 10–12 mg/kg/d in 3–4 doses	0.5–1 mg/kg 'stutter' treatment: 0.2 mg/kg every 10 min (max. 2 mg/kg)	4–7 µg/kg/min

CARDIOLOGY

Class II (Beta-blockers)	Propranolol	SVT, VT Long QT syndrome, sinus tachycardia in hyperthyroidism	1–5 mg/kg/d in 4 doses	0.05–0.1(–0.15) mg/kg slow i.v. (over 10 min)	–
Class III (Primary prolongation of refractory time)	Amiodarone	Treatment, refractory, life-threatening SVES, SVT, VES, VT. First choice in congenital AV nodal tachycardia	10 mg/kg/d in 2 doses for 10 d, then 5 mg/kg/d in 1 dose, then possibly reduce further (Max 200 mg)	1 mg/kg every 10 mins for 10 times then after 12 hours, repeat if necessary (Max 1.2 g in 24 h)	–
	Sotalol (also class II action)	WPW, VES, fibrillation	1–4 mg/kg/dose 12 hourly (Max 200 mg/dose)	0.25–1 (to max. 1.5) mg/kg over 5–15 min	–
Class IV (Calcium antagonist)	Verapamil	SVT (after 1 y of age, not together with beta-blockers)	2–7 mg/kg/d in 3–4 doses	0.1–0.15 mg/kg over 10 min, perhaps repeated once after 5 min	0.005 mg/kg/min
Class V	Digoxin	SVT (not WPW), tachyarrhythmia with irregular ventricular rate	Total loading dose: oral Prematures, 20 µg/kg; neonates up to 6 months, 30 µg/kg; >6 months, 50 µg/kg, after 8 h, 25% of dose. Maintenance dose: 5–10 µg/kg	75% of the oral dose	

(Specifications after Gillette and Garson (1990); Gutheil and Singer (1982).) Many of those drugs should be used with extreme caution in children. SVT = supraventricular tachycardia; VES = ventricular extrasystoles; VT = ventricular tachycardia; SD = single dose; SVES = supraventricular extrasystoles; WPW = Wolff–Parkinson–White syndrome; BS = body surface area.

133

Digitalis treatment

Because of their lower tolerance to digitalis, prematures and neonates are given a daily dose of 0.02–0.03 mg/kg of metildigoxin. After the fourth week of life up to approximately 12 years of age, the full loading dose of 1.0 mg/m² body surface area is given; after that age the full adult loading dose (1.0–1.5 mg) is given. Fifty per cent of the full loading dose can be given on the first two days, then 30% on the third day and 20% on the fourth day. In older children, lower doses than those specified may be given.
In oral administration of digoxin or acetyldigoxin, the specified dosages should be increased by 20%.

Desired serum digoxin levels:

In neonates and infants: 3(–4) mg/ml (3.8–5.1 nmol/l)
In older children: 1–2 mg/ml (1.3–2.6 nmol/l)

A raised digitalis sensitivity is present in:
- prematures and neonates
- myocarditis, cardiomyopathy
- simultaneous administration of corticosteroids
- hypoxia
- hypercalcemia
- hypocalcemia
- reduced hepatic and renal function.

CARDIOLOGY

Digitalis poisoning

The glycoside level is inadequate as a criterion of the presence of poisoning, as toxic symptoms can be produced at therapeutic doses.

Symptoms of poisoning or overdose

Gastrointestinal	Nausea, vomiting, diarrhea, abdominal pain, loss of appetite.
Cerebral	Visual disorders (color vision, double vision, blindness, sensitivity to light); vertigo, hallucination, coma, seizure, headache, neuralgia.
Cardiac	Tachycardic and bradycardic arrhythmias: ventricular extrasystoles and tachycardia, ventricular flutter and fibrillation; atrial tachycardia with and without block, atrial flutter and fibrillation, first to third degree AV block, (active) nodal rhythm, nodal tachycardia.
	Rapid alternation between different arrhythmias is characteristic.
Diagnosis	Blood film, blood sugar, blood gas analysis, serum electrolytes, urea, creatinine, digitalis level. ECG.

Digitalis-induced ECG changes

Ectopic excitation →
- Atrial extrasystoles
- Atrial tachycardia
- Simple AV dissociation
- Rapid AV nodal rhythm
- Ventricular extrasystoles (unitopic, multitopic)
- Extrasystolic salvoes → ventricular flutter or fibrillation.

Depressed excitation →
- PR prolongation (first degree AV block)
- Wenckebach periodicity (second degree AV block)
- Complete AV block (third degree).

Accelerated repolarization →
- Shortening of the QT time (rate-corrected)
- Flattening of the T wave
- Increased height of the U wave (can merge with T wave)
- Discordant ST depression in I, V_5, V_6, aVL; ST elevation in II, V_1–V_3, aVF.

MEMORIX PEDIATRICS

Treatment of digitalis overdose or poisoning

1. Symptomatic
   - In overdose: stop digitalis or reduce the dose
   - In acute poisoning:
     – stomach washout
     – restoration of the electrolytes and water metabolism to normal levels
     – treatment of the rhythm disorders:
       bradycardia → atropine; pacemaker
       ventricular extrasystoles/tachycardia → lignocaine 0.5–1 mg/kg i.v.
         over 1 min, phenytoin 5 mg/kg slow i.v.
       ventricular flutter fibrillation → defibrillation.

2. Causal
   Antidote: digoxin-specific antibodies (Fab fragments)
   80 mg antidote (= 1 amp.) binding 1 mg digoxin/digitoxin
   1 amp. dissolved in 20 ml NaCl 0.9%

   Action: binds the free glycosides

   Indications:
   – severe treatment – refractory arrhythmias
   – intake of a large amount of digoxin

   Contraindications: sheep globulin allergy

   Side-effects:
   – allergic reaction
   – sensitization.

   Dosage
   The dosage is adjusted to the amount (not, as in the adult, to the body weight, body surface, etc.).

CARDIOLOGY

Calculation if serum concentration is known

Amount taken (mg) = (serum concentration µg/l)/1000 × distribution volume (l/kg) × body weight (kg)

Distribution volume is dependent on the glycoside used, but in addition there are important interindividual differences. V_d for digoxin = 5.1–17.1; for digitoxin = 0.46–1.1 l/kg.)

Procedure

a) Pretesting

- Intracutaneous: 0.1 ml of Fab solution +0.4 ml NaCl 0.9%, of which 0.1 ml is injected intracutaneously (inner side of forearm)
- Conjunctivally: one drop of the solution in the conjunctival sac.

b) Infusion

The calculated quantity is given as a rapid infusion in around 30 min. (Total amount is given, even if symptoms recede.)
NB: possibility of shock symptoms at the beginning of the infusion.

c) Electrolytes

The serum potassium level, raised in glycoside poisoning, will be reduced by the antidote, so that hypokalemia may occur; regular potassium checks are therefore necessary.

d) Because of the possibility of sensitivity to sheep globulin, the administration of digoxin antidote should be noted in the patient's records.

e) Treatment follow-up

Rhythm disorders generally regress in 1–3 h after the onset of treatment.

MEMORIX PEDIATRICS

ECG changes in electrolyte disorders

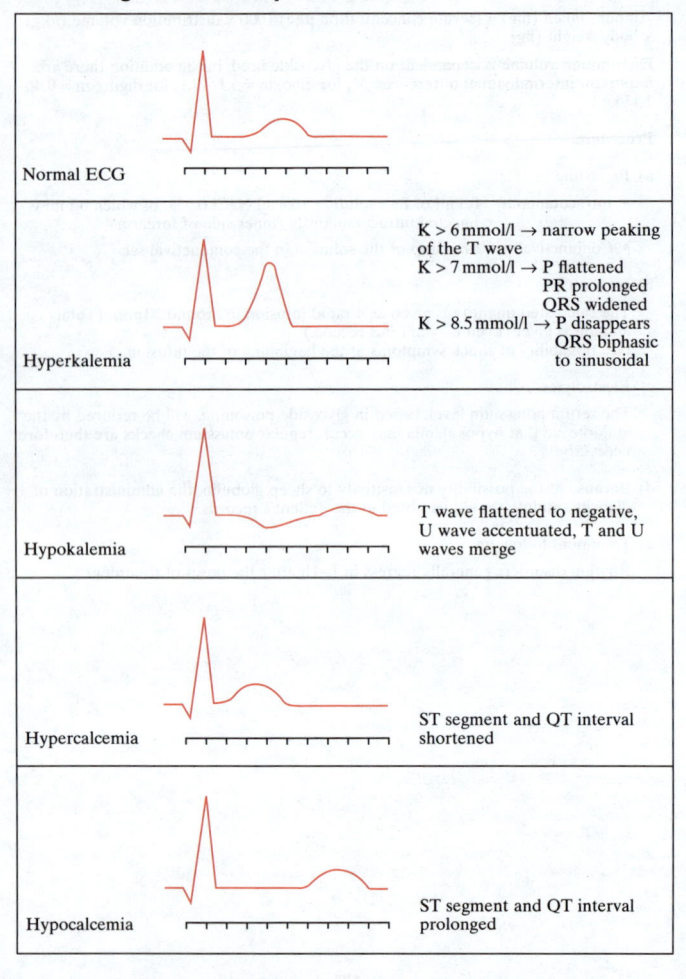

Normal ECG	
Hyperkalemia	K > 6 mmol/l → narrow peaking of the T wave K > 7 mmol/l → P flattened PR prolonged QRS widened K > 8.5 mmol/l → P disappears QRS biphasic to sinusoidal
Hypokalemia	T wave flattened to negative, U wave accentuated, T and U waves merge
Hypercalcemia	ST segment and QT interval shortened
Hypocalcemia	ST segment and QT interval prolonged

CARDIOLOGY

Cardiomyopathies

1. Primary cardiomyopathies
   Primary cardiomyopathies are heart muscle diseases of unknown cause. The World Health Organization definition of 1980 divides them into dilatated cardiomyopathy (DCM), hypertrophic cardiomyopathy with or without obstruction (HOCM, HCM), and restrictive cardiomyopathy (RCM).

2. Secondary cardiomyopathies
   Secondary forms are specific heart muscle diseases of various etiologies. (Compare with tables after Lindinger in Gutheil (1990).)

Causes of secondary cardiomyopathies

Hypertrophic forms

Appearing in neonates and in infancy:
- maternal diabetes during pregnancy (reversible)
- in prematures after catecholamine in high doses
- infants with bronchopulmonary dysplasia and pulmonary hypertension
- Adrenocorticotropic hormone treatment for seizures (reversible)

Metabolic diseases
- glycogen storage disease types I, III and VIII
- subacute necrotizing encephalopathy (of Leigh)
- nesidioblastoses
- alpha-galactoside-A deficiency (Fabry's disease)
- cytochrome-C-oxidase deficiency
- hereditary mitochondrial myopathy with HCM, cataract and lactacidosis

Endocrine diseases
- acromegaly

Neurological diseases
- Friedreich's ataxia

Syndrome associations
- LEOPARD syndrome (multiple Lentigines syndrome)
- Noonan's and Turner's syndromes.

Dilatated forms

After viral myocarditis (enterovirus, Coxsackievirus B, mumps, *Mycoplasma pneumoniae*, etc.)
Bland–White–Garland syndrome
Endocardial fibroelastosis
Toxins (adriablastin > 400 mg/m^2 body surface area)
Metabolic diseases
- carnitine deficiency
- hemachromatoses (β thalassemia major)
- mucopolysaccharidoses (Hurler's disease)
- lysosomal or mitochondrial diseases

Muscular dystrophies
Autoimmune diseases (juvenile chronic polyarthritis, systemic lupus erythematosus)
Arrythmogenic right ventricular dysplasia (Uhl's disease).

MEMORIX PEDIATRICS

Synopsis of idiopathic forms in children and adolescents

Hypertrophic form	Hypertrophy, obstructive form (HOCM)	Dilated form

Definition:

myocardial hypertrophy of left ventricle	Idiopathic hypertrophic subaortic stenosis (HSS) functionally labile	Dilatation of left + right ventricles + left atrium

Histology:
Bizarrely shaped myocardial cells form a disordered tissue pattern. Small branches of the coronary arteries with thickened walls and narrowed lumen. Fibrotic scars in myocardium

Pathophysiology:

Ejection fraction	↑	↓↓↓
Ventricular volume	↔ ↓	↑↑↑
Filling pressure	↑↑↑	↑
Ventricular pumping capacity	↔	↓↓↓

Symptoms:

(rare in children) Infants: poor feeders, dystrophy Older children: reduced energy, dyspnea, angina if arrhythmias	All the signs of cardiac failure: failure to feed and thrive, lack of energy, tachypnea, peripheral cyanosis, edema

Clinical signs:

heaving apex beat, systolic murmur up to 3/6 parasternally (↑ on standing up or Valsalva), frequently third heart sound	Hepato(spleno)megaly, systolic murmur, accentuated third heart sound, moist rales

ECG:

left ventricular hypertrophy, biventricular hypertrophy, pathological ST segment with negative T wave, deep Q wave, rarely bundle branch block, arrhythmias (supraventricular/ventricular extrasystoles, ventricular tachycardia, atrial flutter/fibrillation)	Left ventricular hypertrophy, abnormal repolarization

Echocardiography: (M-mode, 2-D, Doppler)

Ventricular septal hypertrophy > left ventricular posterior wall; small ventricular cavity, systolic motion of the anterior mitral leaflet towards ventricular septum (proportional to the degree of obstruction)	Dilatation of left heart, Shortening fraction (SF) < 25%

Differential diagnosis:

Pulmonary/aortic valvar stenosis, fibromuscular subvalvar aortic stenosis	→ Table on secondary cardiomyopathy (p. 139)

Treatment:

propranolol 2–5 mg/kg/d (Max 80 mg per dose) verapamil 5–7 mg/kg/d (Max 120 mg per dose) Obstruction + symptoms: septal myotomy/myectomy	Digitalis, diuretics, vasodilating sympathomimetics, possibly anticoagulants, antiarrhythmic drugs

CARDIOLOGY

Indirect blood pressure measurement

Approximate age-related sizes of blood pressure cuffs for sphygmomanometry

Age	Dimensions of inflatable cuff (cm)			
	Arm		Leg	
	Width	Length	Width	Length
Neonates	2.5–4	5–9		
Infants	4–6	10–13	8–9	20
Small children	6–9	13–18	12–14	25
Children to 8 y	7–10	17–20	14–16	28
Children to 12 y	1–12	20–24	16–18	30
Adolescents	12–14	22–26	18–20	32–38

Notes: 1. Width of cuff part = 3/4, minimally 2/3, of upper arm length; length of cuff no more than the arm circumference.
2. In borderline cases, the next larger size is selected.
3. The size of the cuff should be adapted to the size of the limb, rather than to the age of the patient.

Phases of blood pressure measurement – changes in the Korotkoff sounds

Phase   Sound quality

1   Sudden onset of knocking sound   → systolic pressure
2   Knocking sound with flow sound
3   Intensity of sound ↑
4   Sound dampened down, no longer knocking → diastolic pressure
5   Sound disappears   → diastolic pressure

Note: Allow for pressure reduction of 2–3 mmHg (0.266–0.399 kPa)/s. If phase 5 cannot be clearly defined, take the pressure in phase 4 as the diastolic pressure (young children).

Definition of hypertension

(Second Task Force on Blood Pressure Control in Children (1987).)

Normal blood pressure → Systolic and diastolic pressure <90th percentile in relation to age and sex

High normal blood pressure → Mean systolic and/or diastolic pressure between 90th and 95th percentile in relation to age and sex

Hypertension → mean systolic and/or diastolic pressure ≥95th percentile in relation to age and sex. Take measurements on at least three occasions.

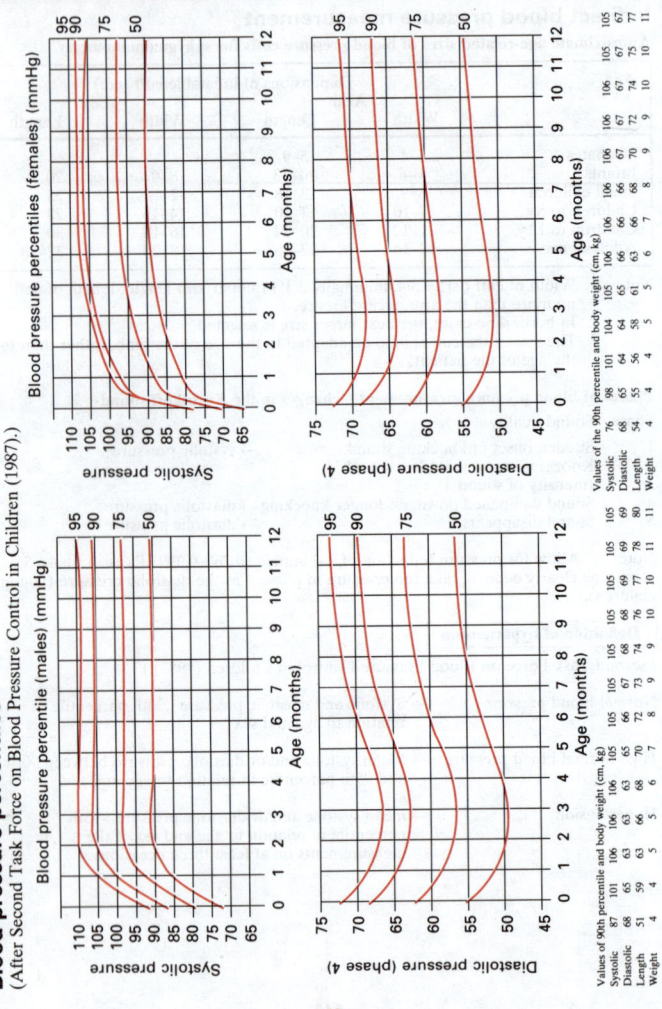

Blood pressure percentiles
(After Second Task Force on Blood Pressure Control in Children (1987).)

Blood pressure percentile (males) (mmHg)

Values of 90th percentile and body weight (cm, kg)

	0	1	2	3	4	5	6	7	8	9	10	11	12
Systolic	87	101	106	106	106	105	105	105	105	105	105	105	105
Diastolic	68	65	63	63	63	65	66	67	68	68	69	69	69
Length	51	59	63	66	68	70	72	73	74	76	78	80	80
Weight	4	4	5	5	6	7	8	9	9	10	10	11	11

Blood pressure percentiles (females) (mmHg)

Values of the 90th percentile and body weight (cm, kg)

	0	1	2	3	4	5	6	7	8	9	10	11	12
Systolic	76	98	101	104	105	106	106	106	106	106	106	105	105
Diastolic	68	65	64	64	65	66	67	67	67	72	74	75	77
Length	54	55	56	58	61	63	66	68	69	70	71	75	77
Weight	4	4	5	5	5	6	7	8	9	9	10	10	11

142

CARDIOLOGY

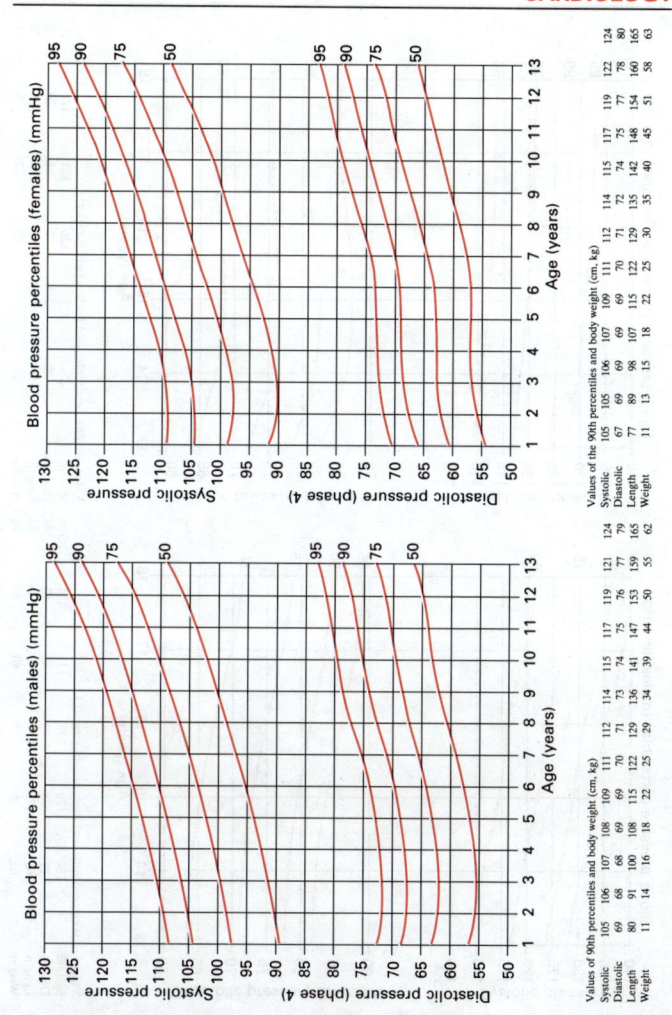

Blood pressure percentiles (males) (mmHg)

Values of 90th percentiles and body weight (cm, kg)														
Systolic	105	106	107	108	109	111	112	114	115	117	119	121	124
Diastolic	69	68	68	69	69	70	71	73	74	75	76	77	77
Length	80	91	100	108	115	122	129	136	141	147	153	159	165
Weight	11	14	16	18	22	25	29	34	39	44	50	55	62

Blood pressure percentiles (females) (mmHg)

Values of the 90th percentiles and body weight (cm, kg)														
Systolic	105	105	106	107	109	111	112	114	115	117	119	122	124
Diastolic	67	69	69	69	70	71	72	74	75	77	78	80
Length	77	89	98	107	115	122	129	135	142	148	154	160	165
Weight	11	13	15	18	22	25	30	35	40	45	51	58	63

MEMORIX PEDIATRICS

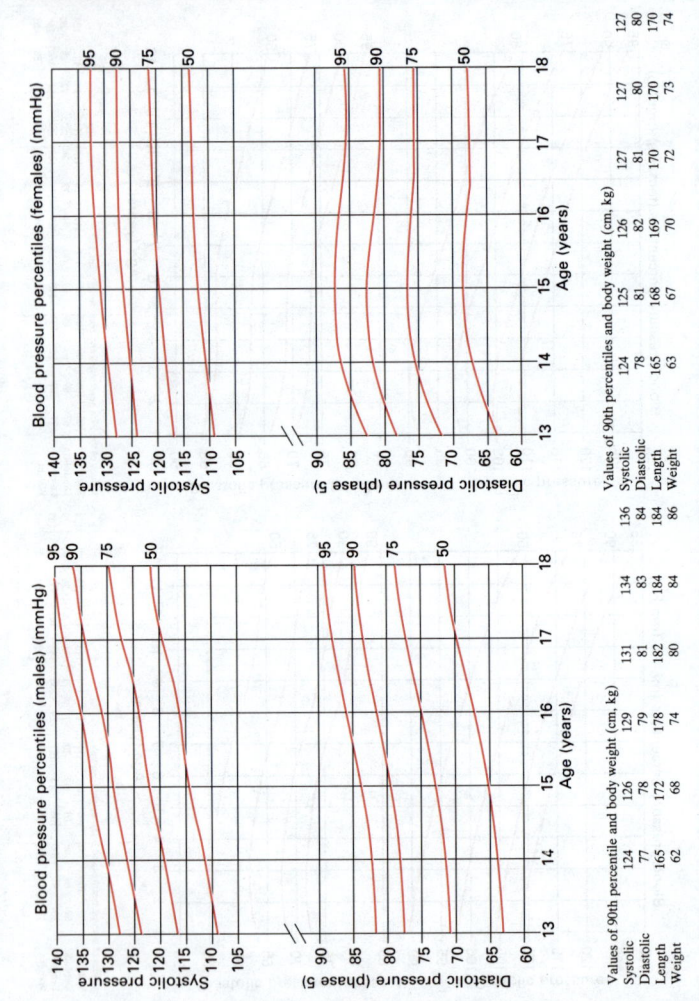

Blood pressure percentiles (males) (mmHg)

Values of 90th percentile and body weight (cm, kg)						
Systolic	124	126	129	131	134	136
Diastolic	77	78	79	81	83	84
Length	165	172	178	182	184	184
Weight	62	68	74	80	84	86

Blood pressure percentiles (females) (mmHg)

Values of 90th percentiles and body weight (cm, kg)						
Systolic	124	125	126	127	127	127
Diastolic	78	81	82	81	80	80
Length	165	168	169	170	170	170
Weight	63	67	70	72	73	74

CARDIOLOGY

Hypertension

Age-related classification of hypertension

(Second Task Force on Blood Pressure Control in Children (1987).)

Age	Significant hypertension Systolic/diastolic (mmHg)	Severe hypertension Systolic/diastolic (mmHg)
7 d	Systolic ⩾ 96	Systolic ⩾ 106
8–30 d	Systolic ⩾ 104	Systolic ⩾ 110
>2 y	⩾112/ ⩾ 74	⩾118/ ⩾ 82
3–5 y	⩾116/ ⩾ 76	⩾124/ ⩾ 84
6–9 y	⩾122/ ⩾ 78	⩾130/ ⩾ 86
10–12 y	⩾126/ ⩾ 82	⩾134/ ⩾ 90
13–15 y	⩾136/ ⩾ 86	⩾144/ ⩾ 92
16–18 y	⩾142/ ⩾ 92	⩾150/ ⩾ 98

Algorithm for the diagnosis of hypertension in children and adolescents

(Modified from Second Task Force on Blood Pressure Control in Children (1987).)

NB: For percentile assignment, the mean value of at least two measurements should be used.

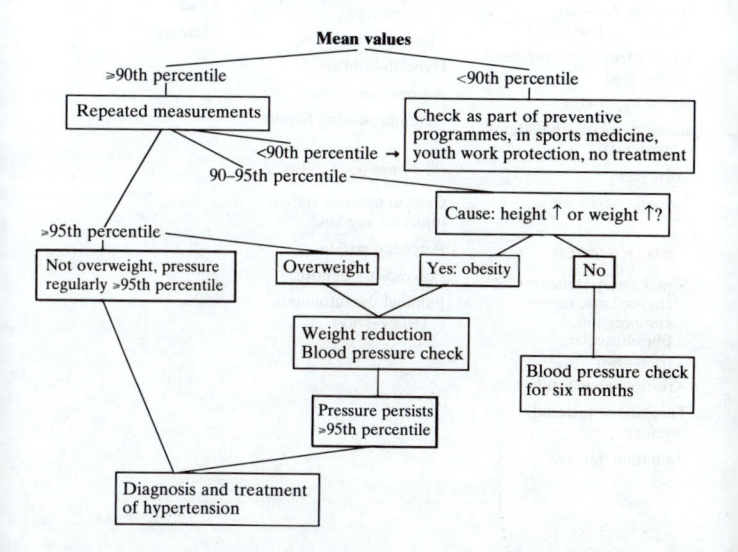

Mean values

- ⩾90th percentile → Repeated measurements
  - <90th percentile →
  - 90–95th percentile → Cause: height ↑ or weight ↑?
    - Overweight → Yes: obesity → Weight reduction, Blood pressure check → Pressure persists ⩾95th percentile → Diagnosis and treatment of hypertension
    - No → Blood pressure check for six months
  - ⩾95th percentile → Not overweight, pressure regularly ⩾95th percentile → Diagnosis and treatment of hypertension
- <90th percentile → Check as part of preventive programmes, in sports medicine, youth work protection, no treatment

MEMORIX PEDIATRICS

Checklist of the underlying diseases in hypertension

① Renal causes

Parenchymal damage

Obstructive uropathies
Reflux nephropathies
Chronic pyelonephritis
Glomerulonephritis
Autoimmune disease
Chronic renal insufficiency
Kidney transplant rejection
Hemolytic-uremic syndrome
Nephrosclerosis
Tubular pathology
Nephrolithiasis
Tumors (Wilms' tumor, tuberous sclerosis, lymphoma, leukemia)
Kidney trauma (+ perirenal hematoma)
Renal hypoplasia
Renal dysplasia (unilateral/bilateral)
Polycystic
Juvenile nephrosis

Vascular damage

Renal artery stenoses (hypoplasia, tumor compression, fibromuscular dysplasia)
Arteriovenous fistula
Thrombosis (arterial, venous)
Radiation damage

② Cardiovascular causes

Aortic coarctation
Generalized aortic hypoplasia
Aortic valvar regurgitation
Arteriovenous fistula
Persistent ductus arteriosus

③ Endocrine causes

Neuroblastoma
Pheochromocytoma
Hyperparathyroidism
Primary aldosteronism
Adrenogenital syndrome (11β and 17-hydroxylase deficiency)
Cushing's syndrome
Hyperthyroidism
Adrenal carcinoma
Renin-producing tumors

④ Neurogenic causes

Central nervous system injury of any kind
Polyneuropathies
Polyradiculoneuritis
Familial dysautonomia (Riley–Day)

⑤ Other causes

Burns
Immobility
Hypernatremia
Hypercalcemia
Porphyria

Drugs

Steroids
Contraceptives
Sympathomimetics

Poisons

Liquorice
Lead
Mercury

CARDIOLOGY

Diagnosis of hypertension

Non-specific suspicious symptoms

Epistaxis	Irritability	Vomiting	Growth retardation	Drowsiness
Headache	Insomnia	Dystrophy	Chest pains	Lassitude

Indicative symptoms and findings

(1) Renal
(1) (3) (5)
Fever
Pallor
Polyuria
Polydipsia
Enuresis
Uremic fetor
Edema
Urolithiasis
Abdominal tumor
Arthralgia
Joint swelling
Café-au-lait spots
Sebaceous adenoma

(2) Cardiovascular
(2)
Calf cramps
Cyanosis (neonates)
Dyspnea (neonates)
Waterhammer pulse (arms)
Slow weak pulse (legs)

(3) Endocrine
(3) (4) (5)
Opsoclonia
Obesity
Perspiration
Striae
Intersexual genitalia ♀
Virilization
Increased longitudinal growth
Tetany (neonates)
Spontaneous fracture

(4) Neurogenic
(1) (4) (5)
Disorders of consciousness
Seizures
Pareses
Hypotension
Paresthesias

(5) Other
(5) (1) (3) (4)
Tachypnea
Tachycardia
Pruritus
Erythema
Colic
Psychosis

Basic diagnostic investigations

Blood: full blood count
ESR
pH
Bicarbonate
Base excess (±)

Serum: Electrolytes
Calcium
Phosphate
Creatinine
Urea
Uric acid
C-reactive protein

Urine: analysis

Vanillylmandelic acid

Plasma renin

Sonography: abdomen
Doppler sonography aortic flow, renal vessels
ECG, radiography: chest and/or **echocardiography**
Static renal scintigraphy (^{99}Tc-dimercaptosuccinate (DMSA))
Ophthalmoscopy
Electroencephalography

MEMORIX PEDIATRICS

> Additional targeted diagnostic procedures

① i.v. excretion urography,
Dynamic renal scintigraphy (^{99}Tc-diethylenetriamine pentaacetic acid (DTPA) or ^{123}I-hippuran)
Glomerular filtration rate
Micturition cystourethrography,
Computed tomography (CT)
Selective renin measurement (inferior vena cava, renal veins)
Renal biopsy.

② Angiography.

③ Vanillylmandelic acid normal, clinically suspicious: other metabolites (methoxytyramine, normetanephrine)
Vanillylmandelic acid ↑: selective catecholemine measurement in inferior vena cava.
^{123}I-metaiodobenzylguanidine (MIBG) scintigraphy

Plasma aldosterone ↑:
- quantification of the mineralocorticoids (24 h urine)
- dexamethasone suppression test
- adrenal scintigraphy (after sonography and CT),

Plasma aldosterone ↓:
- quantification of the mineralocorticoids (24 h urine) quantification of the other plasma mineralocorticoids (corticosterone, desoxycorticosterone and glucocorticoids)
- measurement of plasma cortisol after adrenocorticotropic hormone (ACTH) stimulation or dexamethasone suppression.

④ Electroencephalography, central nervous system magnetic resonance tomography.

CARDIOLOGY

Antihypertensive treatment: three-stage program

(After recommendations of the Second Task Force on Blood Pressure in Children (1987).)

Stage 1 — **One-drug treatment:** beta-blocker
or
diuretic
or
calcium antagonist
or
ACE inhibitor.

Stage 2 — **Two-drug treatment:** beta-blocker
or
calcium antagonist
or
ACE inhibitor
or
alpha$_1$-blocker
plus
diuretic.

Alternatively: calcium antagonist plus beta-blocker
or
calcium antagonist plus ACE inhibitor.

Stage 3 — **Three-drug treatment:**
diuretic plus beta-blocker plus vasodilator
or   diuretic plus calcium antagonist plus ACE inhibitor
or   diuretic plus vasodilator plus alpha$_2$-sympathomimetic.

Treatment of hypertensive crises

Medication	Initial → high dose	Method of administration	Onset of action (min)	Duration of action (h)	Effect (direct, indirect)
Nifedipine	0.5–3 mg/kg (Max 40 mg)	Sublingually	15	2–5	Vasodilatation, tachycardia, edema, flushes
Diazoxide	2–6	i.v. (rapid)	1–2	4–12	Vasodilatation, retention (H_2O, sodium), hyperglycemia
Sodium nitroprusside	0.5–8 µg/kg/min (in 5% glucose)	i.v.: adapt infusion rate	Immediately	Only during infusion	Vasodilatation, tachycardia, cyanide or rhodanide poisoning
Hydralazine	0.2–0.4 mg/kg	i.v.	5–10	3–6	Vasodilatation, tachycardia
Clonidine	2–6 µg	i.v., s.c., i.m.	5–10	8–12	(Anti)sympathomimetics, sedation, bradycardia

CARDIOLOGY

Antihypertensive medication for long-term treatment

Generic name	Daily dose (mg/kg)	No. of doses/day	Action	Side-effects	Indication in renal failure
Diuretics:					
Hydrochlorothiazide	0.5–2	2	Blood volume ↓, vasodilatation	Hypokalemia, hyperuricemia	–
Furosemide	0.5–5	2–3	Blood volume ↓, vasodilatation,	Hypokalemia	+
Spironolactone	1–5	2–3	Blood volume ↓	Hyperkalemia	–
Beta-blockers:					
Propranolol	1–3	2–3	Pulse-time-volume↓, central sympathetic inhibition, vasodilatation	Bradycardia, sedation, bronchospasm	(+)
Alpha₁-blockers:					
Prazosine	0.05–0.5	2	Vasodilatation	Tachycardia, orthostatic collapse	–
Antisympathomimetics:					
Clonidine	0.005–0.03 (Max 300 µg/dose)	2–3	Central excitability of baroceptors	Sedation	+
Methyldopa	10–40	3	As for clonidine	Sedation	–
Calcium antagonists:					
Nifedipine	0.5–3 (Max 40 mg/dose)	2–3	Calcium canal block, vasodilatation	Tachycardia, edema, flushes	+
Vasodilators:					
Dihydralazine	1–5 (Max 50 mg/dose)	3	Vasodilatation	Tachycardia, stroke volume ↑, allergy	(+)
Minoxidil	0.1–0.5	2	Vasodilatation	Salt and water retention, sympathetic counter-regulation, hypertrichosis	+
ACE inhibitors:					
Captopril	Infants <6 months 0.05–0.5 Children >6 months 0.5–2.0 (Max 50 mg/dose)	3 3	Inhibition of angiotensin-converting enzyme, vasodilatation	Leukocytopenia, renal failure after previously reduced function	(+)

Hypotension: active orthostatic test

Upper limit of normal for percentage deviation from resting value
(After Klimt and Rutenfranz (1976).)

Age	3–5 years	6–9 years
Pulse rate ↑	40%	50%
$P_{syst.}$ ↓	10%	10%
$P_{diast.}$ ↑	$-5 \rightarrow +35\%$	$-5 \rightarrow +35\%$
P wave amplitude ↓	40%	50%

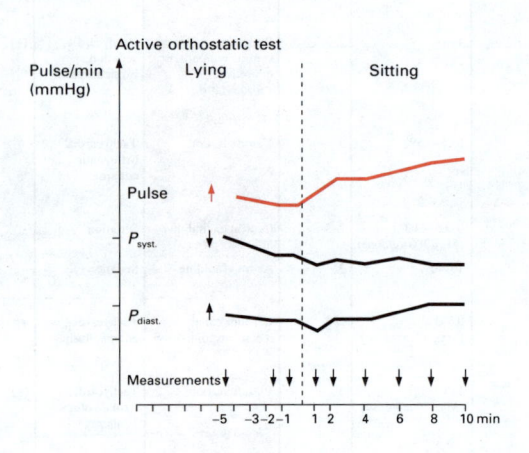

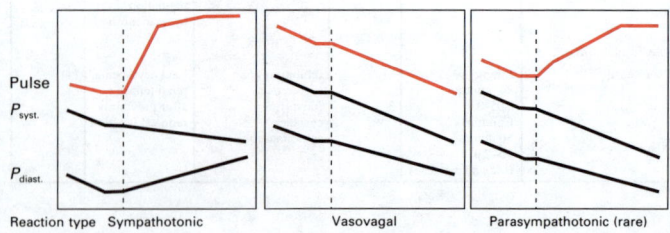

Active orthostatic test

Schellong test (normal reaction)

Reaction type: Sympathotonic — Vasovagal — Parasympathotonic (rare)

CARDIOLOGY

Indications for endocarditis prophylaxis according to degree of risk

(After Schumacher *et al.* (1989/90) and recommendations from the Paul Ehrlich Association for Chemotherapy.)

Minimum risk
- Atrial septal defect (secundum type)
- Mitral valve prolapse without valvar insufficiency
- After closure of a ventricular septal defect without patch material
- After ductus arteriosus ligature
- After aortocoronary bypass

• No prophylaxis

Medium risk
- All congenital heart defects (without atrial septal defect, secundum type)
- All acquired valvar defects
- Mitral valve prolapse with regurgitation (apical systolic murmur)
- Hypertrophic obstructive cardiomyopathy
- After palliative/corrective operations (exceptions: operations with minimal risks)
  a) with residual findings (shunt/stenosis)
  b) without residual findings

• Standard prophylaxis

• Lifetime standard prophylaxis
• Standard prophylaxis only in first postoperative year

Particularly high risk
- Valve prostheses, homografts, valveless aortopulmonary and ventriculopulmonary conduits
- Operated aortic valve stenosis
- After bacterial endocarditis

• High risk prophylaxis

Scheme for endocarditis prophylaxis

Standard prophylaxis:
    Single dose — oral — 60 min — before operation
                — intravenous — 30 min — before operation
                 — intravenous — at beginning of operation under anesthesia

High risk prophylaxis:
    First dose — intravenous — 30 min before the procedure
                            at beginning of operation under anesthesia
    Second dose — intravenous — after 8 h (vancomycin after 10–12 h)
    Third dose — intravenous — after 16 h

Supplementary procedures:
- A dental clean-up should be undertaken before every heart operation
- In proven bacterial infection, antibiotic treatment should be given for 8–12 days (including superinfection with viral bronchitis/pneumonia)

Antibacterial dosages for the prophylaxis of endocarditis

Group 1

Indications	Antibiotic	Dose/kg	Maximum daily dose
Standard prophylaxis	Penicillin V or	50 000 IU	2 mill. IU
	Amoxicillin	50 mg oral 25 mg i.v.	3 g 2 g
Penicillin not tolerated	Clindamycin	15 mg	600 mg
High risk prophylaxis	Penicillin V Penicillin G	{ 55 000 IU after 8, 16 h then 15 000	3 mill. IU
	or		
	Amoxicillin	25 mg i.v. after 8, 16 h then 25 mg	4 g
Penicillin not tolerated	Clindamycin (Infusion lasting over 1 h)	15 mg after 8, 16 h then 10 mg i.v.	1.2 g
	or		
	Vancomycin (Infusion lasting over 1 h)	20 mg i.v. 1 h before and 10–12 h after the operation	1 g

Group 2

Standard risk	Amoxicillin	50 mg oral 25 mg i.v.	3 g 2 g
	or		
	Ampicillin	50 mg i.v.	2 g
Penicillin not tolerated	Vancomycin	20 mg i.v.	1 g
High risk prophylaxis	Amoxicillin	25 mg i.v.	2 g
	or		
	Ampicillin	50 mg i.v. For both: same dose after 8, 16 h	2 g
Penicillin not tolerated	Vancomycin	20 mg same dose after 10–12 h	1 g

CARDIOLOGY

Group 3

Indications	Antibiotic	Dose/kg	Maximum daily dose
Standard risk	Flucloxacillin	30 mg oral or i.v.	2 g
Penicillin not tolerated	Clindamycin	15 mg oral	600 mg
High risk prophylaxis	Vancomycin	20 mg i.v. same dose after 10–12 h	1 g
Note for all high risk prophylaxis: potentiation of penicillin and clindamycin can be achieved with:	Gentamicin	2 mg i.v. plus 1 mg after 8, 16 h	

Endocarditis prophylaxis: commonest organisms

Organism	Affected area	Risk cover procedures/Treatment
Streptococci (viridans group)	Mouth, pharynx, upper respiratory tract	**Group 1** Teeth and gum surgery, root treatment, tooth-scaling, tonsillectomy, adenoidectomy, myringotomy, rigid-tube bronchoscopy, surgery on the respiratory passages, intubation, flexible-tube bronchoscopy, gastroscopy, esophageal bougie
Enterococci	Gastrointestinal and urogenital tracts	**Group 2** All surgical procedures plus bladder catheterization, enema, rectoscopy, lithotripsy (stone infection)
Staphylococci	Skin	**Group 3** Incision of abscess

Cardiac failure: principles of treatment

Aims of treatment	Measures and medication	Observations
Additional cardiac work ↓	Bedrest, sedation, tube/parenteral nutrition, warmth	
O_2-transport ↑	Compensate any anemia, O_2 administration	If necessary, artificial ventilation (PEEP)
Elimination of acidosis	Base deficit × 0.3 × kg body weight = mmol of required sodium bicarbonate	1 mmol = 1 ml of 8.4% $NaHCO_3$ solution Acid–base equilibrium is a prerequisite for the effectiveness of drug treatment
Myocardial contractility ↑	Digoxin (dosage see p. 134) Digitoxin Sympathomimetics in acute cardiac failure: Dopamine 2–10 µg/kg/min	In chronic renal failure administration via a central venous catheter; other effects: vasodilation (kidney), peripheral vasoconstriction
	Dobutamine 3–10 µg/kg/min Suitable combination: dopamine 1.5–3 µg/kg/min + dobutamine 5–10 µg/kg/min Adrenaline 0.05–0.5 µg/kg/min	Only for reinforcement of dopamine or dobutamine, possibly combined with a dilator
Preload ↓	Positioning (trunk ↑, legs ↓)	
Preload ↓ = diuresis ↑	Furosemide 0.5–1 mg/kg Spirolactone 0.5–2 mg/kg/d	Especially in hyperaldosteronism
Preload ↓ + afterload ↓ = venous and/or arteriolar vasodilation	ACE inhibitors: captopril 0.2–0.3 mg/kg/d Alpha-blocker: prazosine 0.03–0.4 mg/kg/d	Previous correction of an intravascular volume deficiency, check central venous pressure Begin with the lowest dosage, adapting this later

CARDIOLOGY

Hypoxemic attack: pathophysiology and treatment

(Red arrows = therapeutic correction)

Occurs in cyanotic cardiac defects, most often in tetralogy of Fallot.

Symptoms: increase in cyanosis, loss of consciousness, convulsions, systolic murmur in second left intercostal space less audible.

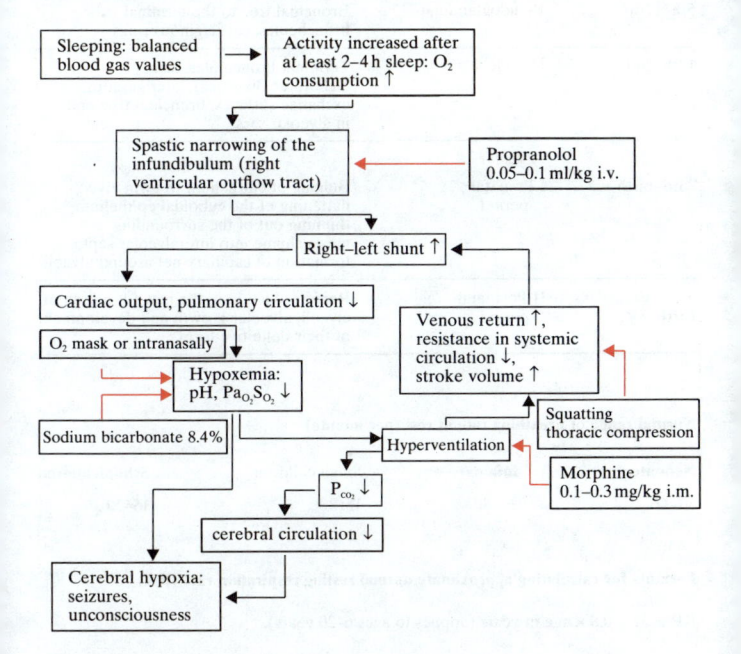

```
[Sleeping: balanced blood gas values] → [Activity increased after at least 2–4 h sleep: O₂ consumption ↑]
                                              ↓
                       [Spastic narrowing of the infundibulum (right ventricular outflow tract)] ← [Propranolol 0.05–0.1 ml/kg i.v.]
                                              ↓
                                   [Right–left shunt ↑]
                          ↙                                    ↘
[Cardiac output, pulmonary circulation ↓]        [Venous return ↑, resistance in systemic circulation ↓, stroke volume ↑]
       ↓
[O₂ mask or intranasally]
       ↓
[Hypoxemia: pH, Pa_O₂ S_O₂ ↓]                      [Squatting thoracic compression]
       ↓
[Sodium bicarbonate 8.4%]     [Hyperventilation] ←
                                      ↓
                                 [P_CO₂ ↓]          [Morphine 0.1–0.3 mg/kg i.m.]
                                      ↓
                           [cerebral circulation ↓]
                                      ↓
[Cerebral hypoxia: seizures, unconsciousness]
```

Note: 50% of the propranolol dose slowly as a single dose, the rest over 5 min i.v.; morphine is effective only after the removal of the base deficit; be prepared for respiratory arrest.

MEMORIX PEDIATRICS

Morphology of lung development

Weeks of pregnancy	Phase	Recognizable signs
4th–7th	Early embryonic	Main, lobar and segmental bronchi, lung arteries and veins
5th–17th	Pseudoglandular	Bronchial tree to the terminal broncheoles, cartilaginous rings
13th–26th	Canalicular	Terminal bronchioles, acini (10 dichotome divisions): later gaseous exchange surfaces; bronchial tree ends in alveolar sacs
	Alveolar	
23rd–birth	I Prenatal period	Bulging of epithelium to form alveoli, flattening of the cuboidal epithelium, thinning out of the surrounding mesenchyme into interalveolar septa, formation of capillary net around alveoli
Birth–8 y	II Postnatal period	Rapid reduction in the new formation of alveoli, alveolar growth and development of their definitive form

Normal range of breathing rate at rest (per minute)

Neonates	Infants	Small children	Schoolchildren
30–60	20–40	15–30	15–20

Formula for calculating approximate normal resting respiration rate (RR)

RR = 31 − 0.8 × age in years (applies to ages 6–20 years).

PULMONOLOGY

Differential diagnosis of rhythmic respiration

Type	Occurs in
Normal	
Biot's (irregular breathing at irregular intervals)	Brain damage
Kussmaul's (extreme hyperpnea)	Acidosis: diabetic coma, acetonemic vomiting, renal tubular failure, asphyxial syndrome, infant toxicosis
Cheyne–Stokes	Prematurity, acute central nervous system injury, cardiac failure, renal failure
Gasping respiration	Preterminal respiration

Oxyhemoglobin binding: partial pressure profile

Variation factors in oxyhemoglobin binding

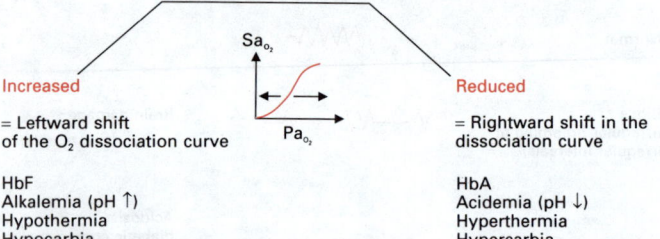

O_2 affinity for hemoglobin

Increased

= Leftward shift
of the O_2 dissociation curve

HbF
Alkalemia (pH ↑)
Hypothermia
Hypocarbia
2,3-diphosphoglycerate ↓

Reduced

= Rightward shift in the
dissociation curve

HbA
Acidemia (pH ↓)
Hyperthermia
Hypercarbia
2,3-diphosphoglycerate ↑

Normal partial pressure profile of respiration

P mmHg (kPa)	Inspiratory air	Alveoli	Arteries	Veins	Exspiratory gas mixture
P_{O_2}	158 (21.0)	103 (13.7)	90–110 (11.0–14.6)	37–42 (4.9–5.6)	116 (15.4)
P_{CO_2}	0.3 (0.04)	40 (5.3)	34–46 (4.5–6.1)	40–52 (5.3–6.9)	28 (3.7)
P_{H_2O}	5 (0.7)	47 (6.3)	–	–	47 (6.3)
P_{N_2}	596 (79.3)	570 (75.8)	574 (76.3)	574 (76.3)	569 (75.7)

PULMONOLOGY

Differential diagnosis of cyanosis

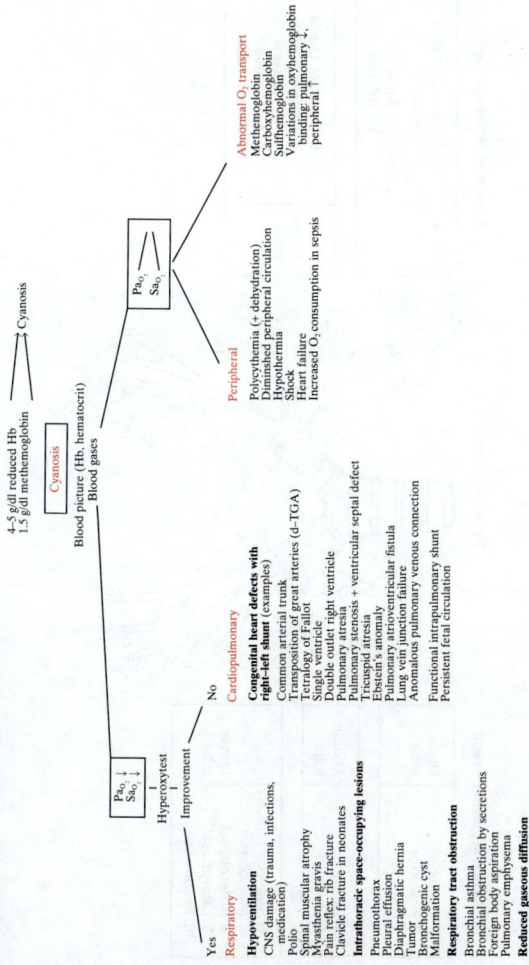

4–5 g/dl reduced Hb
1.5 g/dl methemoglobin → Cyanosis

Cyanosis

Blood picture (Hb, hematocrit)
Blood gases

$Pa_{O_2} \downarrow$, $Sa_{O_2} \downarrow$

Hyperoxytest
Improvement

Yes

No → Cardiopulmonary

$Pa_{O_2} \rightarrow$, $Sa_{O_2} \rightarrow$

Peripheral
Polycythemia (+ dehydration)
Diminished peripheral circulation
Hypothermia
Shock
Heart failure
Increased O₂ consumption in sepsis

Abnormal O₂ transport
Methemoglobin
Carboxyhemoglobin
Sulfhemoglobin
Variations in oxyhemoglobin binding, pulmonary ↓, peripheral ↑

Respiratory

Hypoventilation
CNS damage (trauma, infections, medication)
Polio
Spinal muscular atrophy
Myasthenia gravis
Pain reflex, rib fracture
Clavicle fracture in neonates

Intrathoracic space-occupying lesions
Pneumothorax
Pleural effusion
Diaphragmatic hernia
Tumor
Bronchogenic cyst
Malformation

Respiratory tract obstruction
Bronchial asthma
Bronchial obstruction by secretions
Foreign body aspiration
Pulmonary emphysema

Reduced gaseous diffusion (area, length)
Hypoplasia of one lung
Pneumonia
Infant or 'adult' respiratory distress syndrome
Bronchopulmonary dysplasia
Lung fibrosis

Cardiopulmonary

Congenital heart defects with right–left shunt (examples)
Common arterial trunk
Transposition of great arteries (d-TGA)
Tetralogy of Fallot
Single ventricle
Double outlet right ventricle
Pulmonary atresia
Pulmonary stenosis + ventricular septal defect
Tricuspid atresia
Ebstein's anomaly
Pulmonary atrioventricular fistula
Lung vein junction failure
Anomalous pulmonary venous connection
Functional intrapulmonary shunt
Persistent fetal circulation

Bronchial segments: anatomy

Bronchial segments – right

Upper lobe	1 Apical 2 Posterior 3 Anterior
Middle lobe	4 Lateral 5 Medial
Lower lobe	6 Superior (apical) 7 Mediobasal 8 Anterobasal 9 Laterobasal 10 Posterobasal

Bronchial tree

Bronchial segments – left

Upper lobe	1 + 2 Apicoposterior 3 Anterior
Lingula	4 Superior 5 Inferior
Lower lobe	6 Superior (apical) 7 Usually absent 8 Anterobasal 9 Laterobasal 10 Posterobasal

PULMONOLOGY

X-ray diagnosis: schema of lung segments

Bronchopulmonary segments in the chest film.
Radiological shadows of lung segments.

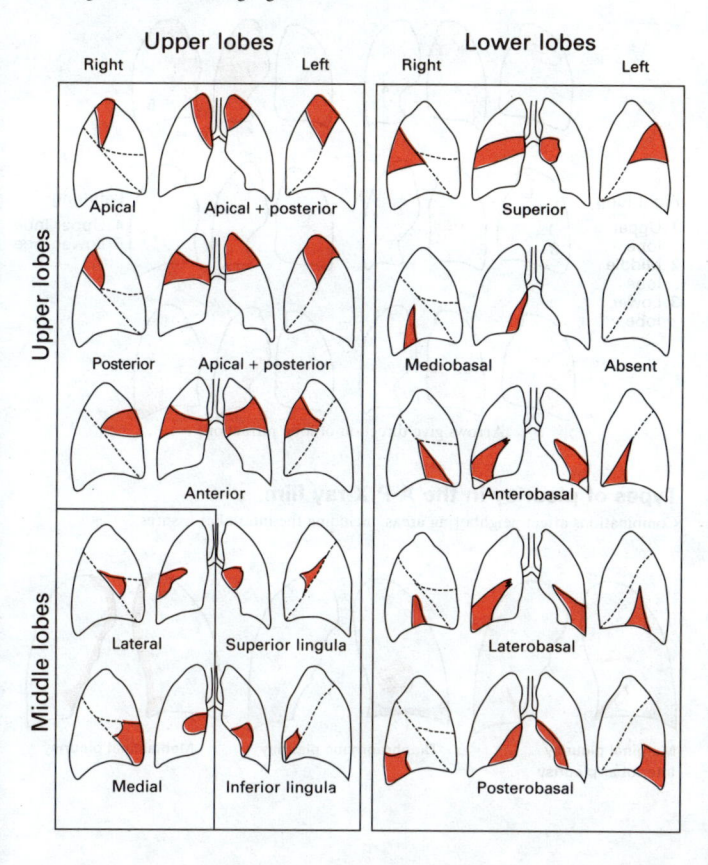

Upper lobes

Upper lobes (Right / Left):
- Apical
- Apical + posterior
- Posterior
- Apical + posterior
- Anterior

Middle lobes:
- Lateral
- Superior lingula
- Medial
- Inferior lingula

Lower lobes

(Right / Left):
- Superior
- Mediobasal / Absent
- Anterobasal
- Laterobasal
- Posterobasal

MEMORIX PEDIATRICS

X-ray diagnosis: appearance of lobar atalectasis

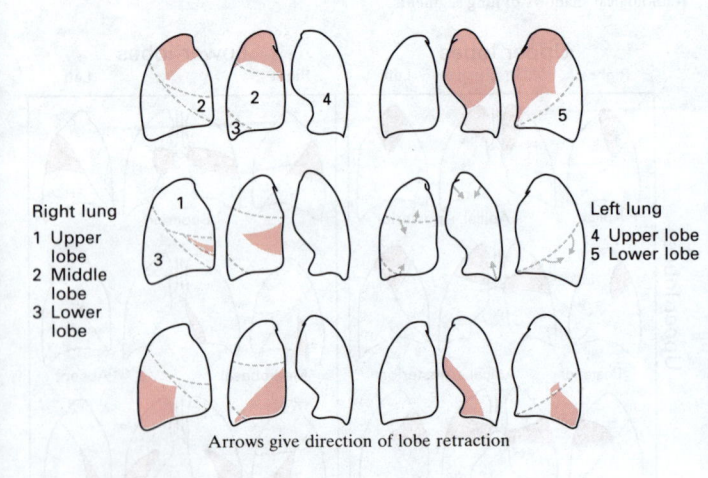

Right lung
1 Upper lobe
2 Middle lobe
3 Lower lobe

Left lung
4 Upper lobe
5 Lower lobe

Arrows give direction of lobe retraction

Types of pleurisy in the A-P X-ray film

Combinations affect neighboring areas, including the interlobar fissures.

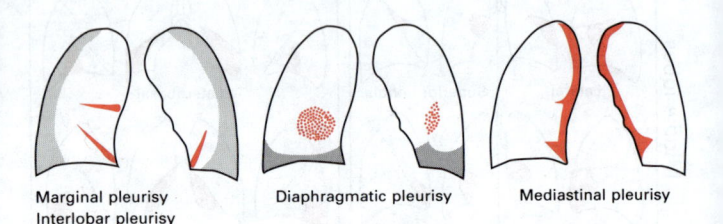

Marginal pleurisy
Interlobar pleurisy

Diaphragmatic pleurisy

Mediastinal pleurisy

PULMONOLOGY

X-ray diagnosis: appearance of pulmonary vessels

(from Schumacher and Bühlmeyer (1989) with permission.)

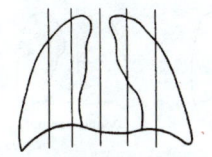

Division of the lung fields into three
to assess the appearance of the pulmonary vessels

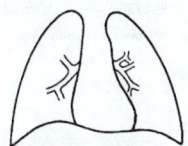

Normal appearance of pulmonary vessels

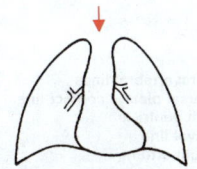

Raduced pulmonary vascular markings

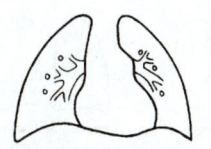

Enlarged pulmonary vascular markings
(Recirculation, active hyperemia)
Dilated pulmonary arteries, sharply delineated contours and cross-sections

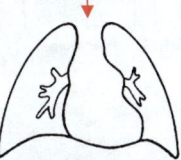

Pulmonary hypertension
(Eisenmenger reaction)
Central pulmonary arteries dilated, decreased vascular markings, lung periphery translucent

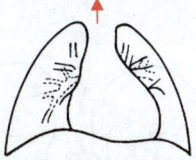

Pulmonary venous obstruction
(passive hyperemia)
Central pulmonary veins dilated poorly defined vascular contours and cross-sections, mainly in upper fields

MEMORIX PEDIATRICS

X-ray diagnosis: appearance of different forms of thymus hyperplasia

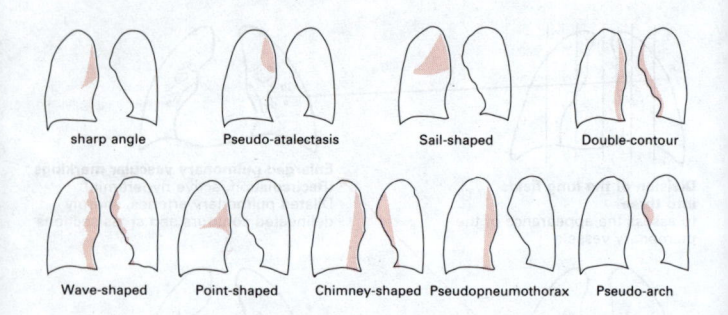

sharp angle Pseudo-atalectasis Sail-shaped Double-contour

Wave-shaped Point-shaped Chimney-shaped Pseudopneumothorax Pseudo-arch

Pleuromediastinal lines in chest film
(After Ball (1990).)

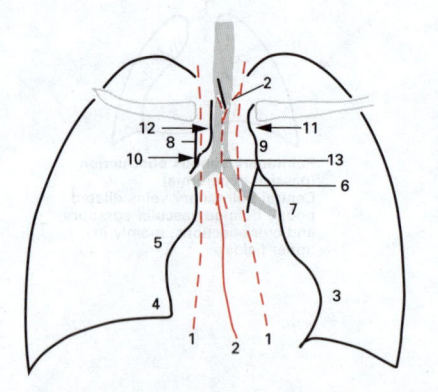

1 Paravertebral lines
2 Dorsal pleural contact line
3 Left ventricle
4 Caval line
5 Right atrium
6 Aortic line
7 Pulmonary arch
8 Superior vena cava
9 Aortic arch
10 Azygos arch
11 Subclavial line
12 Paratracheal line
13 Anterior pleural contact line

PULMONOLOGY

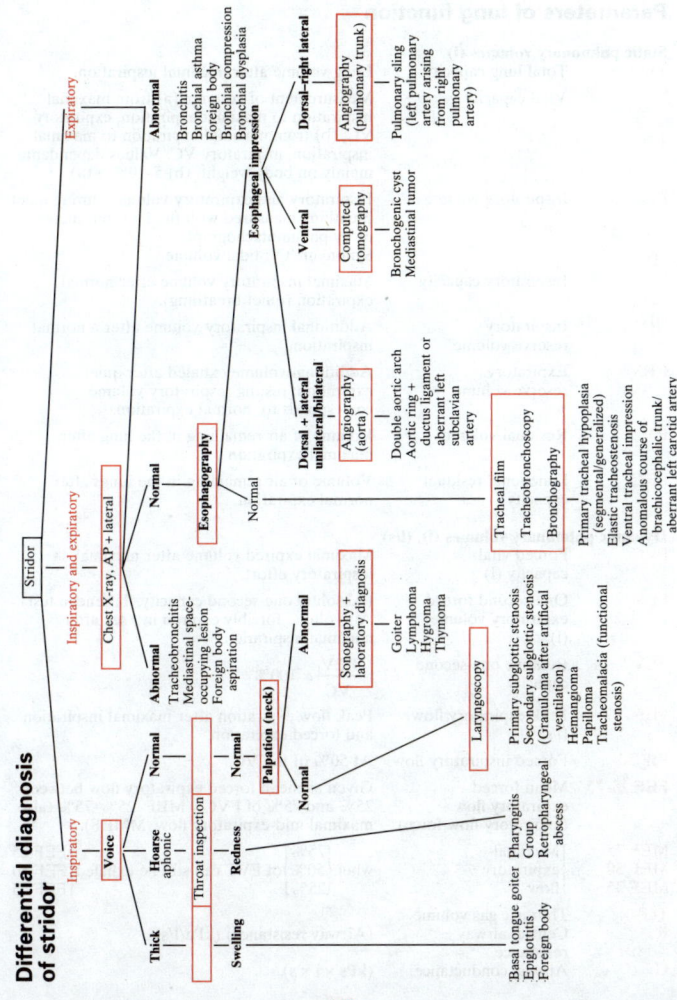

Differential diagnosis of stridor

Stridor

- **Inspiratory**
  - **Voice**
    - **Thick**
      - Basal tongue goiter
      - Epiglottitis
      - Foreign body
    - **Hoarse aphonic**
      - **Throat inspection**
        - **Swelling**
        - **Redness**
          - Pharyngitis
          - Croup
          - Retropharyngeal abscess
    - **Normal**
      - **Palpation (neck)**
        - **Normal**
          - **Laryngoscopy**
            - Primary subglottic stenosis
            - Secondary subglottic stenosis (Granuloma after artificial ventilation)
            - Hemangioma
            - Papilloma
            - Tracheomalacia (functional stenosis)
        - **Abnormal**
          - **Sonography + laboratory diagnosis**
            - Goiter
            - Lymphoma
            - Hygroma
            - Thymoma

- **Inspiratory and expiratory**
  - **Chest X-ray, AP + lateral**
    - **Abnormal**
      - Tracheobronchitis
      - Mediastinal space-occupying lesion
      - Foreign body aspiration
    - **Normal**
      - **Esophagography**
        - **Normal**
          - Tracheal film
          - Tracheobronchoscopy
          - Bronchography
            - Primary tracheal hypoplasia (segmental/generalized)
            - Elastic tracheostenosis
            - Ventral tracheal impression
            - Anomalous course of brachiocephalic trunk/aberrant left carotid artery
        - **Dorsal + lateral unilateral/bilateral**
          - **Angiography (aorta)**
            - Double aortic arch
            - Aortic ring + ductus ligament or aberrant left subclavian artery
        - **Esophageal impression**
          - **Ventral**
            - **Computed tomography**
              - Bronchogenic cyst
              - Mediastinal tumor
          - **Dorsal-right lateral**
            - **Angiography (pulmonary trunk)**
              - Pulmonary sling (left pulmonary artery arising from right pulmonary artery)

- **Expiratory**
  - **Abnormal**
    - Bronchitis
    - Bronchial asthma
    - Foreign body
    - Bronchial compression
    - Bronchial dysplasia

Parameters of lung function

Static pulmonary volumes (l)

TLC	Total lung capacity	Lung volume after maximal inspiration.
VC	Vital capacity	Measurement of volume: (a) from maximal inspiration to maximal expiration, expiratory VC; (b) from maximal expiration to maximal inspiration, inspiratory VC. Values dependent mainly on body weight. (b) 5–10% > (a).
IV	Inspiratory volume	Inspiratory and expiratory volumes during quiet breathing measured with the bell spirometer or by pneumotachograph. Synonym: TV; tidal volume.
IC	Inspiratory capacity	Maximal inspiratory volume after normal expiration (quiet breathing).
IRV	Inspiratory reserve volume	Additional inspiratory volume after a normal inspiration.
ERV	Expiratory reserve volume	Additional volume exhaled after quiet expiration; resting respiratory volume corresponds to normal expiration.
RV	Residual volume	Volume of air remaining in the lung after maximal expiration.
FRC	Functional residual capacity	Volume of air remaining in the lungs after normal expiration.

Dynamic pulmonary volumes (l), (l/s)

FVC	Forced vital capacity (l)	Maximal expired volume after maximal inspiratory effort.
FEV_1	One-second forced expiratory volume (l)	(Absolute one-second capacity, Tiffeneau test). Air volume forcibly expired in 1 sec after maximal inspiration.
FEV%	Relative one-second capacity	$= \dfrac{FEV_1}{VC} \times 100\%$
PEF	Peak expiratory flow (l/s)	Peak flow expiration after maximal inspiration and forced expiration.
FIF 50	Forced inspiratory flow	At 50% of the VC.
FEF 25–75	Mean forced expiratory flow (expiratory flow force)	Given as mean forced expiratory flow between 25% and 75% of FVC = MEF 25%–75% (also maximal mid-expiratory flow, MMEF).
MEF 75 MEF 50 MEF 25	Maximal expiratory flow	when {75%, 50%, 25%} of FVC can still be exhaled {FEF 25, FEF 50, FEF 75}
TGV	Thoracic gas volume	
R	Central airway resistance	(Airway resistance) (kPa/l/s)
G	Airway conductance	(kPs × l × s)

PULMONOLOGY

Normal lung volumes/O₂ treatment

Reference values of static and dynamic respiratory volumes for girls and boys (mean values)
(After Zapletal, Samanek and Paul (1987).)

Height (cm)	VC (l)	TLC (l)	RV (l)	FRC (l)	IC (l)	IRV (l)	ERV (l)	IV (ml)	PEF (l/s)	FEV$_1$ (l)	FVC (l)	MEF 50 (l/s)	R $\frac{kPa}{l \times s}$
115	1.37	1.91	0.52	0.94	0.97	0.67	0.44	280	2.85	1.12	1.37	1.86	0.55
120	1.53	2.13	0.57	1.05	1.08	0.75	0.49	300	3.15	1.27	1.52	2.04	0.50
130	1.89	2.62	0.67	1.30	1.33	0.93	0.62	350	3.80	1.58	1.92	2.43	0.40
140	2.29	3.18	0.79	1.59	1.60	1.14	0.77	400	4.52	1.95	2.38	2.85	0.34
150	2.75	3.80	0.92	1.91	1.91	1.38	0.94	460	5.30	2.37	2.92	3.31	0.29
160	3.26	4.48	1.05	2.26	2.26	1.64	1.13	520	6.18	2.84	3.53	3.81	0.24
170	3.83	5.25	1.20	2.66	2.63	1.94	1.34	580	7.13	3.36	4.22	4.35	0.21
180	4.45	6.08	1.35	3.09	3.05	2.26	1.58	640	8.15	3.95	5.00	4.93	0.18

Oxygen therapy

$$F_{iO_2} = \frac{O_2 \text{ flow} + (0.21 \times \text{airflow})}{\text{flow of gas mixture}} = O_2 \text{ proportion in inspiratory gas mixture}$$

F_{iO_2} of air = 0.21 (21%)

O₂ admixture to respiratory air – attainable inspiratory O₂ proportion
(After Chatburn and Lough (1990).)

Conditions: respiratory volume and breathing frequency normal.

O₂ flow rate (l/min)	Approximate values of attainable F_{iO_2}(%)		
	Nasal tube	Oxygen mask	O₂ mask with breathing bag
1	24		
2	28		
3	32		
4	36		
5	40		
5–6		40	
6	44		60
6–7		50	70
7–8		60	80
9			90
10			~100

MEMORIX PEDIATRICS

Lung function diagnosis

Lung volumes

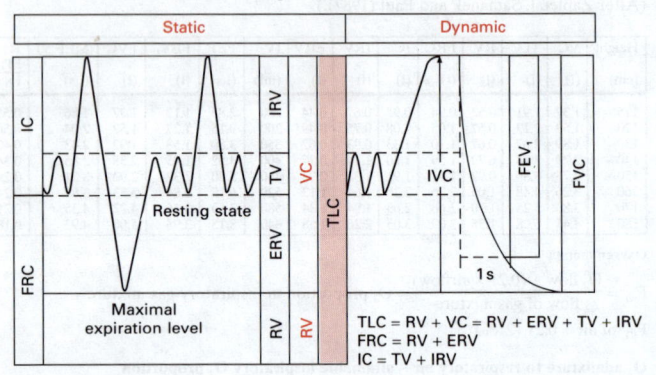

[Static | Dynamic]

Resting state

Maximal expiration level

$TLC = RV + VC = RV + ERV + TV + IRV$
$FRC = RV + ERV$
$IC = TV + IRV$

Flow–volume curve

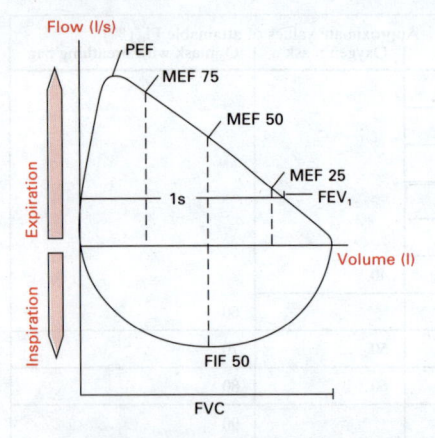

Flow (l/s)
PEF
MEF 75
MEF 50
MEF 25
FEV$_1$
1s
Volume (l)
Expiration
Inspiration
FIF 50
FVC

TV = tidal volume; see p. 168 for definitions of other abbreviations.

PULMONOLOGY

Disorders of lung function

Types of ventilation disorder

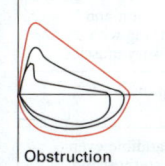

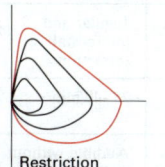

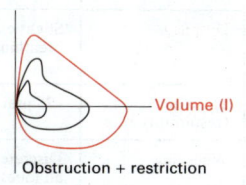

| Obstruction | Restriction | Obstruction + restriction |

Flow (l/s) — Volume (l)

Diagnostic significance of various respiratory patterns

Hyperventilation: → Compensation of a metabolic acidosis (diabetes, lactacidosis, uremia, drug poisoning).
→ Primary respiratory alkalosis (salicylate poisoning, hepatic coma, pulmonary disease, psychogenic).

Hypoventilation: → Compensation of a metabolic alkalosis.
→ Respiratory acidosis (respiratory diseases, neuromuscular diseases, disorder of central respiratory regulation).

Hyper- and hypoventilation are frequently found in coma of metabolic origin.

Cheyne–Stokes breathing: Periodic hyperventilation; crescendo–decrescendo type, followed by apnea.
→ Disorders in both hemispheres with intact brain stem function.

Central hyperventilation: Sustained regular deep and rapid breathing.
→ Midbrain disorder.

Gasping: Irregular sporadic respiration of varying amplitude.
→ Disorder in the region of the medulla and pons.

Bronchial asthma: symptom scores for calculating grade of severity of an asthma attack
(After Von der Hardt (1989).)

Symptoms \ Points	0	1	2
Cyanosis	None	Discrete (lips)	Definite (lips, fingers)
Dyspnea	Slight exertion breathing	Jugular and intercostal retraction	Retraction and breathing with accessory muscles
Tachypnea (respiratory rate)	<25/min	25–40/min	>40/min
Wheezing	Discrete over all lobes	Audible without stethoscope	Not audible even with stethoscope (silent obstruction)
Disorder of consciousness	None	Beginning (closes eyes, still responsive, orientated)	Clouded consciousness to unconsciousness

Calculation   0–3 points   mild asthma attack
              4–5 points   severe asthma attack
              >6 points   danger of respiratory failure.

Grading of bronchial asthma
(After Reinhardt and Berdel (1990).)

Grade 1 Beginning asthma   Occasional breathing difficulty/cough (allergic bronchitis/tracheobronchitis).

Grade 2 Mild asthma   Occasional attacks of dyspnea with (irregular) necessity for bronchodilators.

Grade 3 Moderate asthma   Variable attacks of dyspnea with regular need for antiasthmatics + topical glucocorticoids.

Grade 4 Severe asthma   Frequent, sustained attacks of dyspnea to the severest asthma attacks or continually requiring glucocorticoids.

PULMONOLOGY

Drug treatment
(Modified from Warner *et al.* (1989); Reinhardt (1991).)

Symptoms	Low grade, intermittent	Medium grade, intermittent	Severe intermittent	Medium grade persistent	Severe persistent
Treatment Age (years)	A	B (| If inadequate effect, proceed to next treatment step)	C	D	
≤1	None (possibly mucolysis)	1. Oral beta₂ sympathomimetics or theophylline | 2. Beta₂ sympathomimetics by inhalation Ipratropium bromide alone or combined with 2	B + oral glucocorticoids if getting worse	DSCG alone or combined with B	B + DSCG + glucocorticoids by inhalation | B + DSCG + oral glucocorticoids (alternating doses)
1–3	Oral beta₂ sympathomimetics and/or theophylline	Beta₂ sympathomimetics by inhalation or with ipratropium bromide	B + oral glucocorticoids (3–7 d)	DSCG alone or combined with B	B + DSCG + glucocorticoids by inhalation | B + DSCG + oral glucocorticoids (alternating)
3–5	Inhalation (aerosol with inhalator) or oral beta₂ sympathomimetics	DSCG or ketotifen intermittently, reinforced by A or ipratropium bromide (inhalation)	A + oral glucocorticoids (3–7 d)	B | B + beta₂ sympathomimetics by inhalation or B + theophylline or B + glucocorticoids by inhalation	B + beta₂ sympathomimetics by inhalation + glucocorticoids by inhalation | + beta₂ sympathomimetics in retard form | + oral glucocorticoids (alternating) in lowest effective dosage
5–18	Beta₂ sympathomimetics by inhalation	DSCG alone or + A	A + oral glucocorticoids	B | B + beta₂ sympathomimetics by inhalation or theophylline or B + glucocorticoids by inhalation	B + retard form of beta₂ sympathomimetics/ theophylline | + ipratropium bromide | + high dose glucocorticoids by inhalation | + oral glucocorticoids (alternating)

DSCG = disodium chromoglycate.
NB: adapt the treatment scheme to the individual pathogenesis.

Anti-asthmatic drugs

Drug	Form of administration	Age range	Dose	Number of times per day	Comments
Inhibitors of mast cell degranulation					
Sodium cromoglycate (SCG)	Aerosol inhalation	All ages	10 mg (2 puffs)	4	
	Nebulized solution	All ages	20 mg	4	
Bronchodilators					
β_2-adrenoreceptor stimulants					
Fenoterol	Aerosol inhalation	6–12 years	100 µg (1 puff)	3–4	
		>12 years	100–200 µg (1–2 puffs)	3–4	
Reproterol	Aerosol inhalation	6–12 years	500 µg (1 puff)	3	
		>12 years	0.5–1 mg (1–2 puffs)	3	
Salbutamol	By mouth	<2 years	100 µg/kg	4	
		2–6 years	1–2 mg	3–4	
		6–12 years	2 mg	3–4	
	Aerosol inhalation	Child	100 µg (1 puff)	3–4	Increase to 200 µg (2 puffs) if necessary Prophylaxis
		Child	100 µg (1 puff)		
	Nebulized solution	>18 months	2.5 mg	4	May be increased to 5 mg if necessary, but consider medical assessment

PULMONOLOGY

Terbutaline	By mouth	<7 years 7–15 years	75 µg/kg 2.5 mg	3 2–3
	By s.c./i.m/slow i.v. injection	2–15 years	10 µg/kg (max. 300 µg)	4
	Aerosol inhalation	All ages	250–500 µg (1–2 puffs)	3–4
	Nebulized solution	<3 years 3–6 years 6–8 years >8 years	2 mg 3 mg 4 mg 5 mg	2–4
Tulobuterol	By mouth	6–10 years >10 years	0.5–1 mg 1–2 mg	2 2
Xanthine derivatives					
Theophylline	By mouth	Refer to proprietary product's data sheet	100–200–350 mg	2 (but some brands 3–4)	Effective level (serum) = 8–20 µg/ml 1 mg/kg → increases level by around 1.7–3.5 µg/ml ↑ at ideal weight
Parasympatholytics					
Ipratropium bromide	Aerosol inhalation	<6 years 6–12 years	20 µg (1 puff) 20–40 µg (1–2) puffs	3 3	
	Nebulized solution	3–14 years	100–500 µg	3	First dose inhaled under medical supervision
Glucocorticoids					
Prednisolone	By mouth	All ages	2–8 mg/kg	1	Initial dose in attack
Beclomethasone	Aerosol inhalation	All ages	50–100 µg	2–4	
Budesonide	Aerosol inhalation	All ages	50–200–800 µg	2	Dosage depends on product brand – check data sheets

MEMORIX PEDIATRICS

Renal function

Approximate amount of urine production (ml/kg/h):

Fetuses	10
Neonates	1.5 (0–12 h)
	2 (12–36 h)
	3 (>36 h)

Osmolality (osmol/kg H_2O) = amount of osmotically effective portion of substance per mass (kg) of the solution medium.

Osmolarity (osmol/l H_2O) = osmotically effective amount of material per volume (l) of the solution material.

Approximation formula for calculating plasma osmolality:

$$\text{mosm}/\text{kg } H_2O = 2 \times Na(\text{mmol}) + \frac{\text{glucose (mg/dl)}}{18} + \frac{\text{urea-N (mg/dl)}}{2.8}$$

Osmolar gap = measured osmolality − calculated osmolality.
Normal: mosm/kg H_2O < 10
If value >10, additional osmotically effective substances are present.

Mannitol is added to the above formula: $\dfrac{+ \text{mannitol (mg/dl)}}{18}$

Normal osmolality values (mosm/kg H_2O):

Serum	275–295
Urine	50–650 neonates
	50–1250 infants
	50–1450 older children
	>850 after 12 h without fluid intake

Relation urine : serum = 1 to 3, after 12 h thirst >3.

Estimation of urine osmolality:

mosm/kg H_2O = 2 × (Na + K + NH_4[mmol/l]) + urea NH_4: 20–40 mmol/l
urea = protein supply (g/d) × 5.

Glomerular filtration:

Principle of calculating clearance: $C_x = \dfrac{U_x}{P_x} \times V \text{ (ml/min)}$

x = any filtrate
P = plasma concentration
U = urine concentration
V = urine flow

Osmotic clearance: $C_{Osm}\text{(ml/min)} = \dfrac{\text{urine osmolality}}{\text{plasma osmolality}} \times V$

Clearance of free water: $C_{H_2O} = V \times \left(1 - \dfrac{\text{urine osmolality}}{\text{plasma osmolality}}\right) = V - C_{Osm}$

Creatinine clearance per body surface (BS):

$$C_{cr}\text{ (ml/min/1.73 m}^2\text{)} = \frac{U \times V}{P_{cr}} \times \frac{1.73}{m^2 BS} = \frac{U_{cr}\text{(mg/dl)} \times V\text{(ml)} \times 1.73}{P_{cr}\text{(mg/dl)} \times 1440 \times m^2 BS}$$

Conversion (from 24 h urine): 24 × 60 = 1440 min

NEPHROLOGY/UROLOGY

Calculation of approximate glomerular filtration rate (GFR):

$$\text{GFR} \left(\text{ml/min}/1.73\,\text{m}^2\right) = \frac{k \times \text{body height (cm)}}{P_{cr}\,(\text{mg/dl})}$$

$k = 0.33$ infants (lowest birth weight)
$k = 0.45$ older infants
$k = 0.55$ children 2–12 years
$k = 0.70$ ♂ 13–21 years
$k = 0.57$ ♀ 13–21 years

GFR (ml/min/1.73 m²) = 1.1 × body height (cm) for the mature neonate

GFR – normal values

Age	GFR ml/min/1.73 m²
Prematures:	
27 weeks	2–10
32 weeks	4–12
36 weeks	6–40
40 weeks	8–42
Neonates:	
1 week	20–53
4 weeks	30–90
Infants:	
2 months	42–90
4 months	56–120
6 months	90–145
12 months	63–150
Older children:	
>2 years	100–185

Serum creatinine normal range: (mg/dl (µmol/l))

Age (years)	Girls	Boys
Cord blood	1.2 (106)	
Neonates	1.0 (88)	
Infants	0.4 (35)	
1	0.4 (35)	0.5 (44)
2	0.5 (44)	
3–6	0.6 (53)	
7–10	0.7 (62)	0.8 (70)
11–14	0.7 (62)	0.9 (80)
15–16	0.8 (70)	0.9 (80)
17–20	0.9 (80)	1.1 (97)

Calculation of approximate creatinine value (healthy children):

Serum:
$0.37 + (0.018 \times \text{age in years}) = \text{mg/dl}$ ♀
$0.35 + (0.025 \times \text{age in years}) = \text{mg/dl}$ ♂
Urine:
$15 + (0.5 \times \text{age in years}) \pm 3 = \text{mg/kg/d}$

Proximal tubular functions

Fractional excretion (FE = amount excreted as part of the filtrate)

$$\text{Fe}_x (\%) = \frac{U_x \times V}{P_x \times C_{cr}} = \frac{U_x \times P_{cr}}{U_{cr} \times P_x} \times 100$$

x eg: Na, HCO_3, phosphate
C_{cr} creatinine clearance
P plasma (serum concentration)
U urine concentration
V urine flow (ml/min)

Tubular absorption: $TR(\%) = (1 - FE_x) \times 100$

Functional tubular absorption (T_x)

$$= \frac{\text{filtrate} - \text{excreted amount}}{\text{glomerular filtration rate}\,(C_{cr})} = \frac{C_{cr} \times P_x - U_x \times V}{C_{cr}}$$

Renal function tests: distal tubular function

Urine concentration: testing only required if specific gravity in spontaneously voided morning urine is <1.024.

Thirst trial: 1. Infants on doubly concentrated nutritional feeds (= half fluid volume).
2. Older children given only solid food after midday, collect urine from 19–20 hours onwards four-hourly or next morning.
Weigh before and after the trial. Take temperature during trial.

Acid excretion: loading test only if morning urine pH is >5.4.

1. Net acid excretion = (titratable acidity + $NH_4 - HCO_3$) × urinary flow (V) = mmol/min/1.73 m^2.
   Measurement in spontaneous metabolic acidosis and bicarbonate <17 mmol/l (< one year of age), <20 mmol/l (older children).

Urine anion gap = $Na_u + K_u - Cl_u$
Urinary Cl = indirect measure for the amount of NH_4 in the urine. The urinary ion gap is negative in prerenal acidosis.

2. Ammonium chloride test
   Specimen of urine for measurement of net acid excretion
   (a) NH_4Cl 75–100 mmol/m^2 given in 1 h
   (b) NH_4Cl 100 mg/kg daily orally over three days
   (c) $CaCl_2$ 2 mg/kg instead of ammonium chloride in liver disorder.
   Result: plasma bicarbonate <15 mmol/l, urinary pH < 5.5.

NEPHROLOGY/UROLOGY

Renal tubular acidosis (RTA)
(After Chan (1983).)

Characteristics	RTA type I	RTA type II	RTA type III	RTA type IV
Site of tubular defect	Distal	Proximal	Undefined	Distal
Failure to thrive/retarded growth	+	+	+	+
Nephrocalcinosis	Frequent	Rare	+/−	Rare
Renal failure	−	−	−	+
Blood pH	↓	↓	↓	↓
Serum Cl$^-$	↑	↑	↑	↑
Serum K$^+$	Low	Low	Low	Hyperkalemia
Urine K$^+$	↑	n/↑	↑	n/↓
FE_{HCO_3}, in normal plasma concentration	<5%	>15%	5–15%	<15%
Urine: plasma P_{CO_2} (mmHg)	<15	>20	<15	>20
Net acid excretion after NH_4 loading	↓	Normal	↓	↓
Regulatory urine acidity in acidosis urinary pH	>5.5	<5.5	>5.5	Variable
Urine anion gap	Positive	Normal	+/−	Positive
Citraturia	↓	↑	(↑)	(↑)
Treatment: $NaHCO_3$ (mmol/kg/d)	2–4	2–14	2–14	2–3
Daily K requirement	↓ with correction of acidosis	↑ with correction of acidosis	+/−	+/−

MEMORIX PEDIATRICS

Renal tubular acidosis: diagnostic plan

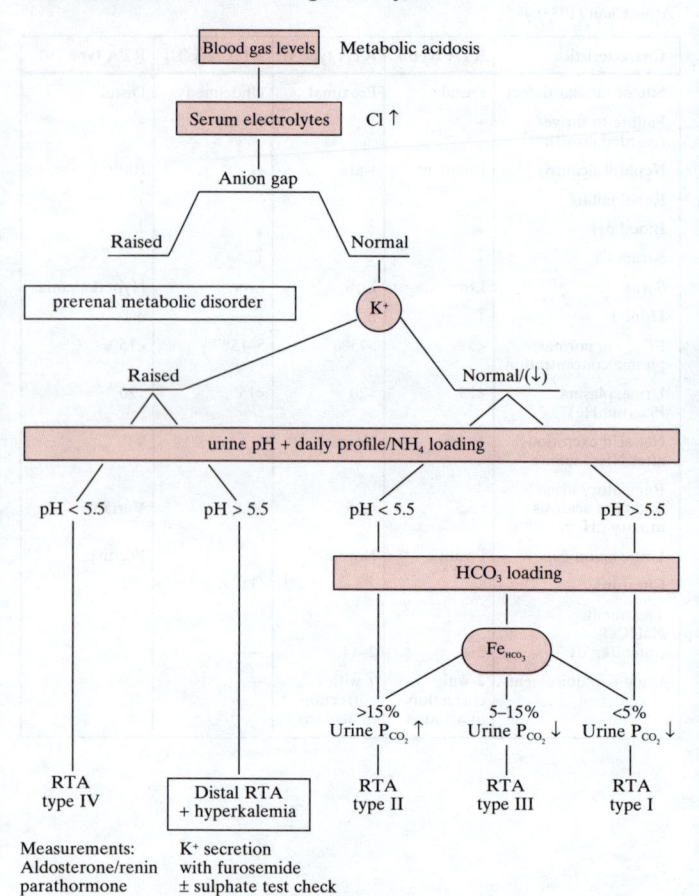

```
                    Blood gas levels ── Metabolic acidosis
                            │
                    Serum electrolytes ── Cl ↑
                            │
                        Anion gap
                       ╱         ╲
                   Raised        Normal
                     │              │
        prerenal metabolic         K⁺
            disorder          ╱         ╲
                          Raised      Normal/(↓)
                            │              │
                    urine pH + daily profile/NH₄ loading
                    ╱         ╲         ╱              ╲
              pH < 5.5   pH > 5.5   pH < 5.5         pH > 5.5
                                                         │
                                                  HCO₃ loading
                                                         │
                                                     Fe_HCO₃
                                              ╱         │         ╲
                                           >15%       5–15%       <5%
                                         Urine P_CO₂↑ Urine P_CO₂↓ Urine P_CO₂↓

    RTA        Distal RTA              RTA         RTA          RTA
    type IV    + hyperkalemia          type II     type III     type I
```

Measurements:	K⁺ secretion
Aldosterone/renin	with furosemide
parathormone	± sulphate test check

Further diagnostic aim: elucidation of the causes of RTA

NEPHROLOGY/UROLOGY

Causes of renal tubular acidosis/tubulopathy

Primary acidosis: (familial, sporadic)

Secondary acidosis:

Kidney

Urinary tract obstruction
Medullary cystic nephropathy
Transplant rejection
Nephrotic syndrome
Nephrocalcinosis
Autoimmune diseases
Cardiac failure

Metabolism

Cystinosis
Galactosemia
Glycogen storage
Fructose intolerance
Lowe's syndrome
Wilson's disease
Fabry's disease
Metachromatic leukodystrophy
Carbonic anhydrase deficiency
Pyruvate carboxylase deficiency
Vitamin D-resistant rickets

Other causes

Liver cirrhosis
Dysproteinemia
Poisoning
  lead
  cadmium
  mercury
  amphotericin B
  gentamicin
  vitamin D
Ehlers–Danlos syndrome
Marfan's syndrome

Primary tubulopathies

(Disorders of absorption)

(Renal glycosuria) — Glucose

(RTA) — HCO_3

(Phosphate diabetes) — Phosphate
(Pseudohypoparathyroidism type I, II)

— Amino acids

Hartnup's disease
Dicarboxylaminoaciduria
Dibasic aminoaciduria
Hyperhistidinuria
Iminoglycinuria
Cystinuria — Multiple substances
  (De Toni–Fanconi syndrome)

Renal hyperuricemia — Uric acid

(Pseudohypoaldosteronism) — Na^+

(Bartter's syndrome) — Cl^-

(RTA) — H^+

(Diabetes insipidus) — H_2O

Secondary tubulopathies

Predominantly combined absorption–secretion disorders as symptoms of:

Inborn metabolic defects, renal diseases

Intoxication (see p. 475)

MEMORIX PEDIATRICS

Potter's pathological classification of cystic kidney diseases

(Osathenondh and Potter (1964).)

Type	Pathogenesis	Morphology Macroscopic	Morphology Microscopic
Potter I	Hyperplasia and dilatation of the interstitial region of the collecting tubules (the area between the dichotomous divisions	Kidneys symmetrically enlarged at birth, fetal lobes preserved. Innumerable cysts, up to 2 mm, on the surface. On section, dilated collecting tubules recognizable in cortex and medulla. Papillae, calyces, pelvis and ureter normal	Collecting tubules dilated, saccular and elongated. Single-layerered, cuboidal epithelium. No atresia, intraluminal pressure normal
Potter II	Disorder of the ampullary part of the developing collecting tubules: no separation, ampulla becomes cystic and fails to produce nephrons. It can affect one, both or only a part of a kidney	Shape of kidneys distorted by cysts. The kidneys can be enlarged or hypoplastic. Papillae defective, pelvis deformed by cysts. Ureter atretic, hypoplastic or dilated proximally. Cysts contain cuboidal epithelium. No primary urine	Numerous thick-walled oval or round cysts; nephron count sharply reduced. Connective tissue partly undifferentiated (cartilage). Vessels dysplasic
Potter III	Developmental abnormality of part of the collecting tubules in the ampullary or interstitial region. In contrast to the normal place of division of the daughter generation of the ureteral bud, the collecting tubules of the previous generation are markedly lengthened. Divisions of the younger generations are increased.	Generally both kidneys affected and enlarged. At birth kidneys preponderantly microcystic. Cysts continue to grow. Papillae mostly absent, calyces deformed, pelvis tubular. Ureter, bladder and urethra normal	Cysts of different sizes can affect nephrons or collecting tubules in every area. Collecting tubules often dilated, dysplasia of connective tissue and vessels
Potter IV	Functional disorder of the ampulla of the collecting tubule buds as a result of raised pressure in early urethral stenosis	Kidneys normal or enlarged. Bladder wall hypertrophied. Ureter dilated and/or elongated	Collecting tubules may be dilated. Small cysts develop in the cortex (dilated glomeruli)

NEPHROLOGY/UROLOGY

Characteristics of cystic nephropathies

Disease	Pathology	Type of inheritance	Diagnostic criteria	Prognosis
Polycystic neuropathy (infantile type)	Kidney shape preserved, size ↑, Potter type I	Autosomal-recessive	Sonography: echogenicity ↑, renal biopsy, liver biopsy obligatory, congenital cholangiodysplastic fibrosis, primary anuria/renal failure	90% die in the neonatal period, variable progression in 10% (kidneys rapidly, liver slowly, or vice versa)
Polycystic nephropathy (adult type)	Potter type III	Autosomal-dominant	Sonography: in adolescence kidney-size ↑, bilaterally almost equal number of different sized cysts. Cysts in other organs (liver, spleen, pancreas) Renal failure. Molecular genetic analysis in the affected families	Chronic renal failure. Final stage usually not reached until adulthood
Medullary cystic disease (juvenile nephrophthisis)	Kidney size ↓, cysts in medulla and cortex (diverticula of the distal tubular convolutions), tubular atrophy, glomerulosclerosis, periglomerular and interstitial sclerosis. Additionally: tapetoretinal dysplasia, coloboma, ataxia, mental retardation	Autosomal-recessive	Sonography: echogenicity ↑, corticomedullary differentiation lost. Biopsy: atrophy, chronic inflammation, sclerosis, hyposthenuria, salt loss	Chronic renal failure
Medullary cystic nephropathy	As for medullary cystic disease. Cysts also in the collecting tubes. No extrarenal disorders	Autosomal-dominant	As for medullary cystic disease	Chronic renal failure, beginning in adulthood

Characteristics of cystic nephropathies (continued)

Disease	Pathology	Type of inheritance	Diagnostic criteria	Prognosis
Dysontogenetic cysts	Two types: 1. Retroperitoneal cysts from metanephrogenic tissue kidney inclusions. 2. Cystic teratomas within the renal fascia, which displace the kidney or grow in a kidney, displacing other tissue	–	Sonography: cysts without renal tissue or cystic tumor in one kidney. Deficiency in the excretory urogram. Histology	Question of malignant degeneration
Pyelogenic cysts	Pyelon diverticuli after recurrent pyelonephritis or congenital calyx stenosis	–	Sonography: cystic ectasia of midechos or cysts of midecho. Excretory urogram: renal pelvic deformity	Can become the cause of a chronic pyelonephritis
Renal pseudocysts ('urinomas')	Perirenal pseudocysts after traumatic kidney rupture or spout rupture of cystically dilated nephrons. Urine collection in the perirenal fascia, no epithelial boundary	–	Sonography: perirenal renal cysts of different sizes	Depends on traumatic kidney damage

NEPHROLOGY/UROLOGY

Hematuria

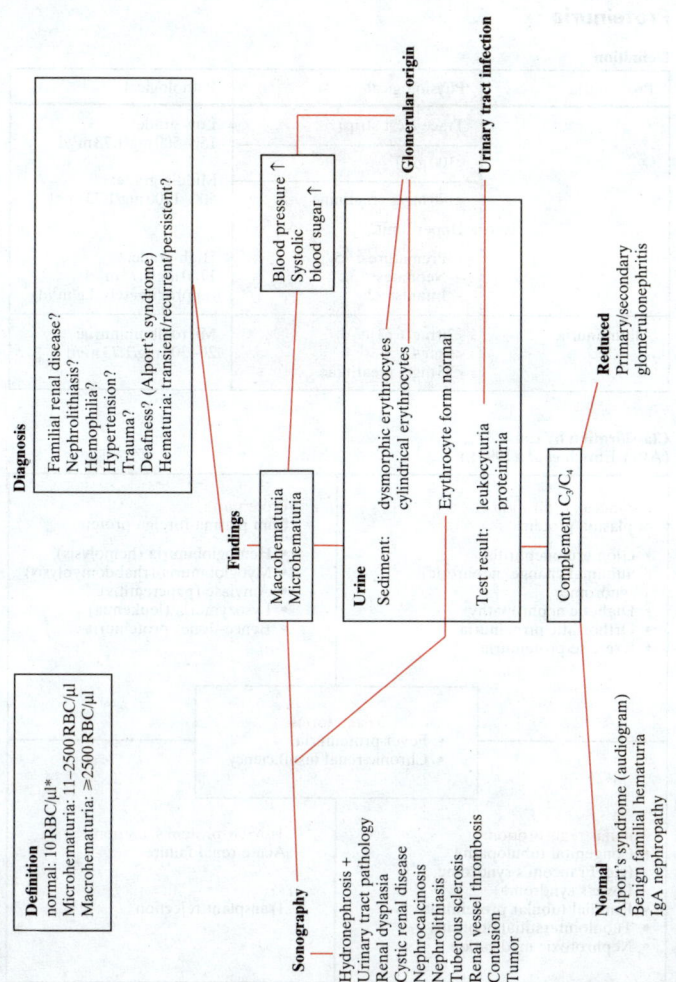

Definition
normal: 10 RBC/µl*
Microhematuria: 11–2500 RBC/µl
Macrohematuria: ≥2500 RBC/µl

Diagnosis
Familial renal disease?
Nephrolithiasis?
Hemophilia?
Hypertension?
Trauma?
Deafness? (Alport's syndrome)
Hematuria: transient/recurrent/persistent?

Findings

Macrohematuria
Microhematuria
→ Blood pressure ↑ Systolic blood sugar ↑

Urine
Sediment: dysmorphic erythrocytes, cylindrical erythrocytes → **Glomerular origin**
Test result: Erythrocyte form normal
leukocyturia, proteinuria → **Urinary tract infection**

Complement C₃/C₄

- **Normal**
  Alport's syndrome (audiogram)
  Benign familial hematuria
  IgA nephropathy

- **Reduced**
  Primary/secondary glomerulonephritis

Sonography

Hydronephrosis +
Urinary tract pathology
Renal dysplasia
Cystic renal disease
Nephrocalcinosis
Nephrolithiasis
Tuberous sclerosis
Renal vessel thrombosis
Contusion
Tumor

* RBC = red blood cell(s)

185

Proteinuria

Definition

Proteinuria	Physiological	Pathological
	Trace (test strip)	Low grade: 150–500 mg/1.73 m²/d
	<100 mg/l	
	<170 mg/g creatinine Upper limit. – Prematures: ×5 – Neonates: ×3.5 – Infants: ×2	Middle grade: 500–1700 mg/1.73 m²/d High-grade: 1700 mg/1.73 m²/d (approximately 1 g/m²/d)
Albuminuria	<20 mg/1.73 m²/d <6 mg/l <35 mg/g creatinine	Microalbuminuria: 20–300 mg/1.73 m²/d

Classification by cause
(After Ehrich *et al.* (1993).)

Glomerular filtration of plasma protein: • Glomerulonephritis 'minimal change' nephrotic syndrome • Diabetic nephropathy • Orthostatic proteinuria • Exercise proteinuria	**Proteinuria** from plasma-foreign protein: • Hemoglobinuria (hemolysis) • Myoglobinuria (rhabdomyolysis) • Amylase (pancreatitis) • Lysozymuria (leukemia) • Bence–Jones proteinuria
Tubular reabsorption: • Congenital tubulopathy (e.g. Franconi's syndrome, Lowe's syndrome) • Familial tubular proteinuria • Tubulointerstitial nephritis • Nephrotoxic medication	**Tubular protein secretion:** Acute renal failure Transplant rejection

Mixed forms:
- Fever proteinuria
- Chronic renal insufficiency

NEPHROLOGY/UROLOGY

Renal diagnosis/renal biopsy

Further diagnostic methods in persistent hematuria and proteinuria

Blood: blood picture, C-reactive protein, pH, bicarbonate, coagulation status

Serum: albumin, antinuclear antibodies (ANA), antinuclear cytoplasmic antibodies (ANCA), electrolytes, calcium, phosphate, electrophoresis, total protein, cholesterol, triglycerides, urea, creatinine, immunoglobulin, gamma-glutamyl transpeptidase, glutamic-oxalacetic transaminase, glutamic-pyruvic transaminase

Serology: Antistreptolysin titer, hepatitis B

24 h urine: total protein, calcium, creatinine, creatinine clearance

Bacteriological culture: (urine, pharyngeal swab), Mantoux test

Imaging procedures, according to sonographic findings

Percutaneous renal biopsy.

Indications for renal biopsy

- Persistent proteinuria
- Nephrotic syndrome (steroid-dependent, steroid-resistant)
- Rapidly progressive glomerulonephritis
- Suspicion of acute interstitial tubular nephritis
- Glomerulonephritis of unknown etiology or pathology
- Recurrent hematuria
- Renal participation in autoimmune disease
- Chronic renal failure of unknown origin
- Suspicion of chronic transplant rejection
- Monitoring of treatment when function tests are not possible
- Suspicion of hereditary nephropathy.

Contraindications to percutaneous renal biopsy

- Single kidney
- Anomalies in vascular supply
- Hemorrhagic diathesis
- Renal tumor.

Nephritic syndrome: morphological description
(Modified from Thoenes (1979).)

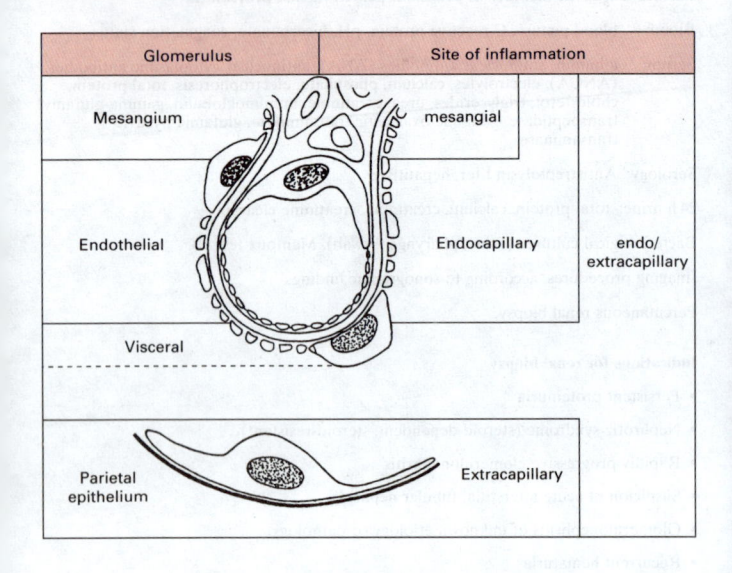

Glomerulus		Site of inflammation	
Mesangium		mesangial	
Endothelial		Endocapillary	endo/extracapillary
Visceral			
Parietal epithelium		Extracapillary	

NEPHROLOGY/UROLOGY

Glomerulonephritis

Microscopic picture

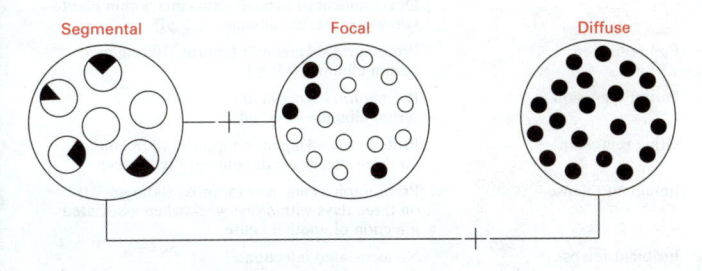

Segmental · Focal · Diffuse

Morphological classification – synonyms
(After WHO (1982); Thoenes (1983).)

WHO classification	Other classification
Diffuse GN	Exudative proliferative GN
Mesangial proliferative GN	Mesangial proliferative GN
Intra-/extracapillary GN	Rapidly progressive, crescentic GN
Membranoproliferative GN	Membranoproliferative GN
Membranous GN	Peri-/membranous GN
Mild glomerular changes (including 'minimal change' nephrotic syndrome)	Minimal change, minimal glomerulitis
Focal segmental accentuated GN	
Focal GN	Focal segmental proliferative GN
Focal segmental glomerulosclerosis	Focal segmental sclerosing GN/glomerulopathy

GN = glomerulonephritis.

Nephrotic syndrome: definitions

Nephrotic syndrome (approx. 1 g/m²/d)	Severe selective proteinuria ≥ 40 mg/m²/h
	Development of hypoalbuminemia within one to two weeks (serum albumin ≤25 g/l)
Full remission	Proteinuria ≤4 mg/m²/h (approx. 100 mg/m²/d) Serum albumin ≥35 g/l
Partial remission	Proteinuria ≥4 mg/m²/d serum albumin 25–35 g/l
Urine remission	Proteinuria ≤4 mg/m²/h (approx. 100 mg/m²/d) on three successive days under prednisone
Imminent relapse	Proteinuria >4 mg/m²/h (approx. 100 mg/m²/d) on three days within one week when associated infection of another cause
Incipient relapse	No associated infection Proteinuria >4 mg/m²/h on two days in one week
Fast relapse	Relapse during or two weeks after alternating prednisone treatment
Frequent relapses	> two relapses within six months or four relapses within one year after successful standard relapse treatment
Infrequent relapses	≤ two relapses within six months
Frequent relapses without steroid dependence	Good reaction to standard relapse treatment, but two further relapses within six months or four within one year afterwards
Steroid sensitivity	Full remission after initial prednisone treatment
Late steroid sensitivity	Full remission after prolongation of the initial prednisone treatment
Steroid dependence	Two successive relapses during standard relapse treatment or within two weeks afterwards, or two of four relapses within six months as rapid relapses
Primary steroid resistance	No full remission during initial prednisone treatment
Late steroid resistance	At first, sensitivity, then steroid resistance during a relapse.

NEPHROLOGY/UROLOGY

Nephrotic syndrome: checklist of causes

Alport's syndrome

Congenital nephrotic syndrome, Finnish type

Nagel–Patella syndrome

Sickle-cell anemia

Alpha$_1$ antitrypsin deficiency

Primary glomerular disease

'Minimal change' nephrotic syndrome

Chronic glomerulonephritis

Secondary systemic diseases

Henoch–Schönlein purpura

Systemic lupus erythematosus

Bacterial infections

Viral infections: hepatitis B, cytomegalic inclusion disease, Epstein–Barr, varicella, AIDS

Protozoa: malaria

Chronic inflammations

Mediterranean fever

Amyloidosis

Cryoglobulinemia

Allergic reactions

Medication (organic gold combinations, penicillamine, mercury, captopril, heroin)

Neoplasias (leukemia, lymphoma)

MEMORIX PEDIATRICS

Nephrotic syndrome: treatment

Variants of the standard initial treatment
(After Arbeitsgemeinschaft für Pädiatrische Nephrologie (APN) (1993).)

Variant I

60 mg/m^2/d prednisone, divided into three single doses for four weeks.

Subsequently:
40 mg/m^2 prednisone every 48 h = 1 morning dose every second day for four weeks.

Total duration: eight weeks

Variant II

As variant I, but treatment duration in both phases is six weeks.

Total duration: 12 weeks

End of treatment

Relapse after variant II is unusual.

Standard prednisone relapse treatment

60 mg/m^2/d prednisone, divided into three individual doses, until the proteinuria over three days is <4 mg/m^2/h (around 100 mg/m^2/d).

Subsequently:
40 mg/m^2 prednisone as one morning dose every second day.

NEPHROLOGY/UROLOGY

Additional recommendations for treatment in minimal change nephrotic syndrome
(After Brodehl (1991).)

Course of disease	Treatment
Relapse unusual	Standard relapse treatment (prednisone)
Frequent relapses without steroid dependence + steroid toxicity	Cyclophosphamide 2 mg/kg/d + prednisone every second day in decreasing dosage (e.g. 60–40–30–10–0) Duration: eight weeks (Leukocytes not <1000/µl)
Frequent relapses with steroid dependence + steroid toxicity	Cyclophosphamide 2 mg/kg/d + prednisone every second day in decreasing dosages (e.g. first four weeks 60 mg/m^2, last four weeks 10 mg/m^2 every 48 h) Duration: 12 weeks (leukocytes not <1000/µl)
Frequent relapses with steroid dependence + relapse after cyclophosphamide + steroid toxicity	Standard relapse treatment ↓ Cyclosporin A: 100–150 mg/m^2/d, initially in two daily doses orally, daily doses adjusted to the whole-blood level of 80–160 ng/ml (monoclonal antibodies) Additionally: prednisone 40 mg/m^2 every 48 h in the first four weeks (serum creatinine check)

Grading of vesicoureteral reflux
(International System of Radiographic Grading of Vesicoureteric Reflux (1985).)

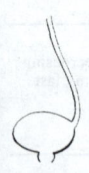

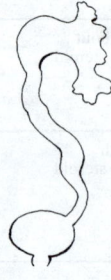

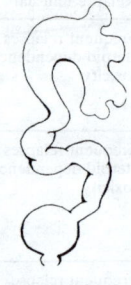

I	II	III	IV	V
Normal appearance of ureter. Reflux only in the ureter of normal appearance.	Normal appearance of ureter; pelvis and fornices of the calyces.	Ureter with mild to medium-grade dilatation and/or tortuosity. Pelvis and calyces dilated mildly to medium-grade. No or at least minimal blunting of the fornices.	Ureter: medium-grade dilatation and/or tortuosity. Pelvis and calyces: dilatation. Fornices not seen. Papillary impressions preserved.	Ureter very much dilated and tortuous. Pelvis and calyces greatly dilated. Loss of papillary impression (majority of the calyces).

NEPHROLOGY/UROLOGY

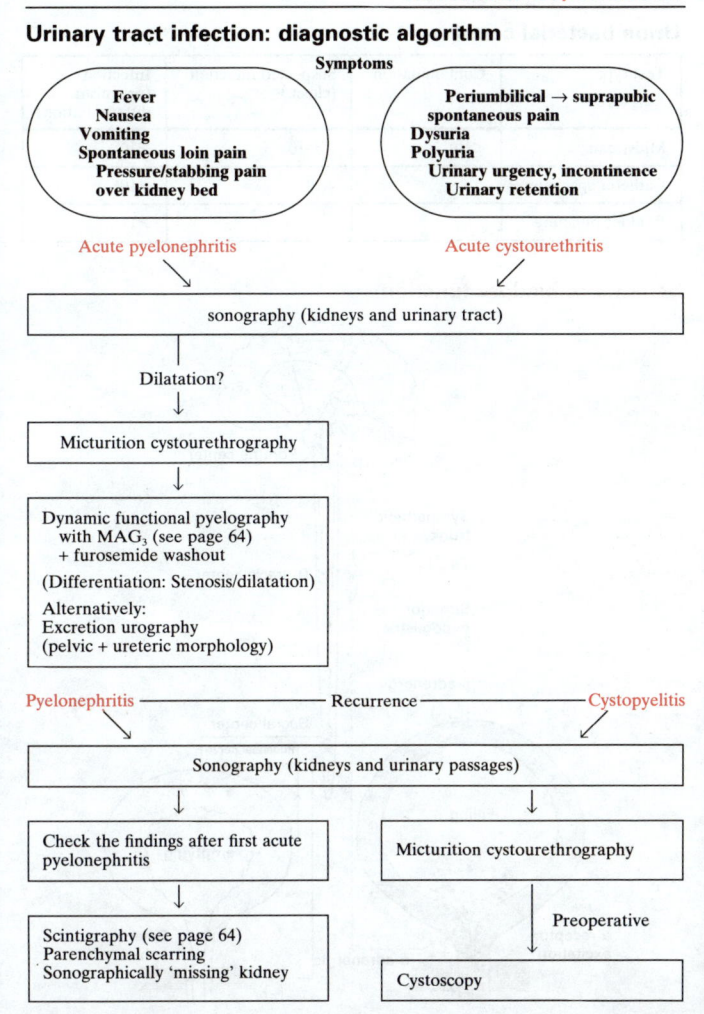

Urinary tract infection: diagnostic algorithm

Symptoms

- Fever
- Nausea
- Vomiting
- Spontaneous loin pain
- Pressure/stabbing pain over kidney bed

- Periumbilical → suprapubic spontaneous pain
- Dysuria
- Polyuria
- Urinary urgency, incontinence
- Urinary retention

Acute pyelonephritis → Acute cystourethritis

↓

sonography (kidneys and urinary tract)

↓ Dilatation?

Micturition cystourethrography

↓

Dynamic functional pyelography with MAG_3 (see page 64) + furosemide washout

(Differentiation: Stenosis/dilatation)

Alternatively:
Excretion urography
(pelvic + ureteric morphology)

Pyelonephritis ——————— Recurrence ——————— Cystopyelitis

Sonography (kidneys and urinary passages)

↓ ↓

Check the findings after first acute pyelonephritis | Micturition cystourethrography

↓ ↓ Preoperative

Scintigraphy (see page 64)
Parenchymal scarring
Sonographically 'missing' kidney | Cystoscopy

MEMORIX PEDIATRICS

Urine bacterial count

Test type	Contamination	Suspected infection (check)	Infection (organism differentiation)
Midstream	$\leq 10^3$	10^4–10^5	$\geq 10^5$
Catheter specimen		$\leq 10^3$	$\geq 10^4$
Bladder puncture			≥ 1

Schema of bladder function

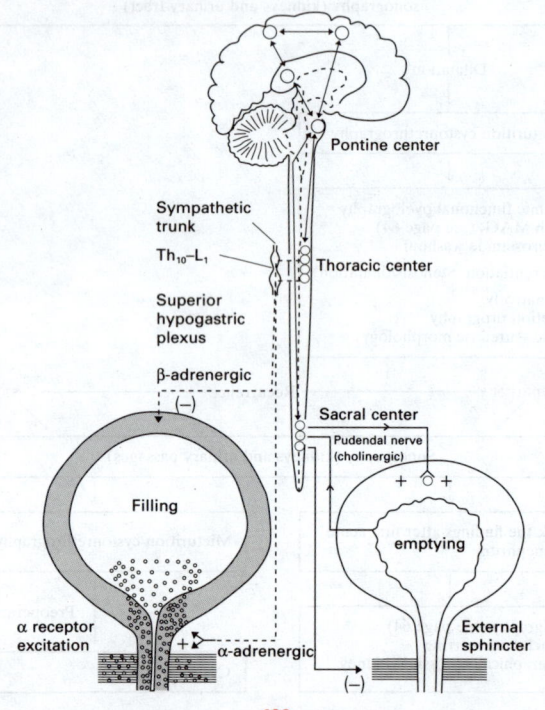

NEPHROLOGY/UROLOGY

Pharmacological treatment of micturition disorders

Problem	Solution principle	Drug treatment	Daily dose (mg)	Frequency
Reduced bladder filling caused by:				
Increased bladder muscle tone	Smooth muscle relaxants			
	Anticholinergics	Oxybutynine	5–10–20	2
Internal sphincter tone	β-sympathomimetics	Ephedrine	0.015–0.15	3
Excess bladder filling (emptying disorder):				
Raised internal sphincter tone	α-receptor blockers	Phenoxybenzamine	0.2–0.4/kg	3–4
External sphincter tone (spasticity)	Muscle relaxants	Baclofen	10–60	3
Bladder muscle tone ↓	β-sympatholytics	Not applicable, too strong an effect on the circulation		

Classification of neurogenic disorders of micturition
(After Bors and Comarr (1971).)

Injury type			
Proximal (upper motor neuron bladder)	Distal (lower motor neuron bladder)	Mixed (mixed motor neuron bladder) A	B
Interruption of conduction above S_2 Peripheral reflex arc preserved	Lesion S_2–S_4 Autonomic bladder	Lesion in area S_2–S_4 Tone of external sphincter preserved (pudendal nerve)	Lesion in area S_2–S_4 Detrusor function preserved (pelvic nerve)
Reflex bladder	Incontinent bladder	Overflow bladder	Incontinent bladder

Formula for approximating bladder capacity:

Bladder capacity (ml) = 32 × age (years) + 73   After age of 9 years there is a tendency to higher values

Normal frequency of micturition:
- Infants
  - ≤6 months   20/d
  - 6–12 months 16/d
- Children
  - ≤2 years   12/d
  - 2–4 years   9/d
  - ≥5 years   4–6/d

NEPHROLOGY/UROLOGY

Urinary stones

Type of stone	Causes	Urine	Treatment (stone removal +)	Prevention
Infection stone:	Anatomic urinary tract anomalies	Bacterial leukocyturia	Antibiotics	
Ammonium urate	Neurogenic bladder			Urine volume ↑
Phosphate: struvite (magnesium ammonium phosphate), carbonate apatite	Reflux Urease-positive organism		Urinary tract correction	Urine pH ↓
Calcium oxalate: Mono-/dihydrate	**Hypercalciuria:** (= >7 mmol Ca per) mmol creatinine			Urine volume ↑
	absorptive: vitamin D	Ca ↑		Diet
	Hypophosphatemia		Sodium cellulosephosphate (resin) magnesium,	
	Renal	Ca ↑	Thiazide	
	Reabsorptive Primary hyperparathyroidism	Ca ↑ Cyclic adenosine monophosphate (cAMP) ↑	Excision adenoma	
	Immobilization			
	Hyperoxaluria			
	Primary: Oxalosis type I (alanine glyoxylate transaminase deficiency)	Oxalic acid ↑ Glycoxalic acid ↑ Glycolic acid ↑	Liver transplant	Vitamin B_6 Diet Urine volume ↑
	Oxalosis type II (D-glycerine acid dehydrogenase deficiency)	Oxalic acid ↑ Glycerine acid ↑		
	Secondary (absorptive):	Oxalic acid ↑	Magnesium	Diet
	Pancreatic insufficiency		Oral calcium	
	Chronic enteritis		Orthophosphate	
	Hyperalimentation		Allopurinol	
Phosphate: Calcium hydrogenphosphate	Renal tubular acidosis (distal type I)	pH > 5.8		Diet
Carbonate apatite		Ca ↑		
Struvite (magnesium ammonium phosphate) (urease + bacteria)		Citrate ↑		

MEMORIX PEDIATRICS

Type of stone	Causes	Urine	Treatment (removal +)	Prevention
Uric acid	Hypoxanthine phosphoribosyl transferase deficiency (Lesch–Nyhan disease)	Uric acid ↑	Allopurinol	Low-purine diet
Xanthine	Xanthine oxydase deficiency, allopurinol treatment of Lesch–Nyhan disease	Xanthine ↑		Urine volume ↑ Diet
2,8-dihydroxyadenine	Adenine phosphoribosyl transferase deficiency	Adenine ↑ Hypoxanthine ↑ 2,8 Dihydroxyadenine ↑	Allopurinol	Urine volume ↑ Diet
Cystine	Cystinuria	Cystine ↑ Ca ↑ Oxalic acid ↑ Uric acid ↑		Urine volume ↑ Diet (low methionine)

Urease-positive urinary tract bacteria:

Proteus, Providencia, Morganella, Klebsiella, Staphylococcus saprophyticus, Enterobacter, Citrobacter, Pseudomonas.

Reaction: $H_2N-C-NH_2 + H_2O \xrightarrow{Urease} 2NH_3 + CO_2 \xrightarrow{+ 2H_2O} 2(NH_4^+OH^-)$

Urinary stones: diagnostic aids

Radiology	Opacity +++	Opacity +	Opacity 0
	Calcium hydrogenphosphate	Cysteine	Ammonium hydrogen urate
	Calcium oxalate		Urate
	Calcium phosphate		2,8-Dihydroxyadenine
	Magnesium ammonium phosphate (struvite)		Xanthine

Sonography: all stones over 2–3 mm in diameter

Physicochemical: infra-red spectroscopy or X-ray diffraction

NEPHROLOGY/UROLOGY

Hypercalciura: calcium loading test
(After Pak, Nicar and Northcutt (1982).)

Preparation: For one week before the test, the patient should take calcium <400 mg and sodium <100 mmol/d.

On the evening before the test, the last meal should be eaten at 6 pm.

Test:

Time	Test	Measurement of
7–9 am	Urine sample (fasting)	Calcium, creatinine, cAMP
9 am	Venous blood	Calcium, phosphate, PTH
9.10 am	Breakfast + loading with 1 g	Calcium/1.73 m^2
9 am to 1 pm	Urine sample	Calcium, creatinine, cAMP
1 pm	Venous blood	Calcium, phosphate, PTH

Assessment:

| Parameter | Hypercalciuria | | |
	Reabsorptive	Renal	Absorptive
Preloading:			
mg Ca/mg creatinine	>0.25	>0.15	≥0.10
cAMP/creatinine (urine)	↑	↓	n, ↓
Afterloading			
mg Ca/mg creatinine	>0.25	>0.25	>0.10
cAMP/creatinine (urine)	↑	↓	↓

cAMP = cyclic adenosine monophosphate; PTH = parathyroid hormone.

Electrolyte disturbances

$$\text{Neuromuscular excitability} = \frac{(K^+) \times (HCO_3^-) \times (HPO_4^-)}{(Ca^{++}) \times (Mg^{++}) \times (H^+)} \text{ (after Szent-Györgyi)}$$

Reduction in the denominators increases neuromuscular excitability.

Calculation of electrolyte substitution
Required electrolyte amount (mmol/l) = (desired value − actual value) × ideal weight* × distribution factor

Distribution factors:	Na	0.6–0.7	* related to actual height
	K	0.2	
	Cl	0.2–0.3	
	HCO$_3$	0.4–0.5	

Hyperkalemia (K > 6 mmol/l)

Symptoms: bradycardia/arrhythmia/ECG: QRS duration ↑, T ↑
muscular hypotonus
blood pressure ↓↓.

Causes: **raised uptake (substitution)**
reduced renal excretion:
    acute/chronic renal failure
    adrenogenital syndrome
    hypoaldosteronism
    Addison's disease

transcellular distribution disturbance
    metabolic/respiratory acidosis
    insulin deficiency
    hemolysis (intravascular)
    rhabdomyolysis
    old conserved blood

pseudohyperkalemia
    in vitro hemolysis.

Treatment:
1. Compensate for the acidosis
2. Glucose i.v. 5 g/kg every 4 h + 1U normal insulin/3 g glucose
3. Resonium A 0.5–1 g/kg oral/rectal
4. Peritoneal dialysis or hemodialysis.

METABOLISM

Hypokalemia (K < 3.5 mmol/l)

Symptoms: tachycardia/arrythmia/ECG: ST ↓, T ↓, (see page 138)
ileus
metabolic acidosis.

Causes: **loss from the gastrointestinal tract:**
vomiting, diarrhea
ureterosigmoidostomy
laxatives

loss from the skin: burns
renal loss: loop diuretics
thiazides
osmotic diuresis
carboanhydrase inhibitors
primary hyperaldosteronism
diabetic ketoacidosis
tubular acidosis
Bartter's syndrome

intracellular transport: (insulin)
alimentation potassium deficiency

Treatment: oral: potassium preparations
parenteral substitution

Blood gases – normal levels
(arterial blood, range 1 SD)
(After Koch and Wendel (1968); Pagtakhan and Pasterkamp (1990).)

Arterial blood values Age	P_{O_2} mmHg	pH	P_{CO_2} mmHg	Standard bicarbonate mmol/l
Birth (umbilical artery)	12.1–19.7	7.18–7.30	43.3–54.9	16.9–20.5
(umbilical vein)	21.7–33.1	7.26–7.37	32.2–43.4	18.6–21.4
5–10 min	39.7–59.5	7.15–7.25	39.1–53.1	15.1–18.3
30 min	42.6–65.6	7.25–7.33	32.0–43.4	16.7–19.7
60 min	52.0–74.6	7.30–7.36	31.9–40.3	18.0–20.4
24 h	63.2–82.2	7.33–7.39	33.3–36.5	18.9–21.5
7 d	63.4–82.8	7.35–7.40	32.8–39.0	20.5–23.1
2 y	80–100	7.35–7.40	32–39	20–22
>2 y	80–100	7.35–7.45	35–45	22–24

Normal levels (base excess): $-2.5 \rightarrow +2.5$ mmol/l (all age groups).

Buffering
Principles of treatment
1. pH range $7.15 \leftarrow 7.35 \rightarrow 7.65$ * Treatment of the basic disease
                                         * If incompletely effective compensation
                                             $NaHCO_3$ buffering (orally if possible).

2. pH range ≤ 7.15 At first, $NaHCO_3$ buffering given diluted, slowly i.v., then treatment of the basic disease.

pH range ≥ 7.65 At first, L-arginine-HCl i.v. over hours, correct the hypokalemia.

Calculation of buffer solution quantity
ml $NaHCO_3$ (8.4%)
 = base deficit   × kg BW × 0.3 (all children)   Bw = body weight.
 (neg. base excess)   Bw × factor
 = base deficit   × kg BW × 0.5 (neonates)   corresponds to
 = base deficit   × kg BW × 0.6 (prematures)   extracellular volume

Note: osmolarity of the 8.4% $NaHCO_3$ solution = 1500 mosmol/l. Dilute with four parts distilled water (300 mosmol/l) and take into account the total volume given.

ml 21% L-arginine-HCl solution
              or   = base excess × kg BW × 0.3.
ml 18.2% lysin–HCl solution

METABOLISM

Acidosis/alkalosis: pathophysiology

Acid–base balance
Definitions
Hypocarbia = $[HCO_3^-] < 21$ mmol/l   Hypocapnia = $P_{CO_2} < 35$ mmHg (<4.67 kPa)
Hypercarbia = $[HCO_3^-] > 28$ mmol/l   Hypercapnia = $P_{O_2} > 45$ mmHg (>6.0 kPa)
Standard bicarbonate concentrations = $[HCO_3^-]$ measured at constant normal P_{CO_2} (40 mmHg)
Actual bicarbonate concentration = $[HCO_3^-]$ measured at actual P_{CO_2}

$$pH = 6.1 + \log\left[\frac{HCO_3^-}{0.03 \times P_{CO_2}}\right] \rightarrow pH \sim \frac{\text{renal work}}{\text{lung work}}$$

Conversion: P_{CO_2} mmol/l = $0.03 \times P_{CO_2}$ mmHg

Disorders and compensation

Disorder	Primary cause	Compensation reference	pH	Gas control findings P_{CO_2}	[HCO$_3^-$] (standard/actual)	Relation $\frac{[HCO_3^-]}{P_{CO_2}}$
Respiratory acidosis compensated noncompensated	$P_{CO_2} \uparrow$	$[HCO_3^-] \uparrow$ $[HCO_3^-] \nearrow$	↓ ↘ ↓	↑ ↑ ↑	n ↑ ↑ / n	<20:1 20:1 <20:1
Respiratory alkalosis compensated noncompensated	$P_{CO_2} \downarrow$	$[HCO_3^-] \downarrow$ $[HCO_3^-] \searrow$	↑ ↗ ↑	↓ ↓ ↓	n ↓ ↓ / n	>20:1 20:1 >20:1
Metabolic acidosis compensated noncompensated	$[HCO_3^-] \downarrow$	$P_{CO_2} \downarrow$ $P_{CO_2} \searrow$	↓ ↘ ↓	n ↓ n	↓ ↓ ↓	<20:1 20:1 <20:1
Metabolic alkalosis compensated noncompensated	$[HCO_3^-] \uparrow$	$P_{CO_2} \uparrow$ $P_{CO_2} \nearrow$	↑ ↗ ↑	n ↑ n	↑ ↑ ↑	>20:1 20:1 >20:1

Combinations (primary + added disorder)
Respiratory metabolic acidosis: at high P_{CO_2} levels pH in normal range
Respiratory metabolic alkalosis: pH levels higher than with individual components
Metabolic respiratory acidosis: blood gas to be checked as in metabolic acidosis, but higher P_{CO_2} levels
Metabolic respiratory alkalosis: P_{CO_2} levels higher than with individual components

---

Normal 20:1 (mmol/l); n = level in normal range; $\nearrow$ = normal or slightly raised;
$\searrow$ = normal or slightly decreased.

MEMORIX PEDIATRICS

Acid–base disorders

Rules for the anticipated compensation of acid–base disorders
(assuming normal pulmonary and renal function)

Disorder	Causes	Compensation	Amount of anticipated compensation
Respiratory acidosis acute	$P_{CO_2} \uparrow\uparrow$	$[HCO_3^-] \uparrow$	• $[HCO_3^-]$ rises around 0.1 mmol/l for each 1 mmHg P_{CO_2} deviating from normal value
chronic	$P_{CO_2} \uparrow\uparrow$	$[HCO_3^-] \uparrow$	• $[HCO_3^-]$ rises around 0.35 mmol/l for each 1 mmHg P_{CO_2} deviating from normal value
Respiratory alkalosis acute	$P_{CO_2} \downarrow\downarrow$	$[HCO_3^-] \downarrow$	• $[HCO_3^-]$ falls around 0.2 mmol/l for each 1 mmHg P_{CO_2} deviating from normal value
chronic	$P_{CO_2} \downarrow\downarrow$	$[HCO_3^-] \downarrow$	• $[HCO_3^-]$ falls around 0.5 mmol/l for each 1 mmHg P_{CO_2} deviating from normal value
Metabolic acidosis	$[HCO_3^-] \downarrow\downarrow$	$P_{CO_2} \downarrow$	• P_{CO_2} falls by around 1–1.3 mmHg for each 1 mmol/l decrease of $[HCO_3^-]$ • $P_{CO_2} = 1.5 \times [HCO_3^-] + 8 \pm 2$ • P_{CO_2} = first two numbers after the decimal point of the pH (e.g. if pH = 7.25, then P_{CO_2} = 25) • $[HCO_3^-]$ + 15 = numbers after the decimal point of the pH (e.g. if $[HCO_3^-]$ = 10, then pH = 7.25)
Metabolic alkalosis	$[HCO_3^-] \uparrow$	$P_{CO_2} \uparrow$	• P_{CO_2} rises by 6 mmHg for each 10 mmol/l increase of $[HCO_3^-]$ • $[HCO_3^-]$ + 15 = first two numbers after the decimal point of the pH (e.g. if $[HCO_3^-]$ = 40, then pH = 7.55)

METABOLISM

Causes of disorders in the acid–base equilibrium

Respiratory acidosis

Central nervous system damage
Sedatives + neuroleptics
Narcotics
Opiates
Respiratory muscle paresis
Foreign body aspiration
Croup
Mucoviscidosis
Bronchial asthma
Bronchiolitis
Preumothorax
Pleural effusion
Pneumonia
Pulmonary edema
Thoracic deformity

Metabolic acidosis

Respiratory alkalosis

Hyperventilation, psychogenic/mechanical
Central nervous system lesions of all types
Hypoxemia

Metabolic alkalosis

Overbuffering with bicarbonate
Milk alkali syndrome (excessive milk ingestion)
} **Addition alkalosis**

Vomiting (checked)
Laxative abuse (low potassium)
Hyperaldosteronism
} **Subtraction alkalosis**

Lactacidosis: Hypoxia
Hypothermia
Methemoglobinemia
CO/CN poisoning
Diabetes mellitus
Glycogen storage type 1
Enzyme defects (see p. 213)
Ketoacidosis: Diabetes mellitus
Starvation, fasting
Maple syrup disease
Isovaleric acidemia
Formic acidosis: Methanol poisoning
} **Addition acidosis** = excess of protons in the extracellular space

Primary renal acidosis
Fanconi's syndrome
Diarrhea
Ileus
Pancreatic fistula
} **Subtraction acidosis** = proton loss

Tubular acidosis
Renal insufficiency
Acute renal failure
Posisoning (vitamin D, mercury, lead)
Hyperparathyroidism
Addison's disease
} **Retention acidosis** = deficient renal tubular proton secretion

Anion gap

Comparable ion loading mmol/l:

Cations				Anions	
Na$^+$	142	Measured ions	Cl$^-$		103
K$^+$	4		HCO$_3^-$		27
Ca^{++}	5		HPO$_4^{--}$		2
Mg^{++}	2	Unmeasured ions	SO$_4^-$		1
Others	1		Organic anions		5
			Proteins		16

| 154 | – | Law of electroneutrality | – | 154 |

Calculation:
Variant 1: $(Na^+ + K^+) - (Cl^- + HCO_3^-)$ normal value = 16 (range 12–20) mmol/l
Variant 2: $Na^+ - (Cl^- + HCO_3^-)$ normal value = 12 (range 8–16) mmol/l

Because of the law of electroneutrality, the measured amounts of ion reflect the quantitative changes in the unmeasured cations and anions.

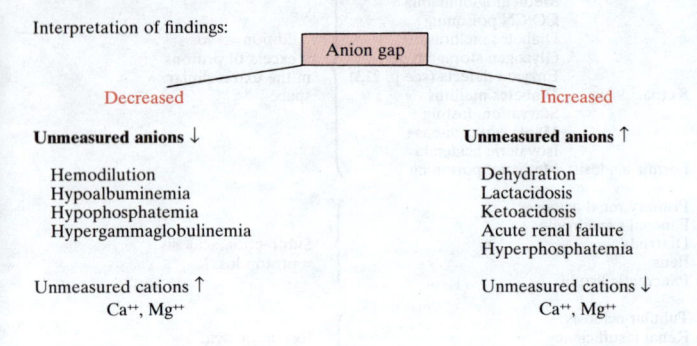

Interpretation of findings:

Anion gap

Decreased   **Increased**

Unmeasured anions ↓   **Unmeasured anions ↑**

  Hemodilution   Dehydration
  Hypoalbuminemia   Lactacidosis
  Hypophosphatemia   Ketoacidosis
  Hypergammaglobulinemia   Acute renal failure
                                                           Hyperphosphatemia

Unmeasured cations ↑   Unmeasured cations ↓
  Ca^{++}, Mg^{++} Ca^{++}, Mg^{++}

Congenital lactacidosis

Primary hyperlactacidemia in:

Glycogen storage types 0, III, IV

Enzyme defect of gluconeogenesis and in pyruvate metabolism

Enzyme defect of the citrate cycle

Respiratory chain defects.

Secondary hyperlactacidemia:

Organic acidurias

Citrullinemia

Enzyme defect of fatty acid oxidation.

Hypolactacidemia:

Defects of muscle glycogenolysis and glycolysis (no rise in lactate after muscular work).

Metabolic acidosis

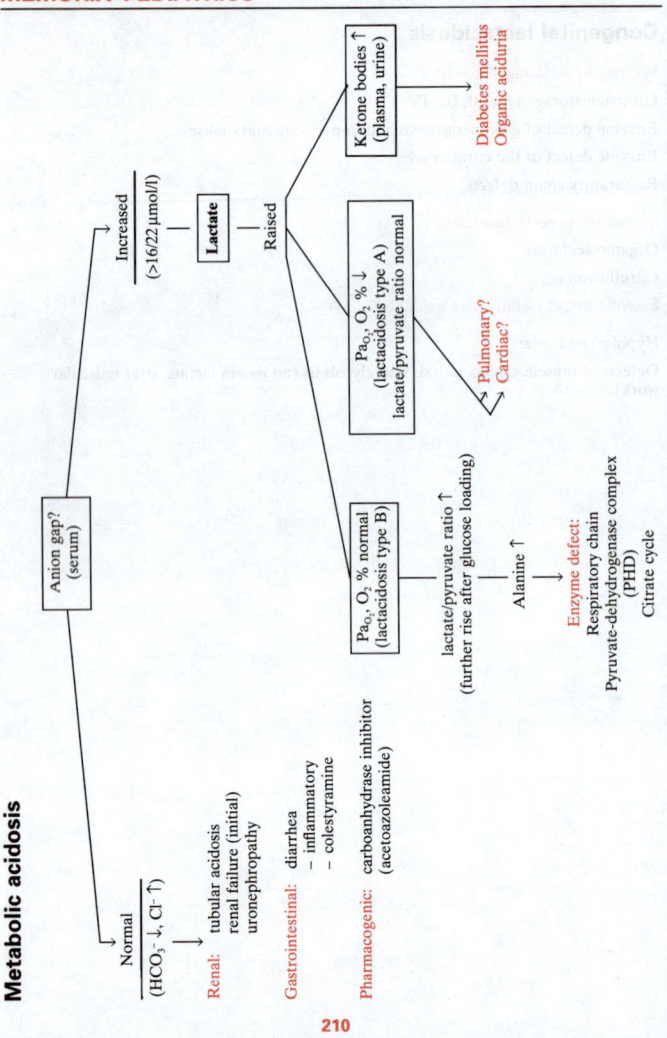

Anion gap? (serum)

Normal
HCO_3^- ↓, Cl^- ↑

- **Renal:** tubular acidosis
  renal failure (initial)
  uronephropathy

- **Gastrointestinal:** diarrhea
  – inflammatory
  – colestyramine

- **Pharmacogenic:** carboanhydrase inhibitor (acetoazoleamide)

Increased (>16/22 µmol/l)

Lactate

Raised

Pa_{O_2}, O_2 % normal (lactacidosis type B)

lactate/pyruvate ratio ↑
(further rise after glucose loading)

Alanine ↑

Enzyme defect:
Respiratory chain
Pyruvate-dehydrogenase complex (PHD)
Citrate cycle

Pa_{O_2}, O_2 % ↓ (lactacidosis type A)
lactate/pyruvate ratio normal

Pulmonary?
Cardiac?

Ketone bodies (plasma, urine)

Diabetes mellitus
Organic aciduria

METABOLISM

Diagnosis of ketoacidosis

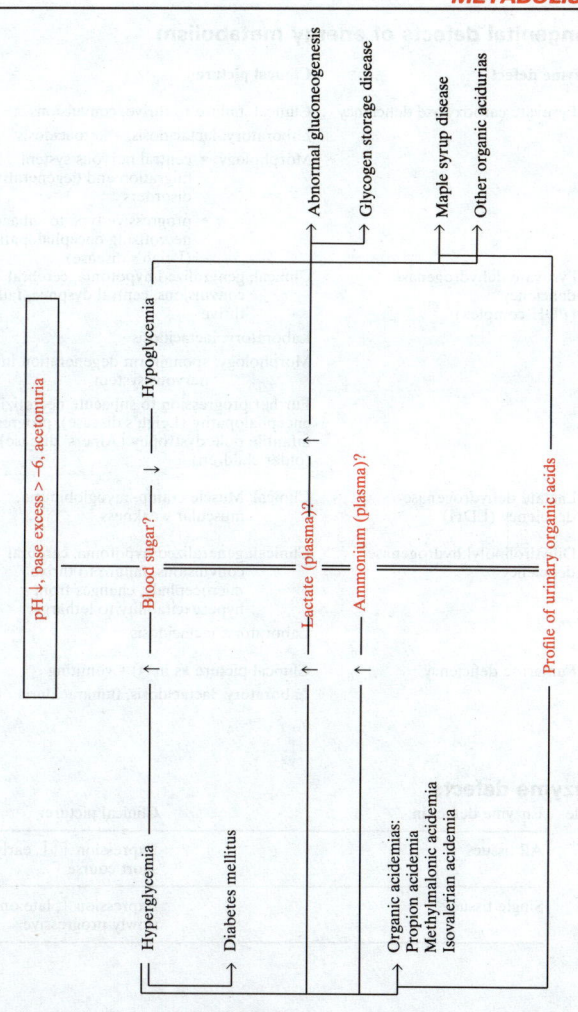

pH ↓, base excess > −6, acetonuria

- Blood sugar?
  - Hyperglycemia → Diabetes mellitus
  - Hypoglycemia
    - → Abnormal gluconeogenesis
    - → Glycogen storage disease
- Lactate (plasma)?
- Ammonium (plasma)?
- Profile of urinary organic acids
  - → Maple syrup disease
  - → Other organic acidurias
  - Organic acidemias:
    - Propion acidemia
    - Methylmalonic acidemia
    - Isovalerian acidemia

Congenital defects of energy metabolism

Enzyme defect	Clinical picture
① Pyruvate carboxylase deficiency	Clinical: failure to thrive, convulsions Laboratory: lactacidosis, + ketoacidosis Morphology: • central nervous system migration and degenerative disorders • progressive type to subacute necrotizing encephalopathy (Leigh's disease)
② Pyruvate dehydrogenase deficiency (PDH complex)	Clinical: generalized hypotonia, cerebral convulsions, central dyspnea, failure to thrive Laboratory: lactacidosis Morphology: spongiform degeneration in central nervous system Further progression to subacute necrotizing encephalopathy (Leigh's disease), progressive infantile poliodystrophy (Alpers' disease), ataxia (older children)
③ Lactate dehydrogenase deficiency (LDH)	Clinical: Muscle cramp, myoglobinuria, muscular weakness
④ Dihydrolipolyl hydrogenase deficiency	Clinical: generalized hypotonia, cerebral convulsions, failure to thrive microcephaly, changes from hyperexcitability to lethargy Laboratory: lactacidosis
⑤ Fumarase deficiency	Clinical picture as in ④ + vomiting Laboratory: lactacidosis, fumaraciduria

Enzyme defects

Rule:

Enzyme defect in:	Clinical picture:
All tissues	Expression ↑↑↑, early onset, short course
Single tissue	Expression ↑, late onset, slowly progressive

METABOLISM

Model of pyruvate metabolism

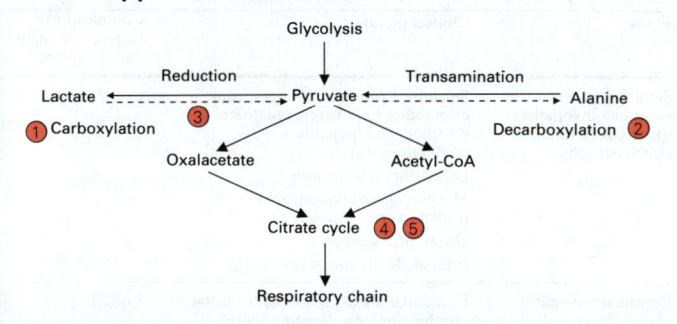

```
                        Glycolysis
                            │
         Reduction          │         Transamination
Lactate ◄──────────────── Pyruvate ────────────────► Alanine
   ① Carboxylation    ③                  Decarboxylation ②
            │                       │
            ▼                       ▼
       Oxalacetate              Acetyl-CoA
                  │         │
                  ▼         ▼
                 Citrate cycle ④ ⑤
                       │
                       ▼
                Respiratory chain
```

Schema of the enzyme complex of the mitochondrial respiratory chain

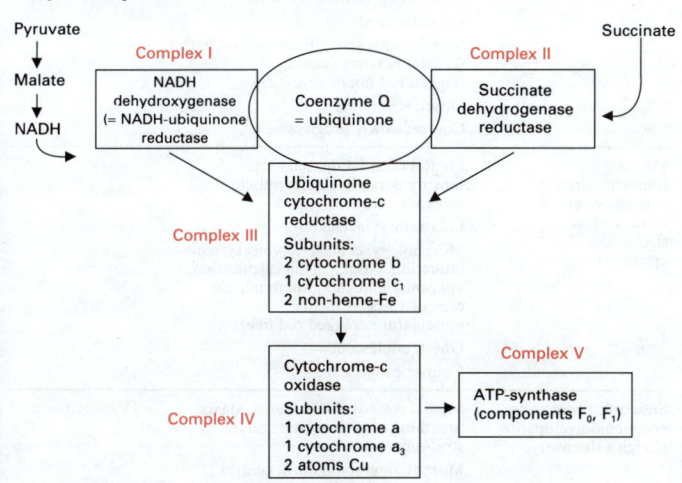

Pyruvate → Malate → NADH →

Complex I: NADH dehydroxygenase (= NADH-ubiquinone reductase)

Coenzyme Q = ubiquinone

Complex II: Succinate dehydrogenase reductase ← Succinate

Complex III: Ubiquinone cytochrome-c reductase
Subunits:
2 cytochrome b
1 cytochrome c_1
2 non-heme-Fe

Complex IV: Cytochrome-c oxidase
Subunits:
1 cytochrome a
1 cytochrome a_3
2 atoms Cu

Complex V: ATP-synthase (components F_0, F_1)

MEMORIX PEDIATRICS

Clinical symptoms of respiratory chain defects

Term	Clinical picture	Complex of the respiratory chain (site of defect)
Fetal infantile encephalomyopathy: (progressive infantile poliodystrophy)	Seizures, hypotonia, changes from excitability to lethargy, breathing disorder + tubulopathy + cardiomyopathy Laboratory: lactacidosis Morphology: poliodystrophy (central nervous system) Onset: first week Course: death after a few weeks	I or III or IV
Encephalomyopathy of childhood and adolescence (Kearns–Sayre syndrome)	Dementia, ataxia, spasticity, external ophthalmoplegia, tapetoretinal degeneration, optic atrophy, sensory nerve deafness, activity muscle pain, muscular weakness, cardiomyopathy Laboratory: lactacidosis after muscular work Morphology: spongiform myelinopathy (central nervous system, 'ragged red fibers' (muscles) Onset: school-age Course: slowly progressive	I or III
MELAS (mitochondrial encephalopathy, lactic acidosis, stroke-like episodes)	Mental retardation, seizures, sensory nerve deafness, muscle weakness, stunted growth Laboratory: lactacidosis Morphology: central nervous system infarction, basal ganglia calcification, abnormal mitochondria in muscle cells of vascular media; musculature: 'ragged red fibers' Onset: adolescence Course: progressive	I
Subacute necrotizing encephalomyelopathy (Leigh's disease)	Mental retardation, seizures, ataxia, breathing disorders, nystagmus, strabismus Morphology: spongiform central nervous system degeneration Onset: first two years, sometimes later Course: rapidly progressive	IV

METABOLISM

Clinical symptoms of respiratory chain defects (continued)

Term	Clinical picture	Complex of the respiratory chain (site of defect)
Trichopoliodystrophy (Menkes' syndrome/ kinky-hair disease/ copper malabsorption)	Mental retardation, spasticity, myoclonic seizures, hypomimicry, hypothermia, stunted growth, abnormal ossification, hair dysplasia, Laboratory: serum Cu, ceruloplasmin ↓ Morphology: central nervous system degeneration Onset: first year of life Course: lifespan 3–14 years	IV
MERRF (myoclonic epilepsy with 'ragged red fibers', Fukuhara's syndrome)	Myoclonus, seizures, ataxia, deafness, muscle weakness Laboratory: lactacidosis	IV
Benign reversible infantile mitochondrial myopathy	Muscle weakness Laboratory: lactacidosis Onset: birth Course: normalization up to 2–3 yr	IV
Myopathy	Muscular activity pain, muscle weakness Onset: childhood to adulthood Course: slowly progressive	I or V
Cardiomyopathy (histiocytoid cardiomyopathy of infancy)	Tachyarrhythmia Morphology: focal myocardial degeneration Onset: from birth Course: variably progressive, usually only months	III

Hyperammonemia: diagnostic plan

Symptoms
Disorder of consciousness, ± hypotension, ± cerebral seizures, seizures, ± cerebral motor disorder, ± vomiting

Ammonia measurement

Exclude: ↑ **Ammonia formation** ↑: muscular work (seizures, tachypnea), cystitis (urease positive bacteria)
↓ **Ammonia poisoning** ↓: Liver failure, portal collateral circulation, arginine deficiency, valproate treatment

Persistent symptoms

From birth — Premature?
Respiratory alkalosis
+ Arginine (P) normal
+ Citrulline (P) normal/↑
+ Argininosuccinase (U) negative
→ **Transitory hyperammonemia of the newborn**

From 2–5 d or on changing from breast to cows' milk
Respiratory alkalosis ↔ metabolic acidosis
± Ketonemia
Anion gap ↑
→ **Organic acidemias / Organic acidurias**

Episodic symptoms

Expression according to enzyme activity
Older children/juveniles
Respiratory alkalosis
Anion gap normal
→ **Urea cycle defect**

Neonates/infants
Arginine (P,U) ↑↑↑
Citrulline (U) ↑
Ornithine (U) ↑
Orotic acid (U) ↑
Lysine (U) ↑
Cystine (U) ↑
→ **Arginase deficiency**

P = plasma
U = urine

METABOLISM

Citrulline (P)

| ≤50 µmol/l | 100–300 µmol/l | >1000 µmol/l |

Orotic acid (U) Argininosuccinate (P) ↑

- (+) → Carbamyl-phosphate synthetase deficiency (CPS)
- +++ → Ornithine transcarbamylase (OTC) (mode: XR)
- → Argininosuccinate lyase (AL)
- → Argininosuccinate synthetase (citrullinemia) (AS)

Ornithine (P) ↑↑↑
Homocitrulline (U) ↑
→ Hyperornithinemia, hyperammonemia, homocitrullinemia syndrome (HHH) (transmitochondrial transport disorder)

L-Alanine loading
|
Arginine (U) ↑
Lysine (U) ↑
Ornithine (U) ↑
Orotic acid (U) ↑
Overflow aciduria

→ Lysinuric protein tolerance (transmembranous transport disorder)

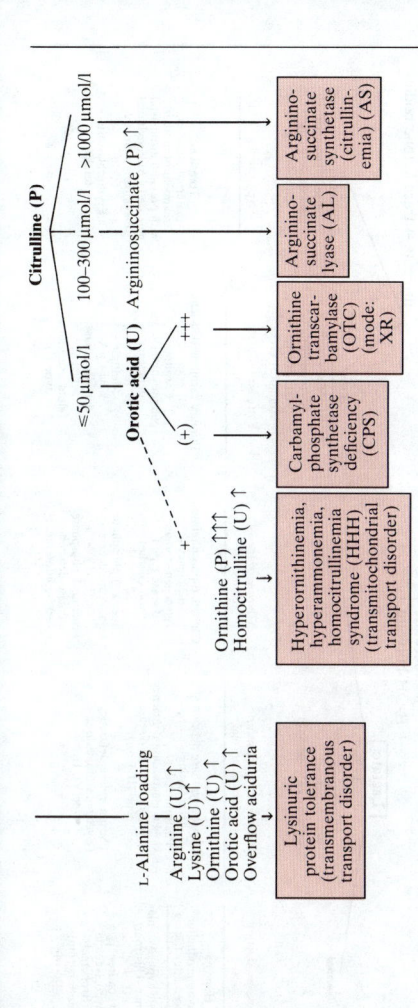

Hyperammonemia

Emergency: ammonia ≥ 250 nmol/l + disorder of consciousness

Acute treatment (After Bachmann (1987).)

Stop protein administration
Measure anion gap and lactate (see p. 212)
Glucose i.v. 6–8 mg/kg/min, if enzyme defect pyruvate dehydrogenase complex (see p. 210)

After 2 h:
initially 1 mmol/kg/h arginine HCl, then 2 mmol/kg/d
L-carnitine 150 mg/kg/d
Na-benzoate (3% solution i.v.) 250 mg/kg in first 2 h, then 250–500 mg/kg/d; maximal effect only after some days; check benzoate serum level (limits 2 mmol/l)
Additionally peritoneal dialysis or hemodialysis

Hypoglycemia

Definition: blood sugar (BS) ≤40 mg/dl (2.22 mmol/l)

Differential diagnosis
(Modified from Böhles (1991).)

24h BS profile
|
BS ≤ 40 mg/dl (2.22 mmol/l)

Ketotic: serum: >2.5 mmol/l
ketone bodies: acetone
acetoacetate
β-OH-butyrate

β-OH-butyric acids

Lactate

Normal

Glucose production reduced

Hypoxia
Glucose production reduced after fasting
Ketotic hypoglycemia (Colle–Ulström) ①↓ ㉒
Hypoadrenergic hypoglycemia (Broberger–Zetterström) ㊳↓⑯

Raised (after carbohydrate loading)

Glycogen synthesis or glycolysis abnormal

Glycogen synthase deficiency
After fasting
Postprandial ⑨↑ ㊴↑
Amylo-1,6-glucosidase deficiency (glycogen storage disease type III, Cori)
Phosphorylase deficiency (glycogen storage disease type VI, Hers)
㉒ ㉓ ㉘d

Raised (after fasting)

Gluconeogenesis abnormal

Glucose-6-phosphatase deficiency (glycogen storage disease type I, von Gierke)
② ㉑ ㉒ ㉓ ㉔
Glucose-6-phosphate translocase deficiency
② ⑲ ㉒ ㉓ ㉔ ↓
Fructose-1-phosphate aldolase deficiency (fructose intolerance)
② ㉓ ㉘d

Hypoketotic: serum <<2.5 mmol/l
urine: 0 → trace ketone bodies

$$\frac{FFA}{\beta\text{-OH-butyric acids}} > 2^{a,b}$$

$$\frac{BS \,(mmol/l) \times}{\beta\text{-OH-butyrate} \,(mmol/l)} < 1.5^{a,c}$$

Fatty acid oxidation abnormal

Primary carnitine deficiency
④ ⑩ ↓⑰m
Carnitine-palmitoyltransferase deficiency
② ㉒ ⑰
Multiple acyl-CoA dehydrogenase deficiency (glutaric aciduria type II)
④ ㊺ ↓㉜

β-OH-butyrate, FFA in plasma – none or inadequately raised after fasting

Hyperinsulinism

Transient:
maternal diabetes, treatment of mother with pre- and intrapartal glucose i.v./sulfonylurea/β-sympathomimetics
Erythroblastosis fetalis ⑨

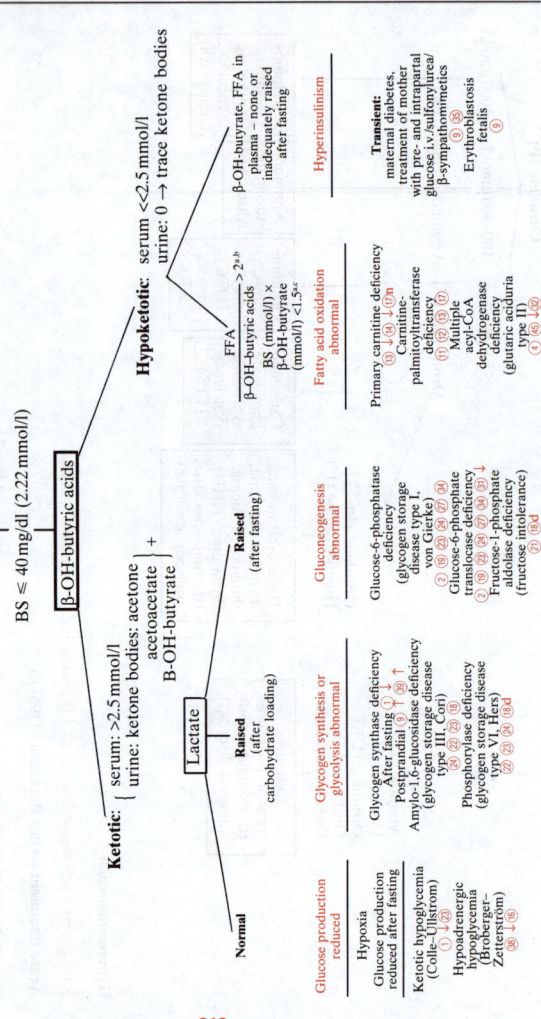

218

METABOLISM

Congenital glucagon deficiency
㉘
Cortisol deficiency (glucocorticoids, adrenogenital syndrome)
① ↓ ⑮
Congenital hypopituitarism
㊴ ↓ ㉓

Phosphorylase-b-kinase deficiency (glycogen storage disease type VIII, Fernandes)
㉒ ㉓ ㉔ ⑱a,b
Galactose-1-phosphate uridyl transferase deficiency
㊿ ⑱b

Fructose-1,6-diphosphatase deficiency
② ① ↑ ㊺ ↑ ㉗
Phosphoenolpyruvate carboxykinase deficiency
① ② ㉓ ⑱d
Pyruvate carboxylase deficiency, multiple carboxylase deficiency
㊻ ⑤ ↑ ㊱ ↑ ㊼ ↑
Methylmalonyl-CoA-apomutase deficiency (methylmalonacidemia)
㊻ ⑤ ↑ ㊶ ↑ ㊼ ↑ ㉛
2-Oxoacid dehydrogenase deficiency (maple syrup disease)
⑤ ↑ ① ↑ ③ ↑ ㊹
Glutaryl-CoA dehydrogenase deficiency (glutaraturia type I)
④ ㊳ ↑ ⑤ ↑ ㊻ ↓ ⑱a,c,d
Ethanol poisoning
⑨ ⑥ ↑

Middle-chain acyl-CoA dehydrogenase deficiency
㊺ ↓ ㉝
Hydroxymethylglutaryl-CoA lyase deficiency
㊺ ↓ ㊷

Beckwith–Wiedemann syndrome
⑨
Persisting:
Nesidioblastosis/insulinoma
⑨ ㊱ ↑ ㉓ ㉜
① ↓
Leucine sensitive hypoglycemia
㊵

Cannot be definitively classified

Hepatitis
⑨
Reye's syndrome
① ↓ ⑤ ↑ ㉙ ↑
㉘ ↑ ㊽ ↑ ㊾ ↑

Special types:
Autoimmune hypoglycemia
㊺ ㊲

Salicylate poisoning
⑨ ㊾ ↑

[a] Measurement at the end of the fasting period; [b] normal value <1; [c] normal value 9–14.

219

MEMORIX PEDIATRICS

Hypoglycemia: diagnostic substances and tests

1. Alanine P, S
2. Alanine loading (oral)
3. Amino acids, double chain (leucine, isoleucine, valine) P, S
4. Amino acid, glutarate P, S
5. Ammonia P
6. Ethanol concentration B
7. Fasting blood sugar
8. Blood sugar day profile
9. Blood sugar monitoring
10. Blood cells
11. β-Hydroxybutyric acid (β-OH-butyrate) P
12. β-OH-butyrate after MCT meal P
13. Carnitine, free P
14. Carnitine ester P
15. Cortisol P
16. 2-deoxyglucose test (i.v.)
17. Dicarbonic acid P
18. Enzyme activity measurement:
    a fibroblasts
    b erythrocytes
    c leukocytes
    d liver
    e muscle
19. Fasting test
20. Free fatty acids (FFA) P
21. Fructose tolerance test (i.v.)
22. Galactose loading test (oral)
23. Glucagon test
24. Glucose tolerance test (oral)
25. Glucose tolerance test (i.v.)
26. Glucose requirement
27. Glycerol loading test (oral)
28. Glycerol loading test (i.v.)
29. γ-glutamyltranspeptidase S
30. Glutarate P, U
31. Granulocyte function test B
32. Urinary metabolites (hexanoyl glycine, phenylproprionyl glycine, octanoyl glycine)
33. Urinary metabolites: Dicarbonic acids
    glutarate
    isobutyryl glycine
    isovaleryl glycine
    α-methylbutyryl glycine
34. Uric acid S
35. HbA_{1C} (maternal) B
36. Insulin/C-peptide P
37. Insulin antibodies
38. Catecholamine P
39. Lactate P
40. Leucine loading
41. Methylmalonate P, U
42. 3-methylglutarylcarnitine U
43. Organic acids P, U
44. 2-oxoacids U
45. pH B
46. Phosphate S
47. Proprionate P, U
48. Prothrombin time B
49. Pyruvate P
50. Reducing substances U
51. Salicylate concentration S
52. Somatostatin suppression B
53. Somatotropic hormone P

(B = blood, U = urine, P = plasma, S = serum medium-chain triglycerides)

METABOLISM

Glycogen metabolic defects (glycogen storage defects)

Type	Name of disease	Enzyme defect (deficiency)	Gene type	Organs participating	Chief symptoms	Enzyme assay
0	(Lewis)	Glycogen synthetase	AR?	Liver	Hypoglycemia	Liver
Ia	von Gierke	Glucose-6-phosphatase	AR	Liver, kidney	Hypoglycemia, hyperuricemia, hyperlipidemia	Liver
Ib	–	Glucose-6-phosphatase translocase	AR	Liver, kidney	as Ia + infections	Liver
II	Pompe	α-1,4-glucosidase (acid maltase)	AR	All tissues, particularly heart, muscles, CNS, liver, granulocytes	Cardiomegaly, muscular weakness	Muscle
III	Cori	Amylo-1,6-glucosidase (debrancher enzyme)	AR	All tissues, particularly liver muscles, blood cells	Hypoglycemia, hepatosplenomegaly, muscular weakness	RBC, WBC, muscle, liver, fibroblasts, chorionic villi
IV	Anderson	α-glucan-6-glucosyl-transferase (brancher enzyme)	AR	All tissues, particularly liver	Hepatosplenomegaly, later cirrhosis of liver	Liver
V	McArdle	Phosphorylase	AR	Musculature	Myalgia myoglobinuria	Muscle
VI	Hers	Phosphorylase	AR	Liver	Hepatomegaly, hypoglycemia	Liver
VII	Tarui	Phosphofructokinase	AR	Musculature, erythrocytes	Myalgia, reticulocytosis	RBC, muscle
VIII	Fernandes	Phosphorylase	XR	Liver, CNS Leukocytes	Hepatomegaly	RBC, WBC

RBC = erythrocytes; WBC = leukocytes.

Diabetes mellitus

Hormone regulation:	Insulin	Glucagon, adrenaline, cortisol, growth hormone
Glucose utilization	↑	↓
Glycolysis/gluconeogenesis	↓	↑
Lipolysis/ketogenesis	↓	↑

Insulin-dependent diabetes mellitus type I: IDDM.
Non-insulin-dependent diabetes mellitus type II: NIDDM.
Maturity onset diabetes of the young (type II disease in the young): MODY.
Gestational diabetes mellitus: GDM (first manifested in pregnancy).
Latent diabetes: previous abnormality of glucose tolerance: Prev AGT.
Impaired glucose tolerance: IGT
Pre-diabetes: potential abnormality of glucose tolerance: Pot AGT.

White's classification of diabetes mellitus in pregnancy

Group A   Glucose intolerance – dietary treatment – independent of age.
Group B   IDDM manifestation after 20 years of age – duration <10 years.
Group C   IDDM manifestation at 10–19 years of age – duration 10–19 years.
Group D   IDDM manifestation <10 years of age – duration > 20 years.
Group R   As for group D + retinopathy.
Group F   Diabetic nephropathy
Group RF As for groups R and F.

Diagnosis

1. Diagnosis possible from criteria:
   polydipsia + polyuria + weight ↓ + acetonuria + blood sugar >200 mg/dl, independent of temporal relation to a meal.
2. Verification of diagnosis: oral glucose tolerance test (OGTT) (procedure, p. 228).

Interpretation

Blood test	Glucose tolerance (blood sugar mg/dl [mmol/l])		
	Normal	Abnormal	Diabetes
Fasting level:			
Capillary blood/venous blood	<115 [6.4]	<120 [6.7]	⩾120 [6.7]
Plasma, venous	<130 [7.2]	<140 [7.8]	⩾140 [7.8]
Level after 120 min:	(+ one level after 30, 60, 90 min):		
Capillary blood	<140 [8.7]	>140 [7.8] <200	⩾200 [11.1]
Venous blood	<120 [6.7]	>120 [6.7] <180	⩾180 [10.0]
Plasma, venous	<140 [7.8]	>140 [7.8] <200	⩾200 [11.1]

METABOLISM

Causes and associated diseases of abnormal glucose tolerance

Dystrophic neonate (delayed β-cell maturation?)
  Signs: rare, intrauterine dystrophy, osmotic diuresis
    Treatment: insulin, improvement after weeks or months
Obesity, glucose tolerance usually improved with weight reduction
Syndromes with obesity (Prader–Willi syndrome, Laurence–Moon–Biedl syndrome)
Chomosomal aberration: trisomy 21 (Down's syndrome), Turner's syndrome,
Klinefelter's syndrome
Isolated growth hormone deficiency
Mucoviscidosis
Friedreich's ataxia
Optic atrophy
Generalized lipodystrophy

Insulin:
U 40 insulin = 40 units/ml
U 100 insulin = 100 units/ml
Normal insulin = old insulin
Basal insulin = retard insulin: delayed release by NPH (neutral protamine Hagedorn)
NPH insulin freely miscible with normal insulin

Treatment principles:
Ascertain the individual insulin requirement:
  Guidelines – start of treatment   1.2–1.5 IU/kg/d
              – transitory recovery stage   0.5–0.1 IU/kg/d
              – one year after manifestation   0.6–0.8 IU/kg/d
              – two years after manifestation 0.8–1.2 IU/kg/d
Intensified insulin treatment = basic requirement + correction requirement
  Basic requirement of normal insulin ← blood sugar remains unchanged before and
    2 h after the injection
  Correction proportion → actual blood sugar measured 2 h after the injection, aim:
    100–120 mg/dl
  Assessment of basic requirement: the difference in blood sugar level before and 2 h
    after the injection of x IU normal insulin = y (mg/dl).
      Compare y with the following blood sugar guiding levels (after Heinze and Holl
      (1991)):
      1 IU insulin lowers the blood sugar by (mg/dl):
      children: 20–30 kg   1 IU by 100 mg/dl
                 40–50 kg   1 IU by 50 mg/dl
      Adults: 1 IU by 30 mg/dl
      How often is the blood sugar guiding level contained in y? Deduct the result as
      IU insulin from the injected x IU = basic requirement

Distribution of amount of insulin into two injections/day: ~2/3 in morning
Distribution of basic requirement according to the nutrition plan:
  Insulin units per bread units (BU): morning ~ 2 IU/BU
                                      midday ~ 1 IU/BU
                                      evening ~ 1.5 IU/BU

Insulin therapy
Soluble insulin

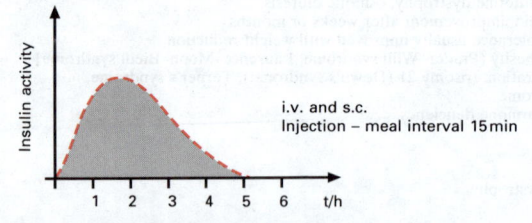

i.v. and s.c.
Injection – meal interval 15 min

Time after s.c. insulin injection

Insulin preparations			
All 100 units/ml	Hypurin Neutral	(B)	CP
(H) Human insulin	Velosulin	(P)	Novo Nordisk, (Glaxo) Wellcome
(P) Porcine insulin	Human Actrapid	(H)	Novo Nordisk
(B) Bovine insulin	Human Velosulin	(H)	Novo Nordisk, Wellcome
	Humulin S	(H)	Lilly
	Pur-In Neutral	(H)	CP

Intermediate- and long-acting insulins

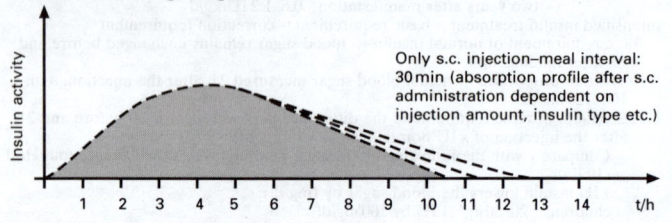

Only s.c. injection–meal interval:
30 min (absorption profile after s.c.
administration dependent on
injection amount, insulin type etc.)

Time after s.c. insulin injection

Insulin preparations			
All 100 units/ml	**Isophane insulin**		
(H) Human insulin	Hypurin Isophane	(B)	CP
(P) Porcine insulin	Insulatard	(P)	Novo Nordisk, (Glaxo) Wellcome
(B) Bovine insulin	Human Insulatard	(H)	Novo Nordisk, Wellcome
	Human Protaphane	(H)	Novo Nordisk
	Humulin I	(H)	Lilly
	Pur-In Isophane	(H)	CP
	Insulin Zinc Suspension (mixed)		
	Hypurin Lente	(B)	CP
	Lentard MC	(B,P)	Novo Nordisk
	Human Monotard	(H)	Novo Nordisk
	Humulin Lente	(H)	Lilly
	Insulin Zinc Suspension (amorphous)		
	Semitard MC	(P)	Novo Nordisk
	Insulin Zinc Suspension (crystalline)		
	Human Ultratard	(H)	Novo Nordisk
	Humulin Zn	(H)	Lilly

METABOLISM

Biphasic insulins

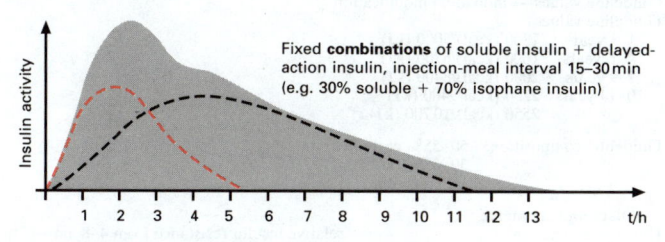

Fixed **combinations** of soluble insulin + delayed-action insulin, injection-meal interval 15–30 min (e.g. 30% soluble + 70% isophane insulin)

Time after s.c. insulin injection

- - - - - Activity of normal insulin
- - - - - Activity of delayed-action insulin
▓▓▓▓▓ Total activity

Insulin preparations
All 100 units/ml
(H) Human insulin
(P) Porcine insulin
(B) Bovine insulin

10% soluble insulin + 90% isophane insulin
Humulin M1	(H)	Lilly
PenMix 10/90	(H)	Novo Nordisk

15% soluble insulin + 85% isophane insulin
Pur-In Mix 15/85	(H)	CP

20% soluble insulin + 80% isophane insulin
Humulin M2	(H)	Lilly
PenMix 20/80	(H)	Novo Nordisk

25% soluble insulin + 75% isophane insulin
Pur-In Mix 25/75	(H)	CP

30% soluble insulin + 70% isophane insulin
Mixtard 30/70	(P)	Novo Nordisk, Wellcome
Humulin M3	(H)	Lilly
PenMix 30/70	(H)	Novo Nordisk
Human Actraphane	(H)	Novo Nordisk
Human Mixtard	(H)	Novo Nordisk, Wellcome

40% soluble insulin + 60% isophane insulin
Humulin M4	(H)	Lilly
PenMix 40/60	(H)	Novo Nordisk

50% soluble insulin + 50% isophane insulin
Initard 50/50	(P)	Novo Nordisk, Wellcome
PenMix 50/50	(H)	Novo Nordisk
Pur-In Mix 50/50	(H)	CP
Human Initard 50/50	(H)	Novo Nordisk, Wellcome

Crystalline bovine in soluble porcine insulin
Rapitard MC	(B+P)	Novo Nordisk

MEMORIX PEDIATRICS

Diabetes: daily energy requirement

Guideline values → individual modification
Guideline values
- 1–3 years   1200 (kcal)/5000 (kJ)
- 4–6 years   1600 (kcal)/6700 (kJ)
- 7–9 years   2000 (kcal)/8400 (kJ)
- 10–14 years   2250 (kcal/9400 (kJ) ♀
-                     2550 (kcal)/10 700 (kJ) ♂

Guideline composition: 50–55% carbohydrate
                              30–35% fat
                                15% protein

Regulation phenomena:
Dawn phenomenon: relative insulin resistance from 4–8 am → higher fasting blood sugar (growth hormone effect?)
Somogyi effect (hyperglycemic rebound): counterreaction after hypoglycemia (glucagon, adrenaline, cortisol, growth hormone): hyperglycemia (headaches)

Hypoglycemia – functional diagnosis
(2) Alanine loading test (oral)
     Principle: checking gluconeogenesis from glucoplastic amino acids
     Fasting levels of alanine, blood sugar, lactate
     0.5 g/kg oral alanine
     Check alanine, blood sugar, lactate after 15, 30, 45, 60, 90 min
     Result: normal: rise in glucose after night-time fast
        abnormal: in fructose-1,6-diphosphatase deficiency, no significant rise in
                   glucose, lactacidosis

     Alanine loading test (i.v.)
     In association with the fasting test
     Excretion levels for alanine, glucose, lactate
     0.3 g/kg of alanine i.v. within 2–3 min
     Check alanine, glucose, lactate after 5, 15, 30, 60, 90 min
     Result: healthy: rise in glucose and lactate
        abnormal: no rise in the parameter in defect of fructose-1,6-diphosphatase,
                   glucose-6-phosphatase, phosphoenolpyruvate carboxykinase,
                   pyruvate carboxylase

(16) 2-deoxyglucose test
     Principle: this substance initiates a hypothalamic adrenergic counterreaction to the fall of intracellular glucose. Effect: blood sugar rise.
     Measure blood sugar 30 min before and immediately before the infusion.
     If blood sugar >60 mg/dl (3.33 mmol/l), give 2-deoxyglucose in 0.9% in NaCl as a 20% solution over 30 min i.v.
     Dosage: 50 mg/kg
     Measure blood sugar every 30 min for at least 3 h after the infusion.
     At the same time, take the pulse and measure blood pressure. Watch out for signs of changed sympathetic tone.
     Result: normal: blood sugar rise ≥35 mg/dl (1.94 mmol/l)
        abnormal: blood sugar rise <35 mg/dl (hypoadrenergic hypoglycemia).

METABOLISM

⑲ Fasting test
Initial measurement of both blood and urinary ketone bodies.
During the test period: no food, water only.
Every two hours, check BS, plus insulin/C-peptide, β-OH-butyrate and free fatty acids if indicated.
Monitor the acid–base equilibrium.
Duration of test: – until onset of hypoglycemia (BS ≤ 30 mg/dl)
  – or BS ≤ 40 mg/dl + symptoms of hypoglycemia
  – or constantly low BS + marked acetonuria.
Fasting time as a rule 4–10 h in neonates and infants, 12–24 h in older children. In a 24 h period, the test provokes as frequently as the 2-deoxyglucose test.
Special indications: suspected hyperinsulinism or abnormal gluconeogenesis.

㉑ Fructose tolerance test (intravenous)
Initial values for fructose, glucose, phosphate, uric acid, magnesium, lactate, alanine in plasma/serum.
Administer fructose (200 mg/kg) within four minutes i.v.
Monitor measurements after 5, 10, 20, 30, 40, 60, 90, 120 min.
Result: in fructose-1-phosphate-aldolase deficiency the concentrations of fructose, glucose, and phosphorus fall 30 min after the injection, while alanine, lactate, uric acid and magnesium levels rise. With continued fructose elimination, the levels rise further for glucose and phosphate, while the concentrations of uric acid and magnesium fall simultaneously. There is a similar concentration profile in fructose-1,6-diphosphatase deficiency, but initially lactate rises higher, as also in enzyme defects in the pyruvate dehydrogenase complex.
Severe hypoglycemia (BS ≤ 20 mg/dl) should be treated daily with i.v. glucose. The glucagon effect is not enough!

㉒ Galactose stress test (oral)
Not to be used in galactosemia.
24 h milk-free diet.
Measure the concentrations of galactose and lactate in blood.
Give galactose (10% solution) in the morning, after fasting.
Dosage: small children   1.75 g/kg ⎫
        preschool-age children 1.5 g/kg ⎬ maximum 40 g
        schoolchildren   1.0 g/kg ⎭
Check galactose and lactate levels after 30, 60, 90, 120 min.
Result: normal: after 30–60 min galactose rises by 20–40 mg/dl, returning to initial value within two hours; parallel with this a transitory rise in lactate
 abnormal: marked increase in galactose and lactate in glycogen storage disease types III, VI, VIII.

MEMORIX PEDIATRICS

(23) Glucagon test
Fasting period 4–10 h (neonates, infants), 10–24 h (older children)
Measure blood sugar (BS), then glucagon (0.1 mg/kg i.m. or 0.03 mg/kg i.v.)
Check BS after 5, 15, 30, 45, 60, 90, 120 min
Results:

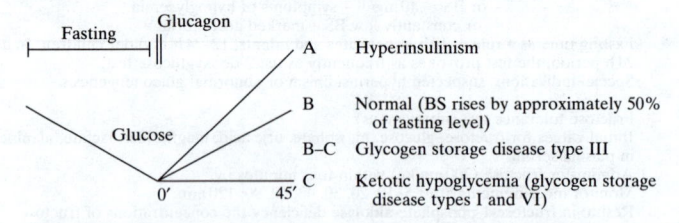

A	Hyperinsulinism
B	Normal (BS rises by approximately 50% of fasting level)
B–C	Glycogen storage disease type III
C	Ketotic hypoglycemia (glycogen storage disease types I and VI)

Postprandial glucagon test: normal BS increase in glycogen storage disease type III
lesser BS increase in phosphorylase deficiency.

Glucose loading test (i.v.)
O value for BS and lactate.
0.5 g glucose/kg i.v. within from 2–3 min.
Measure glucose and lactose levels after 5, 15, 30, 60, 90 min.
Results: healthy subjects: lactate rise to the upper limit of normal defect in pyruvate
dehydrogenase complex: lactate ↑↑
NB: danger of lactacidosis.

(24) Glucose tolerance test (oral (OGTT)
Preconditions: no infection, no disorders of absorption; at least 50 g of
carbohydrate per day for three days before the test; bedrest during the test.
Night-time fast before test of 12–14 h.
Then, on empty stomach give 1.75 g/kg or 50 g/m^2 (maximal dose 100 g) of
glucose or as oligosaccharide mixture, as a solution (maximum 25%) drunk
within 2–5 min.
The 'ideal' weight figure is used to calculate bodyweight.
Measure BS after 30, 60, 90, 120 min (3, 4, 5, 6 h).
Measure the insulin/C-peptide together with the BS.
Results: normal: BS within normal limits after 60 and 120 min
abnormal: BS raised after 60 min and longer (see p. 222)
BS below normal after 4–6 h, simultaneously insulin ↑ =
hyperinsulinism.

METABOLISM

(25) Glucose tolerance test (intravenous)
Night-time fast, bedrest during the test.
Fasting blood sugar (BS).
25% dextrose solution i.v. over 2–4 min, dosage: 0.33 g/kg.
With higher dosage, there is a danger of glycosuria, which simulates a better glucose tolerance (raised glucose level).
BS every 10 min up to 1 h measured in separate venous blood via an indwelling catheter. If there is no glycosuria, calculate the assimilation constant for glucose (GC):

$$GC = \frac{0.693}{t/2\,(h)}$$

Obtaining t/2: entered on half-logarithmic grid (ordinate = logarithmic glucose level), abscissa = arithmetical time. Choose a point along the straight line (diagonal), halve its ordinate and look for the second point at the intersection of half the ordinate level with the diagonal. The difference in the abscissas of both points corresponds to t/2. In glycosuria, transfer must be allowed for (Dost, 1968). Calculation in this case is:

$$\text{Glucose distribution coefficient } \Delta' = \frac{\text{administered glucose (mg)}}{(C_0 - C)\,\text{bodyweight (g)}}$$

C = fasting BS (mg/ml) C_0 = BS (mg/ml) graphically extrapolated to 'zero time'

Glucose pool (Pl) = $\Delta' \times C$ (mg/g)
Glucose transfer (Tf') = Pl $\times$ GC   Tf = Tf' − QH
QH = amount of glucose excreted in the urine per h

No glycosuria: Tf = Tf' or GC = k

Corrected glucose assimilation coefficient $k = \dfrac{Tf}{Pl}$

Normal levels in healthy children

Age	C mg/ml	t1/2 h	k h^{-1}	Δ' mg/ml	Pl mg/g	Tf mg/g/h
1 d	0.43	0.82	0.85	0.44	0.19	0.16
2 d	0.35	0.96	0.72	0.43	0.15	0.11
3 d	0.39	0.87	0.80	0.39	0.15	0.12
4 d	0.29	0.53	1.30	0.42	0.12	0.16
5 d	0.48	0.54	1.29	0.36	0.18	0.23
6–10 d	0.60	0.38	1.81	0.33	0.20	0.36
11–20 d	0.62	0.38	1.83	0.45	0.28	0.51
21–30 d	0.66	0.28	2.47	0.32	0.21	0.52
31–90 d	0.64	0.23	3.01	0.29	0.19	0.56
4–12 mon	0.77	0.16	4.40	0.23	0.18	0.78
1–6 y	0.72	0.32	2.32	0.24	0.17	0.38
7–14 y	0.81	0.34	2.22	0.19	0.15	0.32
>14 y	0.81	0.41	1.70	0.19	0.15	0.26

MEMORIX PEDIATRICS

㉖ Glucose requirement
　Target: a constant blood sugar (BS) of around 80 mg/dl (4.44 mmol/l).
　Lowest possible amount of glucose i.v. (to avoid irritation of veins)
　Requirement: normal ≤6 mg/kg/min
　　　　　　　hyperinsulinism >10 mg/kg/min.

㉗ Glycerine loading test (oral)
　Principle: testing glyconeogenesis.
　Fasting level (morning) of BS, phosphate, lactate and bicarbonate in blood or serum; if possible also pH/bicarbonate in urine.
　Glycerine (1 g/kg) as 20% solution orally.
　Measuring times: 15, 30, 45, 60, 90, 120 min (blood levels)
　　　　　　　　　60, 120 min (urine levels)
　Results: normal: slight rise in glucose, no lactacidosis,
　　　　　abnormal: fall of glucose, bicarbonate and phosphate; rise of lactate in the blood. Bicarbonate excretion in urine (deficiency of fructose-1-phosphate aldolase or fructose-1,6-diphosphatase).

㉘ Glycerine loading test (i.v.)
　0.09 g/kg as 10% solution in 0.9% NaCl solution given i.v. over 4 min.
　Test conditions as in oral loading test.

㊵ Leucine loading test
　Fasting BS
　Glucagon (0.015 mg/kg i.v.) in readiness!
　L-leucine (150 mg/kg) in sweetened tea (only use artificial sweetener).
　Measure BS and insulin after 15, 30, 45, 60, 90 min.
　Results: normal: nor fall in glucose, no insulin rise
　　　　　abnormal: between 15 and 45 min, fall in glucose of more than 50% of the initial level and a rise in insulin = leucine-sensitive hypoglycemia (inject glucagon!).

METABOLISM

Mucopolysaccharidoses

C	Chondroitin sulfate	F	Fibroblasts	Dm	Dysostosis, multiple
D	Dermatan sulfate	L	Leukocytes	HS	Hepatosplenomegaly
H	Heparan sulfate	P	Plasma/serum	M	Mental development
K	Keratan sulfate				

Disease (type)	Lysosomal enzyme defect	Genotype	Chief signs	Diagnosis — Urine excretory products (24 h urine)	Diagnosis — Enzyme assay
Pfaunder–Hurler (I-H)	α-L-iduronidase	AR	Dysmorphia +++, retarded growth, M ↓, corneal opacity, HS, Dm; onset – first year	D, H	F, L
Scheie (I-S)	α-L-iduronidase	AR	Corneal opacity, Dm+, HS, heart valve defects; onset – school age	D	F, L
Hunter (II)	Sulfoiduronate sulfatase	XR	Type II A as I-H corneal opacity rare, Dm++, coarse skin; Type II B less marked, Dm ++	D, H	F, L, P
Sanfilippo (III A)	Sulfamate sulfatase	AR	Dysmorphia +, Dm+, M ↓↓↓, deafness	H	F, L
(III B)	α-N-acetyl-glucosaminidase	AR			
(III C)	Acetyl-CoA-α-glucosaminide-N-acetyl transferase	AR			
(III D)	Glucosamine-6-sulfate sulfatase	AR			
Morquio (IV A)	Galactosamine-G-sulfate sulfatase	AR	Skeletal dysplasia +++, retarded growth		F
(IV B)	specific β-galactosidase	AR	less than IV A	K, C	F, L
Maroteaux–Lamy (VI)	Galactosamine-4-sulfate sulfatase	AR	VI A: Dm +++, retarded growth, corneal opacity VI B: less marked	D	F, L
Sly (VII)	β-glucuronidase	AR	Dm++, retarded growth, M ↓	D, H	F, L, P

Type V not yet elucidated.

Lipid storage diseases
Basic substances

Sphingosine $CH_3-(CH_2)_1 \cdots\cdots (CH_2)_{12}-CH=CH-CH-CH-CH_2O \leftarrow \mathbf{R}$

$+$ $\phantom{CH_3-(CH_2)_{22} \cdots\cdots\cdots\cdots\cdots\cdots (CH_2)}$ OH NH

$|$ Ceramidase

Fatty acids $CH_3-(CH_2)_{22} \cdots\cdots\cdots\cdots (CH_2)_1-C=O$

Ceramide + **R** = storage product ——— blocked breakdown

① Ceramide — H

② Ceramide + Phosphocholine

③ Ceramide + Glu

④ Ceramide + Gal

⑤ Ceramide + Gal-SO_3^-

⑥ Ceramide — Glu — Gal + Gal

⑦ Ceramide — Glu — Gal + Gal-NAc ⟋NS-NS

⑧ Ceramide — Glu — Gal — Gal + Gal-NAc

⑨ Ceramide — Glu — Gal ⟋NS-NS ＼Gal + Gal ＼NAc

Glu = glucose; Gal = galactose; NAc = N-acetyl-; NS = Neuraminic acid.

METABOLISM

Synopsis of lipid storage diseases

Disease	Enzyme defect	Storage substance	Age at manifestation HS, D, BM	Main findings	Diagnostic enzyme assay
Farber (= Lipogranulomatosis)	Ceramidase	Ceramide (R = H) ①	Infants Small children	Lipogranuloma, HS Lipogranuloma, CNS-D	F, L, A
Niemann–Pick	Sphingomyelinase	Type I: sphingomyelin (R = phosphocholine) Type II: Type I + cholesterol ②	Infants Small children, acute and subacute Types I and II	HS, CNS-D	F, L
Gaucher	Glucocerebroside-β-glucosidase	Glucocerebroside (R-glucose) ③	Variable: Type I chronic infants: Type II acute variable: Type III subacute	Type I: HS, BM Type II: HS, CNS-D Type III: type I + II	F, L, A
Krabbe (globoid cell leukodystrophy	Galacto-cerebroside-β-galactosidase	Galactocerebroside (R-galactose) ④	Variable	CNS-D	F, L
Metachromatic leukodystrophy	Arylsulfatase A	Galactosyl-3-sulfate ceramide (R = galactosyl-3-sulfate) ⑤	Variable	CNS-D	F, L
Fabry	Galactosidase	Ceramidetrihexoside (R-Glu-Gal-Gal) ⑥	Childhood	Corneal and lens opacities, acro-paresthesias, vascular diseases, CNS, kidneys, heart	L, plasma
GM1-gangliosidosis	β-galactosidase	GM1-ganglioside ⑦	Infancy, juveniles	CNS-D, HS	F, L, A
Tay–Sachs	β-hexosaminidase A	GM2-ganglioside ⑧	Infancy, juveniles	CNS-D	F, plasma
Sandhoff	β-hexosamidase B	Asialo-GM2-ganglioside Globoside ⑨	Infancy	CNS-D	F, plasma

HS = hepatosplenomegaly; D = degeneration; BM = bone marrow affected; A = amniotic cells; F = fibroblasts; L = leukocytes.

233

Properties of serum lipoproteins

Density class	Chylomicrons	VLDL (very low density lipoproteins)	LDL (low density lipoproteins)	HDL (high density lipoproteins)
Density g/ml	0.95	0.95–1.006	1.019–1.063	1.063–1.21
Shape	◯ (large)	◯	◯ (small)	✧
Diameter (nm)	100–1000	30–70	15–25	7.5×10
Lipoprotein electrophoresis (serum)	Start			
Position (= serum fraction)	Mobility	Pre-β-fraction	β-Globulins	α_2-Globulins
Lipid:protein ratio	99:1	90:10	78:22	50:50
Apolipoprotein	A I, A IV, C I to C III, E, B 48	C I to C III, E, B 100	B 100	A I, A II, C I to C III, E
Synthesis site	Mucosal cells Duodenum	Liver (duodenum)	Intravascular endothelium	Liver

Function of the apoproteins

Lipoprotein binding

Lipoprotein transport

Recognition of specific cell membrane receptors for lipoprotein uptake

Enzyme activation (lipoprotein lipase, lecithin–cholesterol–acetyltransferase)

Basic lipoprotein structure

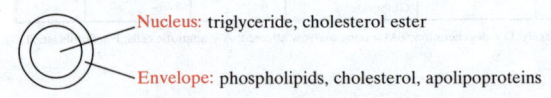

Nucleus: triglyceride, cholesterol ester

Envelope: phospholipids, cholesterol, apolipoproteins

METABOLISM

Hypercholesterolemia: diagnosis and screening according to history

(After Recommendations of the American Academy of Pediatrics (1992).)

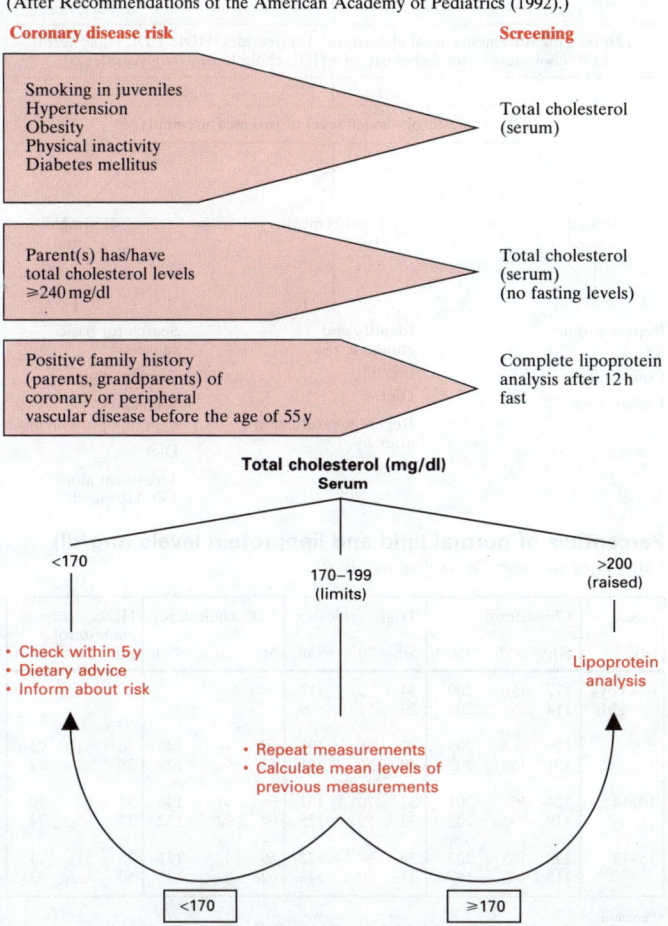

Coronary disease risk   **Screening**

Smoking in juveniles
Hypertension
Obesity
Physical inactivity
Diabetes mellitus

→ Total cholesterol (serum)

Parent(s) has/have total cholesterol levels ≥240 mg/dl

→ Total cholesterol (serum) (no fasting levels)

Positive family history (parents, grandparents) of coronary or peripheral vascular disease before the age of 55 y

→ Complete lipoprotein analysis after 12 h fast

Total cholesterol (mg/dl) Serum

- **<170**
  - Check within 5 y
  - Dietary advice
  - Inform about risk

- **170–199 (limits)**
  - Repeat measurements
  - Calculate mean levels of previous measurements
  - <170 → (back to <170 branch)
  - ≥170 → Lipoprotein analysis

- **>200 (raised)**
  - Lipoprotein analysis

Lipoprotein analysis

Lipoprotein analysis

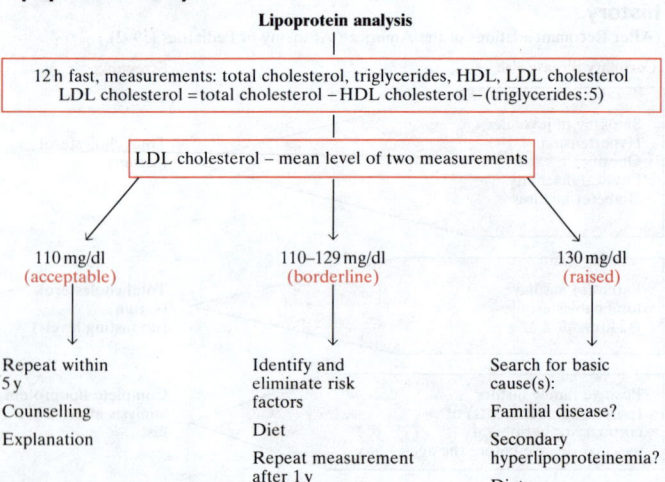

12 h fast, measurements: total cholesterol, triglycerides, HDL, LDL cholesterol
LDL cholesterol = total cholesterol − HDL cholesterol − (triglycerides:5)

LDL cholesterol − mean level of two measurements

110 mg/dl (acceptable)

Repeat within 5 y

Counselling

Explanation

110–129 mg/dl (borderline)

Identify and eliminate risk factors

Diet

Repeat measurement after 1 y

130 mg/dl (raised)

Search for basic cause(s):

Familial disease?

Secondary hyperlipoproteinemia?

Diet

Treatment aim: 130–110 mg/dl

Percentiles of normal lipid and lipoprotein levels (mg/dl)

(After Lipid Research Clinics Program (1980).)

Age (y)	Cholesterol 5th[a]	50th[a]	95th[a]	Triglycerides 5th	50th	95th	LDL cholesterol 5th	50th	95th	HDL cholesterol 5th	50th	95th
0–4 boys	112	156	200	34	59	112						
girls	114	151	203	29	51	99						
5–9	126	163	205	32	55	105	68	98	140	36	52	73
	121	159	203	30	51	101	63	90	129	38	54	74
10–14	124	158	201	37	70	131	68	94	136	37	52	70
	119	155	202	32	59	125	64	94	132	37	55	74
15–19	120	155	203	39	68	132	59	93	137	35	51	74
	113	146	197	37	69	148	62	93	130	30	46	63

[a] Percentile.

METABOLISM

Familial hyperlipoproteinemia

Designation	Type	Cause defect	Lipid and lipoprotein findings	Associated findings	Mode of interitance
Lipoprotein lipase (LPL) deficiency	Ia	Extrahepatic LPL	C ↑, TG ↑, Chylomicrons ↑↑↑, Apo-B₄₈ ↑, LDL n, HDL ↓	Pancreatitis, xanthoma	AR
Apo-C-II deficiency	Ib	LPL cofactor C-II	C ↑, TG ↑, chylomicrons ↑↑, LDL n, HDL ↓	As Ia	AR
Hypercholesterolemia homozygous form	IIa	LDL receptor	C ↑↑↑, LDL ↑↑↑, HDL↓	Xanthoma CA 20y	AD
heterozygous form			C ↑↑↑, LDL ↑↑	Xanthoma CA 60y	
Hypercholesterolemia	IIb	Apo-B-100	C ↑↑, TG ↑, LDL ↑↑, VLDL ↑, HDL n (↑)	Xanthoma CA 60y	AR
Dysbetalipoproteinemia	III	Apo-E-2	C ↑, TG ↑, LDL ↑, IDL ↑↑, VLDL ↑↑, HDL n	Xanthoma CA, PA	AR
Hypertriglyceridemia	IV	Overproduction Apo-B-100, VLDL	C ↑, TG ↑ ↑↑ VLDL ↑↑, LDL n HDL n(↓)	CA	AD
Hypertriglyceridemia	V	VLDL breakdown ↓	C ↑, TG ↑, chylomicrons ↑, VLDL ↑↑, LDL n, HDL ↓	Pancreatitis CA	AR
Hyperalphalipoproteinemia	–		C n, TG n, LDL n, HDL ↓, Apo-AI ↑	–	

C = cholesterol; TG = triglyceride; CA = coronary artery disease; VLDL = VLDL cholesterol; PA = peripheral arterial disease; IDL = intermediate density lipoproteins; n = normal; AR = autosomal recessive; AD = autosomal dominant.

Familial hypolipoproteinemia

Designation	Lipids Cholesterol	Triglyceride	Lipoproteins HDL cholesterol	LDL cholesterol	Apolipoproteins	Associated findings	Mode of inheritance
A-α-lipoproteinemia	n	n	∅	n	AI↓↓, AII↓	CA	AD
Hypo-α-lipoproteinemia	n (↓)	n (↑)	↓↓	n (↑)	AI↓, AII↓	CA	AR
Tangier disease	→	n (↑)	↓↓↓	→	AI↓, AII↓	Corneal opacities, hepatosplenomegaly, peripheral neuropathies, cholesterol storage in RES	
A-β-lipoproteinemia (apolipoprotein-B deficiency, Bassen–Kornzweig)	↓↓	→	n	∅	B 100 ↓↓	Retinitis pigmentosa, ataxia	AR
Hypo-β-lipoproteinemia	↓↓↓	n	n	→	B 100 ↓↓	homozygous: as in A-β-lipoproteinemia heterozygous: no symptoms	AD

RES = reticuloendothelial system.

METABOLISM

Functions of the peroxisomes

① β-oxidation of over long-chain fatty acids
② Plasmalogen biosynthesis
③ β-oxidation of bile acid biosynthesis
④ 1-pipecolic acid breakdown (= bypass in 1-lysin breakdown)
⑤ Glyoxylate metabolism
⑥ Phytic acid oxidation
⑦ H_2O_2-splitting (catalase)

Defect of all functions ①–⑦:

– Zellweger syndrome (ZS)
– Neonatal adrenoleukodystrophy (NALD)
– Infantile Refsum's disease (IR)

Multiple enzyme defects:

– Punctate rhizomele chondrodysplasia (PRCD) ② ⑥
– Zellweger-like syndrome (ZS-like) ① ②

Single enzyme defects:

– adrenoleukodystrophy (ALD) ①
– pseudo-Zellweger's syndrome (pseudo-ZS) ① ④
– pseudoneonatal adrenoleukodystrophy (pseudo-NADL) ①
– hyperpipecolic acidemia (HPA) ④

MEMORIX PEDIATRICS

Synopsis of peroxisomal diseases
(After Schutgens *et al.* (1986).)

Symptoms	ZS	NALD	IR	HPA	PRCD	ALD	Pseudo-ZS	Pseudo-NALD
Onset at birth	+	+	1–6 months	+	+	childhood	+	+
Craniofacial dysmorphism								
– high forehead	+++	++	+	+	+++	–	+++	–
– epicanthus	+++	++	++	+	+++	–	+++	–
– high palate	+++	++	+	++		–	+++	–
– ear dysmorphism	+++	++	+	++	++	–	+++	–
Ocular								
– cataract	+++	+	–		+++		+++	
– abnormal retinal pigmentation	+++	+++	+++	+++			+++	+++
– optic hypoplasia/atrophy	+++	+++		+++		++	+++	+++
Neurological								
– hypotonia	+++	++	+	++	–	–	+++	+++
– hyporeflexia	+++	++	+	+	–	–	+++	+++
– seizures	+++	++	+	++	–	++	+++	+++
– nystagmus	+++	++	+	++		+	+++	+++
– hearing disorders	+++	+++	+++	+++	+++	+	+++	+++
Others								
Hepatomegaly	+++	++	+	++			+++	+
Renal cysts	+++	–	–				+	
Adrenal cortical atrophy	+	+++		–		+++	+	
Extra-epiphyseal calcification	++	–	–	–	+++			
Mode of inheritance	AR	AR	AR	AR	AR	XR		AR

See p. 239 for key to disease names; – missing; + occurs; ++ frequently present; +++ almost always present.

ENDOCRINOLOGY/GROWTH

Calcium phosphate metabolism: hormone regulation

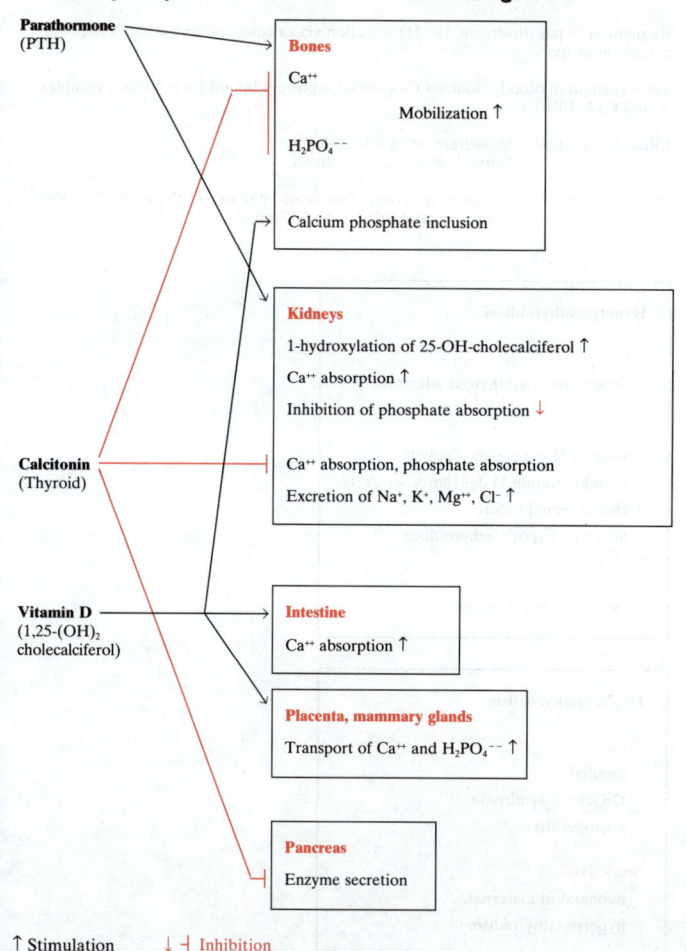

Parathormone (PTH)

Bones
- Ca^{++}
- Mobilization ↑
- $H_2PO_4^{--}$
- Calcium phosphate inclusion

Kidneys
- 1-hydroxylation of 25-OH-cholecalciferol ↑
- Ca^{++} absorption ↑
- Inhibition of phosphate absorption ↓
- Ca^{++} absorption, phosphate absorption
- Excretion of Na^+, K^+, Mg^{++}, Cl^- ↑

Calcitonin (Thyroid)

Vitamin D ($1,25-(OH)_2$ cholecalciferol)

Intestine
- Ca^{++} absorption ↑

Placenta, mammary glands
- Transport of Ca^{++} and $H_2PO_4^{--}$ ↑

Pancreas
- Enzyme secretion

↑ Stimulation ↓ ⊣ Inhibition

Parathormone: regulation/disorders

Regulation of parathormone (PTH) secretion via calcium concentration in the extracellular space.

Total calcium in blood = ionized Ca (~50%) + protein-bound Ca (~40%) + complex-bound Ca (~10%).

Clinical chemistry: Measurement of total calcium.
Normal range: 2.1–2.6 mmol/l.

Protein binding: A change in serum albumin of 1 g/dl causes the same directional change in total calcium by 0.17 mmol/l.

Hyperparathyroidism

Primary:
  hyperplasia/parathyroid adenoma

Secondary:
  vitamin D deficiency – rickets
  pseudo-vitamin D deficiency – rickets
  chronic renal failure
  maternal hypoparathyroidism

Tertiary:
  chronic hypocalcemia

Hypoparathyroidism

Primary:
  familial
  DiGeorge syndrome
  postoperative

Secondary:
  neonatal in maternal
  hyperparathyroidism

ENDOCRINOLOGY/GROWTH

Vitamin D metabolism and rachitogenic disorders

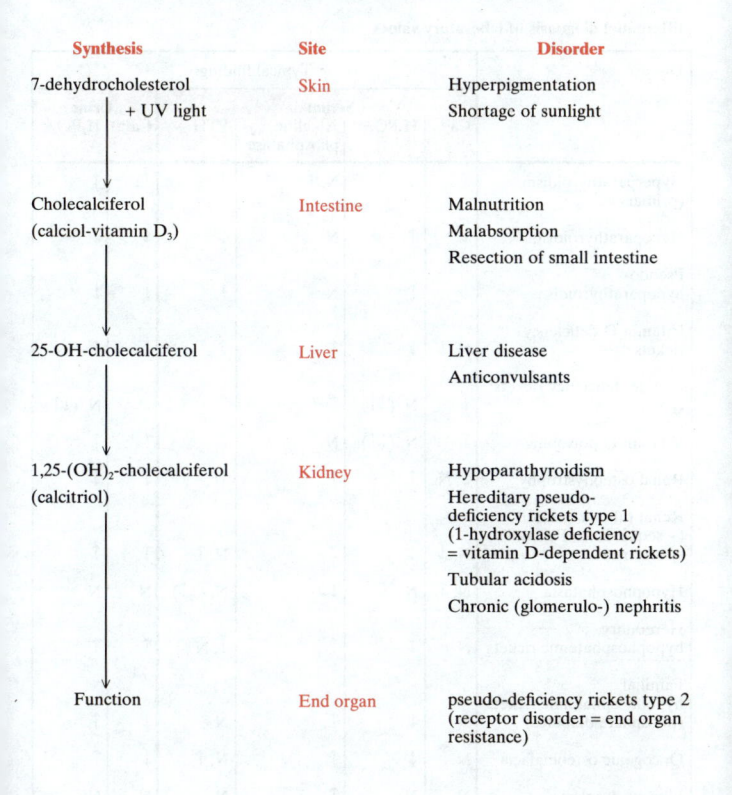

Synthesis	Site	Disorder
7-dehydrocholesterol + UV light	Skin	Hyperpigmentation Shortage of sunlight
↓		
Cholecalciferol (calciol-vitamin D_3)	Intestine	Malnutrition Malabsorption Resection of small intestine
↓		
25-OH-cholecalciferol	Liver	Liver disease Anticonvulsants
↓		
1,25-$(OH)_2$-cholecalciferol (calcitriol)	Kidney	Hypoparathyroidism Hereditary pseudo-deficiency rickets type 1 (1-hydroxylase deficiency = vitamin D-dependent rickets) Tubular acidosis Chronic (glomerulo-) nephritis
↓		
Function	End organ	pseudo-deficiency rickets type 2 (receptor disorder = end organ resistance)

Calcium phosphate metabolic diseases

Differential diagnosis of laboratory values

Disease	\	\	Typical findings	\	\	\
	Serum				**Urine**	
	Ca^{2+}	H$_2$PO$_4{}^{2-}$	Alkaline phosphatase	PTH	Ca^{2+}	H$_2$PO$_4{}^{2-}$
Hyperparathyroidism (primary)	↑	↓	N, ↑	↑	↑	↑
Hypoparathyroidism	↓	↑	N	↓	↓	↓
Pseudo-hypoparathyroidism	↓	↑	N	↑	↓	↓
Vitamin D deficiency rickets	N, ↓	↓	↑	↑	↓	↑
Pseudo-deficiency rickets type 1	↓	N, (↓↑)	↑	↑	↓	N, (↓↑)
Vitamin D poisoning	↑	N, (↓↑)	N	↓	↑	↑
Renal osteodystrophy	↓, N	↑	↑	↑	↓	↓
Renal tubular acidosis (+ sequence to Fanconi's syndrome)	N, ↓	↓	↑	N, ↑	↑	↑
Hypophosphatasia	N, ↑	N	↓↓	N, (↓↑)	N	N
Hereditary hypophosphatemic rickets	N	↓	↑	↓, N	↑	↑
Familial hypophosphatemic rickets (phosphate diabetes)	N	↓	↑	N	↓	↑
Oncogenic osteomalacia	N	↓	↑	N, ↑	↓	↑
Fibrous dysplasia	N	N	↑	N	N	N
Osteopetrosis	N	N	N		↓	N

ENDOCRINOLOGY/GROWTH

Growth

Short stature	= Height <3rd percentile (growth curve)
Decreased growth rate	= Rate of growth <10th percentile (rate of growth curve)
Enhanced growth	= >97th percentile (growth curve)
Tall stature	= >97th percentile
Catch-up growth (growth spurt)	= Increased growth rate after removal of the cause of retarded growth while still in growing phases
Slow down growth	= Decreased growth rate after stopping hormone substitution. With growth outside percentile limits, conversion to the standard deviation score (SDS):

$$SDS = \frac{\text{Height as measured} - \text{mean value according to age}}{\text{standard deviation from the mean}}$$

Mean target size (after Tanner):

$$SDS = \frac{\text{Height as measured} - \text{mean value according to age}}{\text{standard deviation from the mean}}$$

$$\text{Boys} = \frac{\text{height (father)} + \text{height (mother)} + 13}{2} \pm 8.5 \, (2\,SD)$$

Range of target height: Boys = From height of mother + 13 cm to height of father

Girls = From height of mother − 13 cm to height of father

Determination of bone-age (Greulich and Pyle method)

Comparison of X-ray film of the left hand with age-normalized standard films

Assessment: according to the presence of the wrist bones and epiphyseal centres (ulna + distal radius, phalanges)

according to the degree of fusion of epiphyses and shaft

according to the stage of development of form and shape of the ossification centers

Dwarfism: history/investigation
Principal data of child's own and family history in dwarfism/retarded growth

Family:

Final height of siblings, parents and grandparents

Target height of the child or adolescent

Pubertal development of parents

Child (patient):

Course of pregnancy and birth

Length, weight, head circumference at birth

Somatic development

Mental development

Conditions of social development

Previous and present illnesses

Medication

Investigations in dwarfism/retarded growth

General examination

Physical proportions:
   upper/lower body lengths, trunk–limb proportions

Height, weight, head circumference

Estimation of target height

Pubertal development

Voice broken?

Dysmorphic signs (facies, ears)

Goiter

Neurological status

Radiological investigation:
   skull, antero-posterior, lateral
   bones of the left hand
   + others, according to findings

Hormone status:

Screening, HGH (human growth hormone), somatomedin C, sleep pulses of HGH

Provocation test: insulin test

ENDOCRINOLOGY/GROWTH

Skeletal development

Radiograph of the hand: determination of bone age from the postnatal ossification centers
(After Schmid)

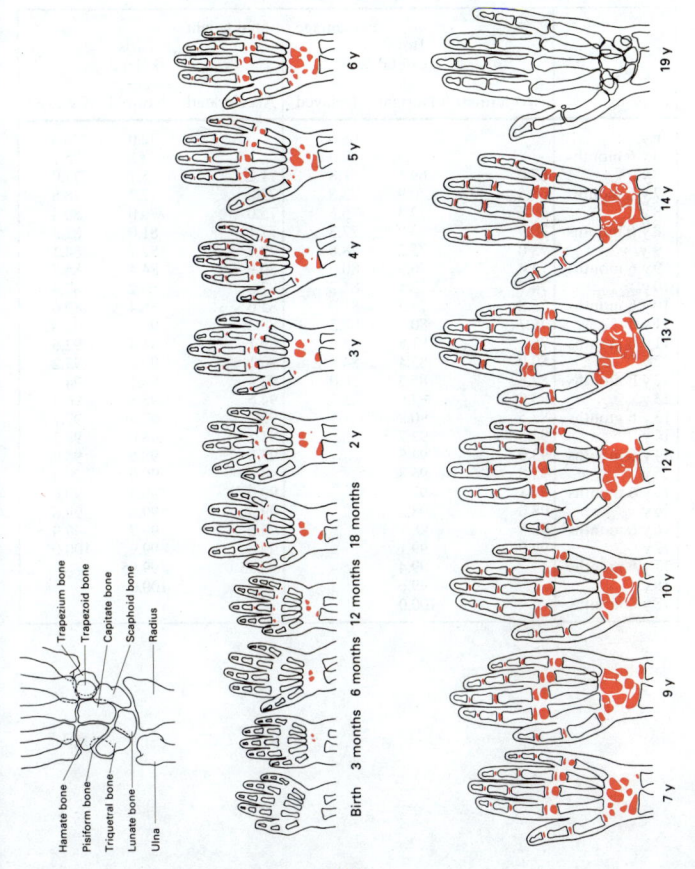

Growth: estimation of final height

Estimation of likely final height from the skeletal age reached and actual body height (after Bayley and Pinneau, 1952).

$$\text{Final height} = \frac{\text{present height (cm)} \times 100}{\text{skeletal age, percentage of final height}}$$

Bone age	Boys Accelerated	Boys skeletal age Normal	Boys Delayed	Girls Accelerated	Girls skeletal age Normal	Girls Delayed
6 y			68.0		72.0	73.3
6 y 6 months			70.0		73.8	75.1
7 y	67.0	69.5	71.8	71.2	75.7	77.0
7 y 6 months	68.5	70.9	73.8	73.2	77.2	78.8
8 y	69.6	72.3	75.6	75.0	79.0	80.4
8 y 6 months	70.9	73.9	77.3	77.1	81.0	82.3
9 y	72.0	75.2	78.6	79.0	82.7	84.1
9 y 6 months	73.4	76.9	80.0	80.9	84.4	85.8
10 y	74.7	78.4	81.2	82.8	86.2	87.4
10 y 6 months	75.8	79.5	81.9	85.6	88.4	89.6
11 y	76.7	80.4	82.3	88.3	90.6	91.8
11 y 6 months	78.6	81.8	83.2	89.1	91.4	92.6
12 y	80.9	83.4	84.5	90.1	92.2	93.2
12 y 6 months	82.8	85.3	86.0	92.4	94.1	94.9
13 y	85.0	87.6	88.0	94.5	95.8	96.4
13 y 6 months	87.5	90.2		96.2	97.4	97.7
14 y	90.5	92.7		97.2	98.0	98.3
14 y 6 months	93.0	94.8		98.0	98.6	98.9
15 y	95.8	96.8		98.6	99.0	99.4
15 y 6 months	97.1	97.6		99.0	99.3	99.6
16 y	98.0	98.2		99.3	99.6	99.8
16 y 6 months	98.5	98.7		99.5	99.7	99.9
17 y	99.0	99.1		99.8	99.9	100.0
17 y 6 months		99.4		99.95	99.95	
18 y		99.6			100.0	
18 y 6 months		100.0				

ENDOCRINOLOGY/GROWTH

Growth and weight percentile curves (girls 0–18 years)

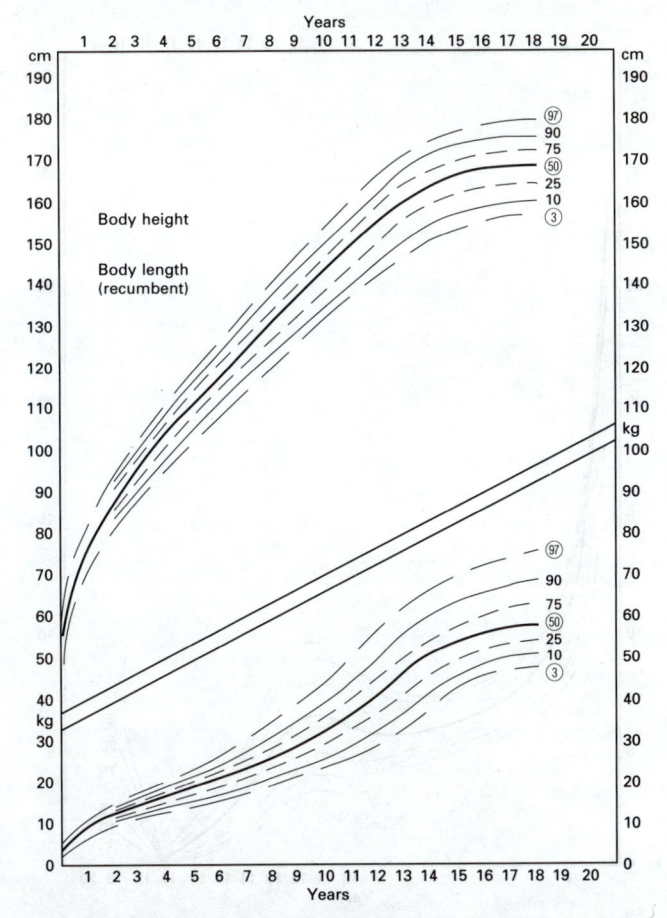

(Source: Reinken *et al.*, 1980; Brandt, 1980; Brandt, 1966. Reproduced by kind permission of Kabi Pharmacia GmbH, D-91054 Erlangen.)

MEMORIX PEDIATRICS

Growth velocity percentiles (girls 0–18 years)

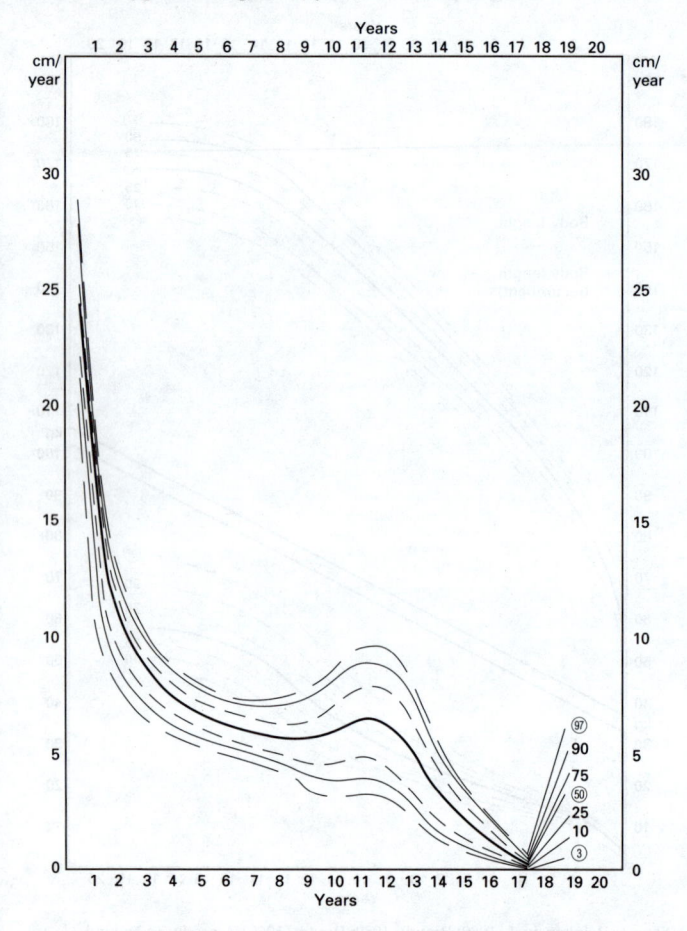

(Reproduced by kind permission of Kabi Pharmacia GmbH, D-91054 Erlangen.)

ENDOCRINOLOGY/GROWTH

Growth and weight percentile curves (boys 0–18 years)

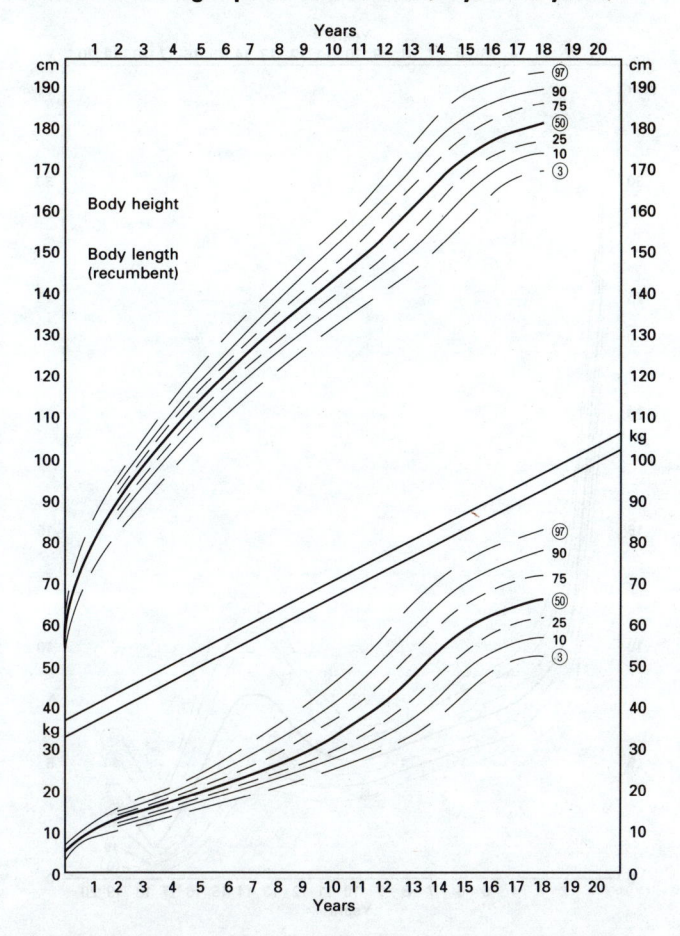

(Reproduced by kind permission of Kabia Pharmacia GmbH, D-91054 Erlangen.)

MEMORIX PEDIATRICS

Growth velocity percentiles (boys 0–18 years)

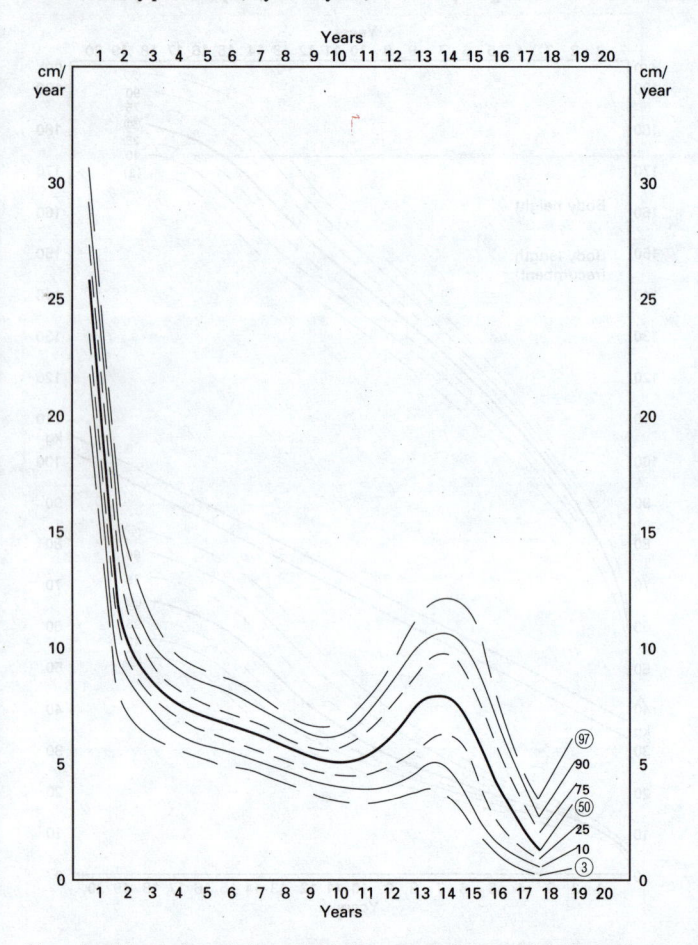

(Reproduced by kind permission of Kabi Pharmacia GmbH, D-91054 Erlangen.)

ENDOCRINOLOGY/GROWTH

Typical growth curves

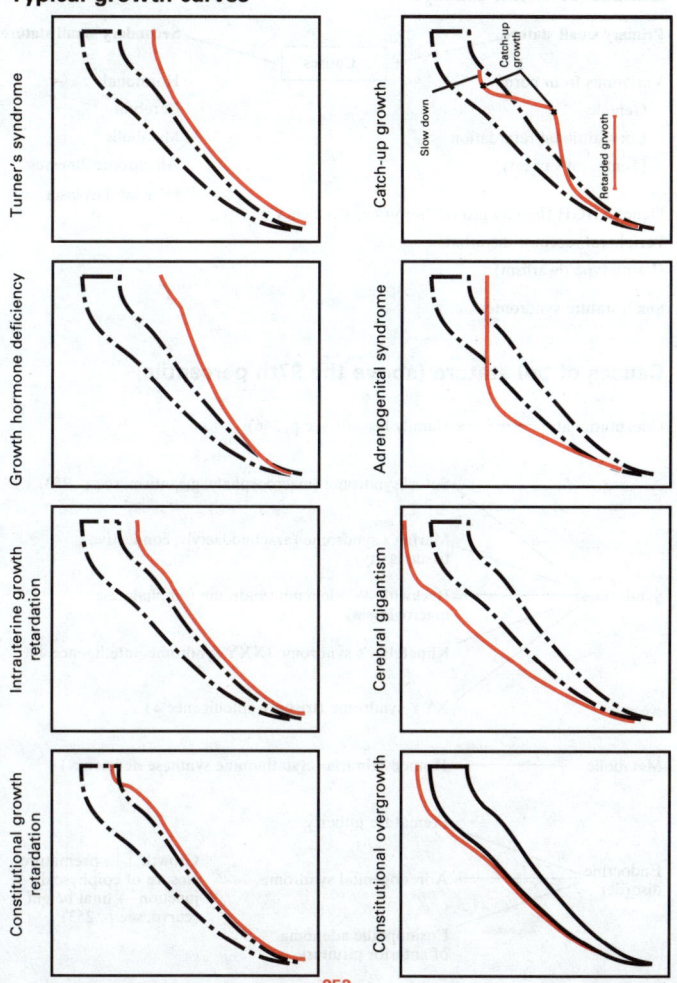

- Turner's syndrome
- Growth hormone deficiency
- Intrauterine growth retardation
- Constitutional growth retardation
- Catch-up growth (Slow down, Catch-up growth, Retarded growth)
- Adrenogenital syndrome
- Cerebral gigantism
- Constitutional overgrowth

MEMORIX PEDIATRICS

Causes of small stature

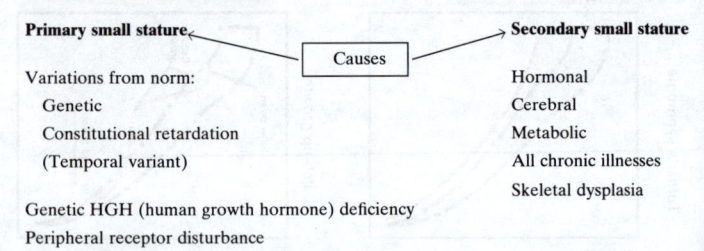

Primary small stature ← Causes → **Secondary small stature**

Variations from norm:
  Genetic
  Constitutional retardation
  (Temporal variant)

Genetic HGH (human growth hormone) deficiency

Peripheral receptor disturbance
(Laron type dwarfism)

Small stature syndromes

Hormonal
Cerebral
Metabolic
All chronic illnesses
Skeletal dysplasia

Causes of tall stature (above the 97th percentile)

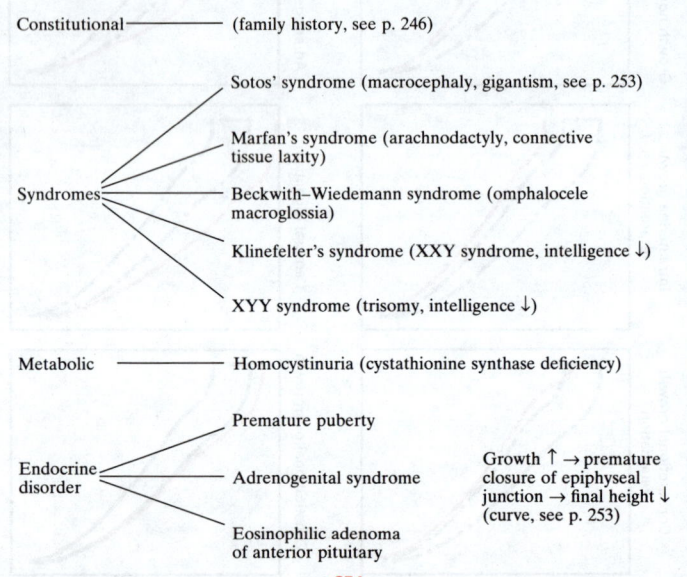

Constitutional —— (family history, see p. 246)

Syndromes:
- Sotos' syndrome (macrocephaly, gigantism, see p. 253)
- Marfan's syndrome (arachnodactyly, connective tissue laxity)
- Beckwith–Wiedemann syndrome (omphalocele macroglossia)
- Klinefelter's syndrome (XXY syndrome, intelligence ↓)
- XYY syndrome (trisomy, intelligence ↓)

Metabolic —— Homocystinuria (cystathionine synthase deficiency)

Endocrine disorder:
- Premature puberty
- Adrenogenital syndrome
- Eosinophilic adenoma of anterior pituitary

Growth ↑ → premature closure of epiphyseal junction → final height ↓ (curve, see p. 253)

ENDOCRINOLOGY/GROWTH

Developmental stages of secondary sex characteristics
(After Tanner (1962).)

Breast development ♀

Stage 1 No glands palpable. No change until beginning of puberty.

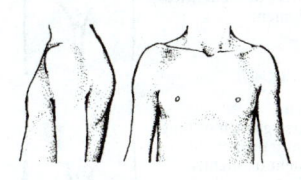

Stage 2 Breast bud stage: start of breast development. Areola diameter increases, elevation of breast and papilla, the areola bulges forward (breast bud).

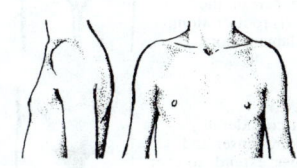

Stage 3 Breast and areola both enlarged and more elevated than in stage 2. Symmetrically round contour of the breast.

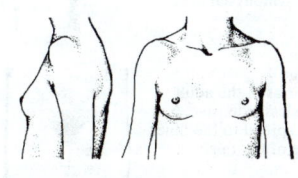

Stage 4 Further breast enlargement. Areola and papilla form a secondary mound projecting above breast contour.

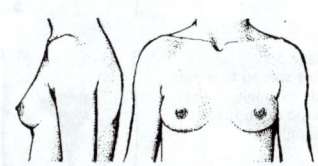

Stage 5 Mature breast: only papilla projects, with areola recessed to general contour of breast.

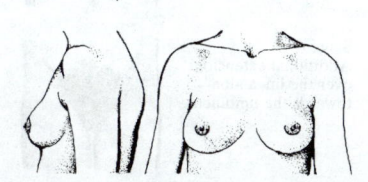

MEMORIX PEDIATRICS

Development of pubic hair ♀

Stage 1
No more hair than on the rest of the hairless abdomen.

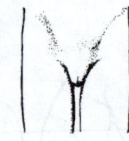

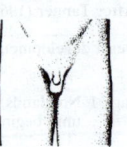

Stage 2
Sparse growth of long, slightly pigmented straight or slightly curly hair on the clitoris root or along the labia majora.

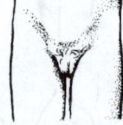

Stage 3
Hair considerably darker, denser and curlier; extends to over the symphysial area.

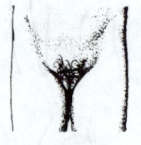

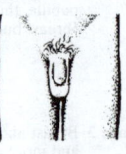

Stage 4
Hair as in the adult but less extensive. Not yet spread to the inner side of the thigh.

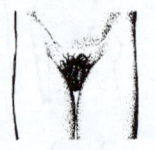

Stage 5
Hair spread to inner side of thigh, in the shape of an inverted triangle.

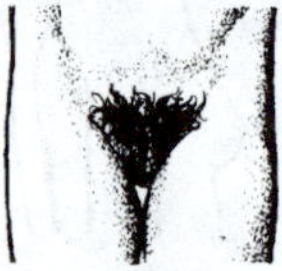

Stage 6
Additional extension over the linea alba towards the umbilicus.

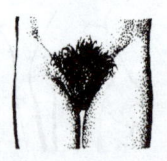

Development of pubic hair/genitalia ♂

Stage 1
Little growth of testes, scrotum and penis from early childhood to onset of puberty.

Stage 2
Scrotum and testes enlarge. Scrotal skin reddens and coarsens. Penis unchanged.

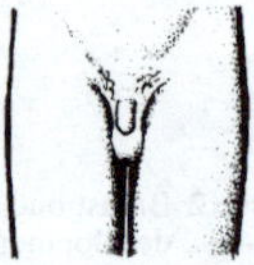

Stage 3
Srotum further enlarged. Penis larger, more in length than breadth.

Stage 4
Scrotum larger and darker than in stage 3. Penis further enlarged in length and breadth. Development of glans.

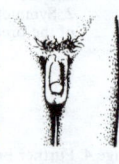

Stage 5
Genitalia have attained adult shape and size.

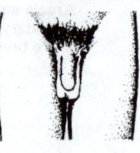

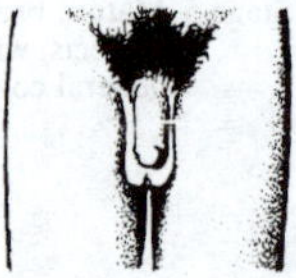

ENDOCRINOLOGY/GROWTH

Pubertal development and age of onset
(After Largo and Prader (1983).)

Stage of development		Age (years) 8–18
Girls		
Pubic hair begins	Stage 2	9–11.5, X at ~10.5
Breast bud	Stage 2	9–12, X at ~11
Greatest growth in height (peak height velocity)	PHV	10–13, X at ~12
Menarche	M	11–14.5, X at ~13
Mature breast	Stage 5	12–16, X at ~14
Boys		
Testicular growth begins	Stage 2	9.5–12.5, X at ~11
Pubarche	Stage 2	10.5–13.5, X at ~12
Penis growth begins	Stage 3	10.5–14, X at ~12.5
Greatest growth in height	PHV	12–15.5, X at ~14
Penis growth ends	Stage 5	13.5–16.5, X at ~15
Pubic hair border horizontal	Stage 5	14–17, X at ~15.5

MEMORIX PEDIATRICS

Phenotypical course of puberty
(After Prader (1986).)

Girls		Boys	
Age (years)	Signs	Age (years)	Signs
<8	None	<10	None
10–11	Thelarche: stage 2 Growth velocity Maturing of vaginal mucosa	11–12	Testicular growth begins
11	Pubarche: stage 2 First thumb sesamoid bone	12–13	Pubarche stage 2 Growth in height ↑ Growth of penis ↑
11–12	Growth of internal and external genitalia ↑	13–14	Slight breast swelling Pubic hair growth stage 3 Marked growth of testes and penis First thumb sesamoid bone
12–13	Greatest growth in height Breast development stage 3 Pubic hair growth stage 3	14	Marked growth in height
13	Menarche Axillary hair Breast development stage 4 Pubic hair growth stage 4	14–15	Upper lip hair growth begins Axillary hair growth Pubic hair growth stage 4
14–15	Ovulatory menses regular	15–16	Voice breaks Pubic hair growth stage 5 Testes (sperm) + penis mature Reduction of breast swelling
16–17	Epiphyseal closure (growth end)	17–19	Increase in facial and body hair Masculine forehead hair line Pubic hair growth stage 6 Epiphyseal closure (end of growth)

ENDOCRINOLOGY/GROWTH

Onset of puberty

Normal onset	Girls	Boys
Chronological age	8–13 years	9½–15 years
Bone age	≥11 years	≥13 years

Variants	Premature	On time	Hormone status
Premature pubarche	Sexual hair	All other characteristics	Premature adrenarche = DHE (plasma) ↑, 17-ketosteroids (urine) ↑ LH, FSH n, 17-hydroxyprogesterone (plasma) n
Premature thelarche	Breast development	All other characteristics	LH, FSH, estradiol (plasma) n, ↑

DHE = dehydroepiandrosterone; LH = luteinizing hormone; FSH = follicle-stimulating hormone.

Causes of delayed puberty

+ Short stature	Normal/tall stature
Ullrich–Turner's syndrome	Isolated gonadotrophin deficiency
Every chronic disease	Anorchidism
Malnutrition	True gonadodysgenesis
Disorders of the hypothalamic-pituitary system	
Constitutional	

Synopsis of premature puberty

Causes	External genital development Girls	External genital development Boys	Hormone status in relation to age norm DHE	Hormone status in relation to age norm FSH, LH	17-keto-steroids (urine)	Estrogen
Constitutional	↑	(↑), n	n	↑	↑	↑
Hypothalamic-pituitary disorder (tumors, hydrocephalus, deformities, hypothyroidism, adrenocortical deficiency)	↑	↑	n, (↓)	↑	↑	↑
Chorionepithelioma Teratoma	↑	n, (↑)	n	↑↑↑	↑↑	↑↑
Adrenocortical hyperplasia (pseudo-premature puberty)	↑ heterosexual	↑ isosexual	↑↑	n	↑↑	↑
Ovarian tumors	↑		n	n	↑	↑↑
Testicular tumor (Leydig cell tumor)		↑ (unilateral)	n	n	↑↑	n

DHE = dehydroepiandrosterone; FSH = follicle-stimulating hormone; LH = luteinizing hormone.

ENDOCRINOLOGY/GROWTH

Normal sexual development

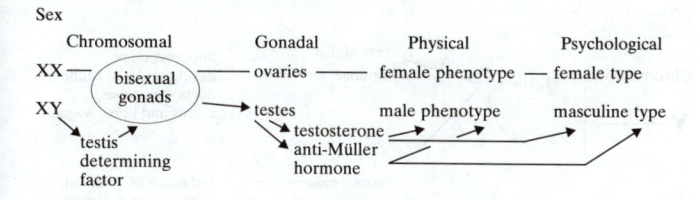

Sex

Chromosomal	Gonadal	Physical	Psychological
XX → bisexual gonads → ovaries		female phenotype	female type
XY → testis determining factor → bisexual gonads → testes	testosterone, anti-Müller hormone	male phenotype	masculine type

Clinical picture	Karyotype	Gonads (T = testes, O = ovaries)	Genitalia (M = masculine, F = feminine)
True hermaphroditism	XX, XX/XY	T + O	Intersex type III–IV
Female pseudohermaphroditism	XX	O	M/intersex type II–V
Male pseudohermaphroditism	XY	T	F/intersex type I–V

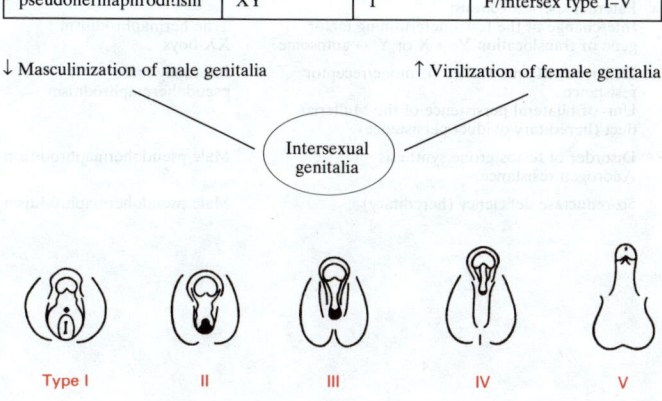

↓ Masculinization of male genitalia → Intersexual genitalia ← ↑ Virilization of female genitalia

Type I II III IV V

Disorders of masculine differentiation and development

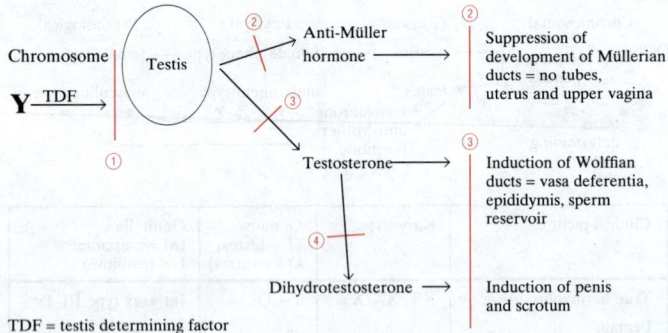

```
                    ② → Anti-Müller          ②  Suppression of
Chromosome  Testis      hormone      →          development of Müllerian
                                                ducts = no tubes,
Y —TDF→             ③                           uterus and upper vagina
            ①
                    → Testosterone    →      ③  Induction of Wolffian
                                                ducts = vasa deferentia,
                    ④                           epididymis, sperm
                                                reservoir
                    → Dihydrotestosterone →     Induction of penis
                                                and scrotum
```

TDF = testis determining factor

Causes

① Paternal spermiogenesis:
Interchange of the testis determining factor
gene or translocation Y → X or Y → autosome

② Deficiency of anti-Müller hormone/receptor
resistance
Uni- or bilateral persistence of the Müllerian
duct (hereditary oviduct persistence)

③ Disorder of testosterone synthesis
Androgen resistance

④ 5α-reductase deficiency (hereditary)

Results

True hermaphroditism
XX-boys

Internally male
pseudohermaphroditism

Male pseudohermaphroditism

Male pseudohermaphroditism

ENDOCRINOLOGY/GROWTH

Congenital disorders of steroid biosynthesis

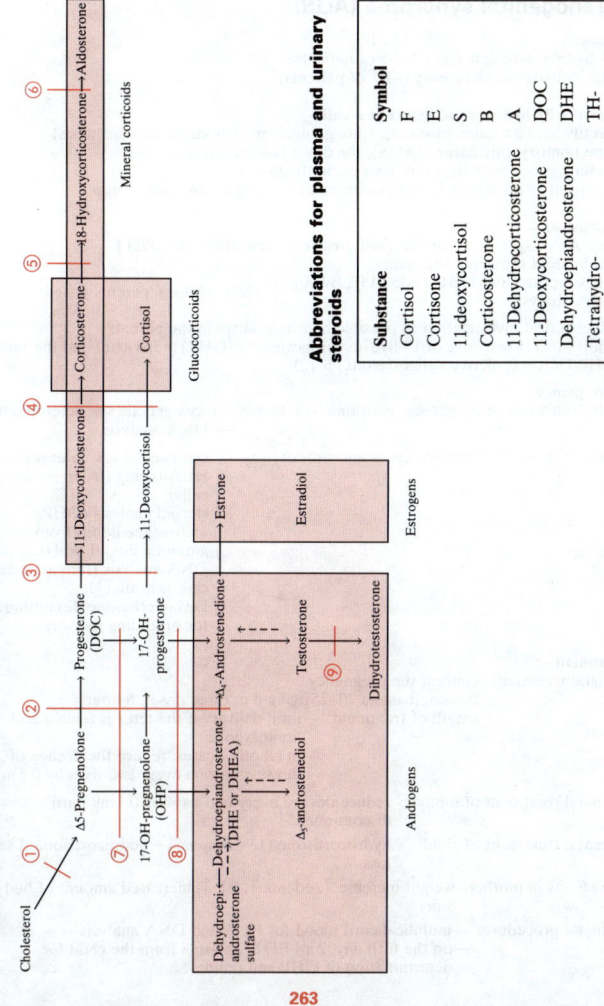

Cholesterol —①→ Δ5-Pregnenolone —②→ Progesterone (DOC) —③→ 11-Deoxycorticosterone —④→ Corticosterone —⑤→ 18-Hydroxycorticosterone —⑥→ Aldosterone

Mineral corticoids

Progesterone —→ 17-OH-progesterone —→ 11-Deoxycortisol —→ Cortisol

Glucocorticoids

Δ5-Pregnenolone —⑦→ 17-OH-pregnenolone (OHP) —⑧→ Dehydroepiandrosterone (DHE or DHEA) —→ Δ4-Androstenedione —→ Testosterone —⑨→ Dihydrotestosterone

Dehydroepiandrosterone sulfate ←— Dehydroepiandrosterone ---→ Δ5-androstenediol ---→ Testosterone

Δ4-Androstenedione —→ Estrone —→ Estradiol

Estrogens

Androgens

Abbreviations for plasma and urinary steroids

Substance	Symbol
Cortisol	F
Cortisone	E
11-deoxycortisol	S
Corticosterone	B
11-Dehydrocorticosterone	A
11-Deoxycorticosterone	DOC
Dehydroepiandrosterone	DHE
Tetrahydro-	TH-

263

Adrenogenital syndrome (AGS)

Causes
21-hydroxylase deficiency (~4/5 of patients)
11β-hydroxylase deficiency (~1/5 of patients)

Risks of a 21-hydroxylase defect in a child
Family with an index case (sick sibling, biochemically confirmed diagnosis)
One homozygotic parent (AGS), the other heterozygotic
Heterozygotic parents, no index case in the family
A parent of an affected child (index case) forming a new relationship

Diagnosis
(After Arbeitsgemeinschaft für pädiatrische Endokrinologie (1992).)
From birth of the index children:
HLA typing (Bw47, B14, B35, B51, Bw60) ⎫
DNA analysis ⎬ child, siblings, parents tested

Biochemical investigation of possible heterozygotism in the parents
Short ACTH test (rise of 17-hydroxyprogesterone (OHP) > 260 ng/dl and the ratio OHP/DOC (11-deoxycorticosterone) > 12)

In pregnancy:
9th–10th week of pregnancy, chorionic villi biopsy → cytogenetic sex determination
→ DNA analysis

13th–16th week of pregnancy, amniocentesis → cytogenetic sex determination
→ HLA typing (from amnion cells)
→ steroid analysis (OHP, androstenedione) from amniotic fluid if no HLA or DNA analysis from an index case is available. Dexamethasone discontinued for preceding five days

Treatment
Prenatal treatment: confirm the pregnancy
dexamethasone 20–25 µg/kg/d in three doses, 8 hourly
length of treatment: – until delivery if the fetus is female and homozygotic
– in all other cases, reduce the dosage of dexamethasone every two days by 0.5 mg

Postnatal treatment of mother: reduce dosage every two days by 0.5 mg until discontinued

Postnatal treatment of child: hydrocortisone (12–15 mg/m^2) + fludrocortisone if salt loss

Side effects in mother: weight increase ↑, edema ↑, BP ↑, increased amount of body hair

Postnatal procedure: – umbilical cord blood for HLA and DNA analysis
– on the fifth day, 2 ml EDTA plasma from the child for determination of OHP and renin

ENDOCRINOLOGY/GROWTH

Steroid biosynthesis: enzyme defects

Enzyme defect	External genitalia Karyotype XX (f = feminine, m = masculine, i = intersexual)	Karyotype XY	Adrenals Cortisol synthesis	Cortical hyperplasia	Salt loss	Clinical signs Hypertension	Virilization	Diagnostic lead steroids (S = serum, U = urine)
① Congenital lipoid hyperplasia of the adrenal cortex 20-hydroxylase 22-hydroxylase 20,22-desmolase	f	i	↓	+	+	–	–	Adrenocortical insufficiency, all steroids (S,U) ↓
② 3β-hydroxysteroid-dehydrogenase/ isomerase deficiency	f,i	i	↓	+	±	–	+	S: pregnenolone ↑, 17-OH-pregnenolone, dehydroepiandrosterone ↑ U: Δ₅-pregnenetriol ↑
③ (AGS): 21-hydroxylase deficiency – without salt loss – with salt loss	i	m	↓	+	– +	–	+	S: 17-OH-progesterone ↑ U: Pregnanetriol ↑
④ 11β-hydroxylase deficiency	i	m	↓	+	(+)	+	+	S: 11-deoxycorticosterone ↑, 11-deoxycortisol ↑ U: Tetrahydrodeoxycorticosterone Tetrahydro-11-deoxycortisol
Hypoaldosteronism: ⑤ Corticosterone-methyloxidase type I ⑥ Corticosterone-methyloxidase type II			n	–	+	–	–	S: Aldosterone ↓, renin ↑
⑦ 17-hydroxylase deficiency	f	f	↓	+	–	+	–	S: 11-deoxycorticosterone ↑, corticosterone ↑ U: Tetrahydrodeoxycorticosterone, Tetrahydrocorticosterone
⑧ 17,20-desmolase deficiency	f	f,i	n	–	–	–	–	U: Pregnanetriol ↑
⑨ 17-ketosteroid reductase deficiency	f	i	n	–	–	–	–	PHm

AGS = adrenogenital syndrome: ①②④⑦, most frequently ③
PHm = male pseudohermaphroditism

265

Treatment of undescended testis
(After Arbeitsgemeinschaft für Pädiatrische Endokrinologie (1991).)

Definition	Illustration	Treatment indication
Retractile testis	Testes either in scrotum or inguinal canal. Follow-up necessary, as secondary non-descent possible	None (normal variant)
Sliding testis	Never spontaneously found in scrotum. Prescrotal testes can be pulled into the scrotum, slipping back immediately into the initial position	Always given
Inguinal testis	Lie in the inguinal canal, only slightly mobile, but can be pulled into the scrotum. Clinically no differentiation possible from epifascial ectopy	Always given
Cryptorchidism	Uni- or bilateral. Testes not palpable. Causes: Abdominal retention Anorchism: if bilateral, diagnosis made by the HCG test (see p. 274)	Always given None if anorchism bilateral

Treatment

Hormone therapy: **HCG (human chorionic gonadotropin)**
  1st year of life   500 IU/week, five times in total i.m.
  2nd–6th year   1000 IU/week, five times in total i.m.
  >6th year   2000 IU/week, five times in total i.m.
  Side-effects: HCG stimulates Leydig cells to secrete testosterone → enlargement of genitalia, more frequent erections, raised aggressiveness
  Little effect in the first year of life.

  GnRH (gonadotropin releasing hormone):
  Three times two spray doses (single dose 0.2 mg) intranasally per day over four weeks
  None of the side-effects seen with HCG.

  Combined GnRH–HCG treatment
  GnRH as above + 1 injection 1500 IU HCG/week, three times in total.

Relapse after treatment frequent, so follow-up desirable.
Age at treatment: at the end of the first year of life.

Surgical treatment: Indications: failure of hormone treatment
        ectopic testis
        undescended testis with sliding hernia
        undescended testis at puberty
        undescended testis after previous inguinal operation.

ENDOCRINOLOGY/GROWTH

Causes of hypothyroidism

Causes	Functional disorder	Diagnosis
Primary hypothyroidism:	For all primary types and as basic diagnosis if abnormal TSH screening: goiter? (sonography) + TSH, T3, T4, free T4 (FT4), thyroglobulin (Tgb) in serum	
Dysgenesis: athyroidism / ectopic thyroid	No hormone / Too little hormone	Tgb absent
Synthesis defects (autosomal recessive)		
Iodination	Iodine pump in the cells	
Iodization	Iodine incorporation in tyrosine: Mono-/diiodothyronine	+ Perchlorate test
Coupling	T2 + T2 → T4	
Protease deficiency	Separation of T4 from Tgb	
Deiodase deficiency	Iodine supply from mono-/diiodothyronine, 'internal thyroid deficiency'	
Thyroglobulin		
Abnormal synthesis (acquired):		
Iodine deficiency (alimentary)	Prenatal: mother → child	T4 normal, T3 ↑, or T4 ↓, T3 normal. Iodine excretion in urine ↓
Iodine superimposition	Wolff–Chaikoff effect: with increasing plasma-iodide concentration, the thyroid takes up less iodine until actually blocked	History, iodine in urine ↑, TSH ↑, T4 ↓
Thyrostatic agents in a wider and stricter sense	Iodination, iodization, thyroxine release	History
Hashimoto's thyroiditis Thyroidectomy	Autoimmune disease	Thyroid antibodies
Secondary (hypophyseal) hypothyroidism	TSH deficiency	Basic diagnosis + TRH test (+ pituitary function tests)
Tertiary (hypothalamic) hypothyroidism	TRH deficiency	CNS diagnosis after exclusion of primary or secondary hypothyroidism
Peripheral hormone receptor disorder	Thyroxine resistance	TSH n/↑, FT4 ↑, T3 ↑
Hormone loss	Protein loss syndrome	e.g. exudative enteropathy

TSH = thyroid-stimulating hormone; TRH = thyrotropin-releasing hormone; CNS = central nervous system.

Goiterogenic substances

Medication: antidiabetic drugs (sulfonyl urea)
resorcinol
paraaminosalicylic acid, aspirin
phenytoin
lithium
bromine, fluoride

Dietary substances: maize
millet
cauliflower
cabbage
beets (some varieties)

Screening for hypothyroidism

Results of thyroid-stimulating hormone (TSH) screening

Test result	Action to be taken
TSH < 10 µU/ml	Normal
TSH 10–20 µU/ml	Check (e.g. test card) Treat until receipt of the result mature neonates 25 µg/d prematures 10 µg/kg/d
TSH 20–100 µU/ml	Suspect transient or permanent hypothyroidism: complete basic diagnosis essential (see p. 269) Treatment
TSH > 100 µU/ml	Suspect permanent hypothyroidism: complete basic diagnosis Treatment

Treatment: Always with sodium levothyroxine.
Maintenance dose based on T4 and TSH serum levels in the individual case. If symptoms of overdosage, reduce by 25%.

Guiding values:
Prematures 25 µg/d
Mature neonates 50 µg/d
Infants to 6 months 10 µg/kg/d
Infants over 7 months 8 µg/kg/d
Children over 1 year 100–150 µg/m^2/d

Recommended oral iodine doses
(After Deutsche Gesellschaft für Ernährung e.V. (1991).)

Age	Iodide (µg/d)	Age	Iodide (µg/d)
0–4 months	50	10–13 y	180
4 months–1 y	80	13–18 y	200
1–4 y	100	Pregnant	230
4–7 y	120	Breast-feeding	260
7–10 y	140		

ENDOCRINOLOGY/GROWTH

Aftercare program in congenital hypothyroidism

Important maternal data: thyroid-stimulating hormone (TSH), T4, T3, antithyroid antibodies, microsomal antibodies

Laboratory programme	Investigation time	Development data
Hormones (TSH, T3, T4, FT4), thyroglobulin, iodine excretion	Initial investigations at onset of treatment	Body measurements (height, weight, head circumference), X-rays of left knee and foot, Motor development
Hormones, thyroglobulin	Two weeks after beginning treatment	Body measurements, Screening for hearing (AEP)
Hormones	3rd, 6th, 9th months	Body measurements, psychomotor development
Hormones	12th month	Body measurements, X-ray of left hand, psychomotor development, objective hearing test
Hormones	18th month	Body measurements, psychomotor development
Hormones	2nd year	Body measurements, psychomotor development, dentition

> **Insert:** Etiological diagnosis
> Preparation: three weeks beforehand change to T3 ($20-40\,\mu g/m^2$), stop treatment for one week and institute diagnosis.
> Scintigraphy with ^{123}iodine.
> Continue treatment with thyroxine.

| Hormones | At $2^1/_2$ and at yearly intervals until age $5^1/_2$ y | Body measurements, psychomotor development, dentition |
| Hormones | 3rd year and at yearly intervals until 18th year | Body measurements, psychomotor development, dentition. In preschool age children, at least one basic intelligence test |

AEP = auditory evoked potential.
The body measurements should not fall below the 25th percentile. Radiological diagnosis (left hand) of bone maturation only if hormone substitution and if serum hormone levels and/or growth abnormal.

Skeletal changes in primary hypothyroidism (with no or incomplete treatment)
  Retarded skeletal maturation
  Kyphosis (ventral flattening)
  Dysplasia of epiphyseal centers, Perthes-like changes in femoral head, bilaterally equal
  Skull: small base, sella relatively large, delayed pneumonatization, delayed closure of fontanelles.

MEMORIX PEDIATRICS

Stages of goiter

0   No goiter, thyroid lobes ≃ size of distal digit

1a Goiter not seen with normal head posture, but palpable

1b Goiter visible with maximum dorsiflexion of throat, independent of goiter size

2   Goiter visible with normal head position

3   Very large goiter, visible from a distance

Upper limits of normal thyroid volume (by sonography)

Age (years)	ml
6	–4
13	–8
15–18	–18

ENDOCRINOLOGY/GROWTH

Growth function tests
(Adapted from Girard (1990).)

Investigation of growth hormone secretion

Hypoglycemia test (insulin-induced)

Principle: Insulin → hypoglycemia = stress → secretion of human growth hormone (HGH) and ACTH → cortisol ↑

Measurement: HGH (plasma), ACTH (plasma), cortisol (plasma), blood sugar (BS)
Quantity of blood: approximately 5 ml per sample.
Blood sugar (at bedside) measured with the appropriate calibrated instrument.

Procedure: In the morning, after night fasting, insert indwelling needle i.v.
Glucose (20%) with 1 amp. of glucagon ready for use.
blood sample: 30 min before and immediately before the injection (0 min).
Insulin injection strictly i.v. Extravasation can cause hypoglycemia up to six hours afterwards!

Insulin: 0.1 IU/kg normal insulin.
0.05–0.075 IU/kg if abnormal counterregulation suspected (applies to glucagon, cortisol and adrenaline).
0.15–0.175 IU/kg in suspected 'insulin resistance' (Cushing's syndrome, diabetes mellitus, obesity); this mixture is best given as an infusion.
Dilute the insulin with 0.9% NaCl.

Sampling times:

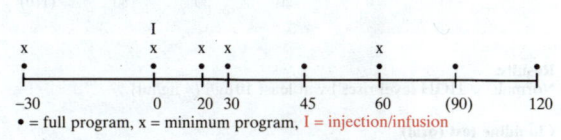

```
              I
     x        x   x  x             x
     •        •   •  •      •      •      •       •
    -30       0  20 30     45     60    (90)    120
```
• = full program, x = minimum program, I = injection/infusion

NB: the 20-min blood sugar serves as a test control.
BS must be <40 mg/dl (<2.2 mmol/l). If it is not, check again in 10 min.
If BS >40 mg/dl and hypoglycemic symptoms (sweating, pallor, shivering, hunger) are absent, start a new test at 30 min with 0.05 IU/kg normal insulin.

Observe patient for six hours for signs of hypoglycemia.

Normal: **HGH:** rises after 30–60 min to at least 10 µg/l.
  Cortisol: rises a minimum of 10 µg/dl (280 nmol/l).
  Maximum level at least 20 µg/dl after 60 min.
  ACTH: Rise to ≥200 pg/ml after 45 min.
  Glucose: Possible fall by 30 to 0-level = venepuncture stress.

MEMORIX PEDIATRICS

HGH secretion profile during sleep

Principle: HGH is physiologically secreted in several pulses on the way to deep night sleep (EEG sleep stages III–IV).

Procedure: insert indwelling needle.
Sampling times: from the beginning of sleep, every 30 min for a minimum of six hours.

Result: Increased pulses.
Amplitude >10 µg/l.

Arginine loading test (i.v.)

Principle: Arginine stimulates the secretion of HGH, insulin, glucagon.

Procedure: Indwelling needle inserted 30 min before the injection.
Amount: arginine 0.5 g/kg; infusion duration 20 min.

Solution:
L-arginine hydrochloride (21.07% = unimolar solution)
1 ml of the solution = 1 mmol/l = 0.21 g arginine HCl.
0.5 g arginine ≙ 2.9 ml.
Maximum dose = 30 g.

Sampling times:

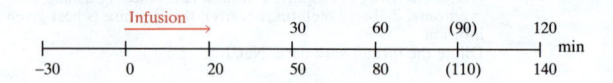

```
                Infusion →
                              30        60       (90)      120
    |-----------|------|------|---------|--------|---------|---- min
   -30          0     20      50        80      (110)     140
```

Results:
Normal: HGH level rises by at least 10 µg/l (= ng/ml)

Clonidine test (oral)

Principle: α_2-receptor-stimulation increases HGH secretion.
Clonidine = centrally active α_2-adrenoceptor agonist.

Procedure: (a) 0-level
25 µg oral clonidine,
sample after 90 min.
(b) In case of no definite rise in HGH concentration:
repeat test with 75–150 µg/m².
Watch out for a fall in blood pressure or an asthma attack.

Result:
normal: increased HGH secretion.

ENDOCRINOLOGY/GROWTH

HGH secretion suppression test

Principle: Raised blood glucose concentration suppresses HGH secretion.

Procedure: See oral glucose loading (p. 228) or glucose tolerance test (p. 228). Additionally, measure cortisol as a stress hormone.

Results: HGH half-life in plasma ~20 min.

Normal: HGH falls to nonmeasureable level.

Abnormal: No suppression (gigantism), inadequate suppression in response to stress.

TRH test (TSH-releasing hormone)

Principle: Synthetic TRH (thyrotropin-releasing hormone) stimulates the pituitary to secrete TSH (thyroid-stimulating hormone) and prolactin.

Procedure: Independent of time of day, >2 h postprandial.
5 ml of blood for the 0-level of TSH, T3, T4 (prolactin if adenoma suspected).

TRH by slow i.v. injection:
infants   TRH 100 µg
older children   TRH 200 µg.

Check TSH after   30 (60) min.

Results:
Normal: TSH elevation to 5–20 mU/l.

Note: No rise → hyperthyroidism, secondary hypothyroidism.
In HGH and steroid treatment, and in obesity, diminished rise; T3 and T4 are normal.

Excessive rise → primary hypothyroidism.

delayed rise → pituitary (secondary) or hypothalamic (tertiary) hypothyroidism.

Luteinizing hormone releasing hormone (LHRH) test

Principle: synthetic LHRH stimulates the pituitary to secrete LH (luteinizing hormone) and FSH (follicle-stimulating hormone).

Procedure: Independent of time of day, >2 h postprandial.
Insert indwelling needle.
5 ml of blood for basic levels of LH and FSH.
Inject 100 µg LHRH over 1 min.
Dilute ampule of LHRH with 5 ml of NaCl (0.9%).

Samples:

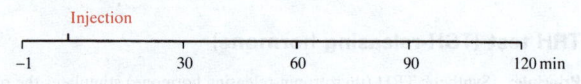

```
                    Injection
   -1          30         60         90        120 min
```

Results:
Normal: Prepubertal: LH rises by 5 U/l ♀ and ♂.
FSH rises by 3 U/l ♀, can be absent in ♂.

Pubertal: LH rise higher, dependent on degree of development.
FSH rise: ♀ unchanging
♂ measurable.

Abnormal: Excessive rise in LH and FSH in primary hypogonadism.

HCG test

Principle: HCG (human chorionic gonadotropin) stimulates the Leydig cells of the testes to secrete testosterone; same effect as LH.

Procedure: Take blood for basal levels of testosterone, FSH and LH.
Inject 5000 U HCG/m^2 i.m.
Measure testosterone after 48 and 72 h.

Results:
Normal: Testosterone in plasma rises above the age- and sex-specific normal levels.

Conversion of testosterone values: µg × 3.47 = nmol
µg = nmol × 0.28.

Indication examples: primary hypogonadism, delayed puberty.

ENDOCRINOLOGY/GROWTH

Dexamethasone test

Principle: Dexamethasone inhibits ACTH secretion → cortisol ↓ (suppression test).

Procedure: Indwelling needle necessary because blood-taking stress inhibits suppression.

Two-step suppression (2 + 8 mg)

0-levels: 24 h urine, blood tests (5 ml) at 8 h and 16 h for ACTH + cortisol. A further check at 24 h if possible.

Oral dexamethasone: 5 mg four times per day for two days, then 2 mg four times per day for three days.

Measure daily: blood (ACTH + cortisol) at 8 h
urine (24 h) (ketosteroids, hydroxysteroids).

One-step suppression (short test)

0-levels for ACTH + cortisol (plasma) at 8am the day before the test.

0-levels measured at 24 h (if possible).

Oral dexamethasone 1 mg at 24 h.

Check ACTH + cortisol (plasma) in the morning (8am, fasting).

Results:

Two-step test

Normal: After 2 mg dexamethasone, complete suppression of ACTH and cortisol; urinary hydroxysteroids about ≥50% ↓.

Note: After 2 mg dexamethasone incomplete suppression, after 8 mg almost or complete suppression → hypothalamic or pituitary disorder (Cushing's disease).

No suppression, ketosteroids and dehydroepiandrosterone in urine ↑ → adrenocortical carcinoma.

One-step test

Normal: ACTH + cortisol below measurable level.

Note: As for two-step test.

ACTH test

Principle: Synthetic adrenocorticotropic hormone (ACTH) stimulates the adrenal cortex.

Procedure:

Variation I: 0-level for cortisol (+ ACTH).
Injection of 250 µg ACTH (1–24) i.v. (s.c., i.m.).
Measure cortisol (plasma) after 30, 60, 120 min.

Variation II: 0-level at 8 am for cortisol (plasma), ACTH (plasma)
Inject 1 mg/m² of depot preparation i.m.
Measure cortisol (plasma) after 8 h.

Variation III: 0-level = 24 hour urine specimen for 17-OH-steroids.
Inject 1 mg/m² depot preparation i.m.
24 hour urine specimen twice after the injection.
In suspected primary adrenocortical deficiency, 0.5 mg/kg prednisone by mouth at the end of the test.

Results:

Normal:

Variation I: Cortisol (plasma) rise to ≥ three times the morning excretory level.

Variation II: Cortisol rise to ≥ 8.3 µmol/l

Variation III: Rise to two to three times the initial level.

Note: Rise absent → primary adrenocortical insufficiency.
Rise absent or little → secondary adrenocortical insufficiency.
Marked rise → Cushing's disease (high 0-levels).

Metyrapone test

Principle: Metyrapone (propyl-/ethyl-4-hydroxybenzoate) inhibits cortisol synthesis via 11β-hydroxylase = reduction of the negative feedback → ACTH stimulation → stimulation of steroid biosynthesis up to block of 11-deoxycortisol (substance S) and 17α-hydroxyprogesterone in plasma.

Procedure: 0-level of ACTH, 11-deoxycortisol, cortisol.
Oral metyrapone 15 mg/kg (600 mg/m²) around midnight with a light meal.
Measure again after 7–8 h.
Give prednisone 0.5 mg/kg prophylactically at end of test.

Results:

Normal: ACTH ↑ to ≥ 200 µg/l.
Substance S ↑ above ≥ 170 µg/l.
Cortisol ↓.

Note: Rise of ACTH + substance S reduced = secondary adrenocortical deficiency.

ENDOCRINOLOGY/GROWTH

Test combinations for the multiple diagnosis of pituitary functions

Principles of tests and evaluation of the results as in individual tests. If there is failure of one function, confirm this by the individual test.

Insulin–LHRH–TRH test

Procedure: Preparation as in the insulin-induced hypoglycemic test (p. 271).

Pretest levels for glucose, ACTH, cortisol, TSH, T3, T3 uptake, T4, HGH, LH, FSH, testosterone, estradiol.

Blood volume: 10 ml.
Injection sequence: 1. insulin
2. TRH
3. LHRH.

Check times from the LHRH injection or from the second insulin injection (if necessary):
0, 3, 45, 60 min.

Results: as in single tests.

Arginine–LHRH–TRH test

Preparation: As in arginine test.

Pretest levels for glucose, TSH, T3, T3 uptake, T4, LH, FSH, testosterone, estradiol, HGH.

Procedure: Arginine infusion.

Give TRH and then give LHRH at the beginning of the infusion.

Check times: as in the arginine test.

Metyrapone–TRH–arginine–LHRH test

Procedure: Insert infusion line (0.9% NaCl).

Sample for pretest levels. Program as in insulin–LHRH–TRH test, plus 11-deoxycortisol.

Give metyrapone and TRH orally.

LHRH injection and, immediately afterwards, arginine infusion over 20 minutes.

Sampling times after beginning of infusion:
30, 60, 120, 180 min.

Vasopressin (desmopressin) test

(After Yared, Foose and Ichikawa (1990).)

Principle: After a thirst test, additional administration of adiuretin-vasopressin (ADH) or desmopressin (1-desamino-8-arginine-vasopressin, DDAVP), to test the different antidiuretic effect in neurohormonal or renal diabetes insipidus.

Procedure:

Thirst test

In the early morning, weigh the test subject after he or she has emptied the bladder. Only dry bread may be eaten by the subject.

Insert indwelling needle.

Check hourly:

Body weight; amount, specific gravity and osmolarity of urine;

Na and osmolarity in serum.

The trial is stopped if:

– serum sodium is >150 mmol/l

– body weight has fallen by ≥3%

– serum osmolarity is 300 mosmol/kg

– specific gravity and osmolarity in the urine differ only slightly (30 mosmol/l) from one another in two consecutive tests.

ADH test immediately after thirst test

Pretest levels for vasopressin and serum osmolarity.

s.c. injection of 5 IU vasopressin or 10 IU of intranasal desmopressin.

Check: osmolarity (serum + urine), specific gravity (urine).

Results:

Normal: Thirst test:

urine osmolarity ↑ (500–1400 mosmol/kg)

urine production ↓

serum osmolarity remains normal

change of levels by ADH

ENDOCRINOLOGY/GROWTH

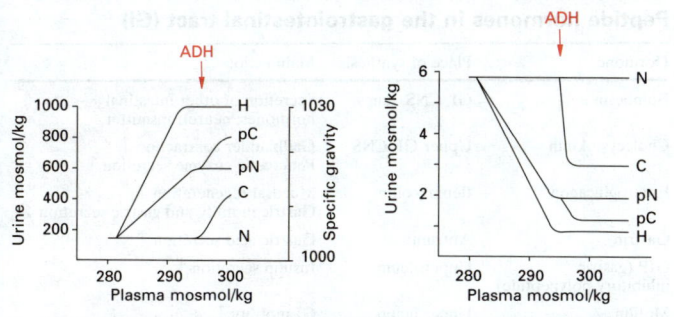

H = healthy child; pC = partial central diabetes insipidus; pN = partial nephrogenic diabetes insipidus; C = central diabetes insipidus; N = nephrogenic diabetes insipidus.

Note:

	Urine volume		Urine osmolarity	
	Thirst	ADH	Thirst	ADH
Central diabetes insipidus (C)	↑	↓	↓	↑ (>50%)
Nephrogenic diabetes insipidus (N)	↑	↑	↓	↓

Approximate calculation

Specific gravity (urine) → osmolarity:

   mosmol/kg = last two numbers of the specific gravity × 35.

Example: specific gravity (urine) 1020: 20 × 35 = 700 mosmol/kg.

Peptide hormones in the gastrointestinal tract (GI)

Hormone	Place of synthesis	Main action
Bombesin	GI, CNS, lungs	Secretion of other intestinal hormones, neurotransmitter
Cholecystokinin	Upper GI, CNS	Gallbladder contraction ↑ Pancreatic enzyme secretion ↑
Enteroglucagon	Ileum, colon	Mucosal regeneration ↑ Gastric motility and gastric secretion ↓
Gastrin	Antrum	Gastric acid secretion ↑
GIP (gastric inhibitory polypeptide)	Upper ileum	Insulin secretion ↑
Motilin	Upper ileum	GI motility ↑
Neurotensin	Ileum, CNS	Gastric emptying and gastric secretion ↓ Neurotransmitter
Pancreatic polypeptide	Pancreas	Pancreatic enzyme secretion ↓ Gallbladder contraction ↓
Peptide Y	GI, CNS	Gastric acid secretion ↓ Intestinal motility ↓
Secretin	Upper ileum	Pancreatic bicarbonate secretion ↑
VIP (vasoactive intestinal polypeptide)	GI, nervous system	Relaxation of smooth muscles ↑ General stimulation of secretion ↑

GASTROENTEROLOGY/NUTRITION

Hypertrophic pyloric stenosis

Cardinal symptoms: projectile vomiting, failure to thrive, dehydration.

Ultrasound
Image characteristics: poor muscle echo, irregular peristalsis, reverse peristalsis

Transverse (rosette formation)

Longitudinal (tubular canal)

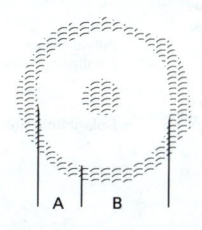

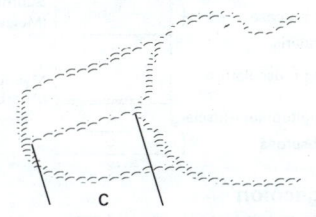

Hypertrophic measure	Muscle wall (A) > 4 mm Diameter (B) > 15 mm	Length (C) > 16 mm

X-ray pictures taken in horizontal position lying on right side after filling the duodenal bulb with contrast material

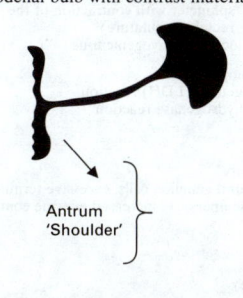

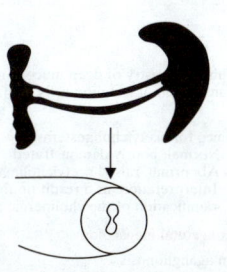

Antrum 'Shoulder'

Laboratory levels: pH ↑, HCO_3^- ↑, base excess ↑, Na^+ n → ↓, K^+ n → ↓, Cl^- ↓

Measurements:
- Gastric sounding (gastric residue ?).
- Preoperative: parenterally 150 ml/kg daily of 0.45% NaCl plus 20 mmol/l KCl plus 10% glucose. Regulate the potassium requirement.
- Postoperatively: change the parenteral to oral feeding.
- Check electrolytes and blood gases until normalization occurs.

Intestinal innervation

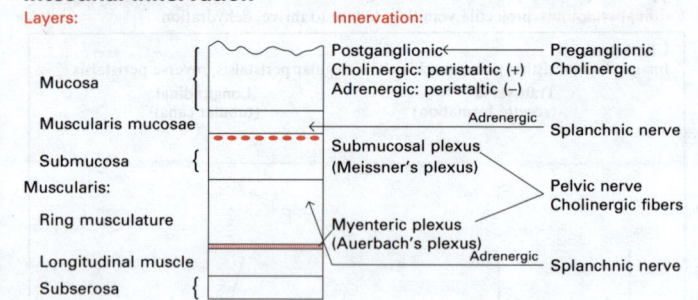

Layers:

Layer	Innervation
Mucosa	Postganglionic ← Preganglionic Cholinergic: peristaltic (+) Cholinergic Adrenergic: peristaltic (−)
Muscularis mucosae	Adrenergic → Splanchnic nerve
Submucosa	Submucosal plexus (Meissner's plexus)
Muscularis: Ring musculature	} Pelvic nerve Cholinergic fibers
Longitudinal muscle	Myenteric plexus (Auerbach's plexus) Adrenergic → Splanchnic nerve
Subserosa	

Megacolon

Principal diagnostic aids in neurogenic motility disorders

Contrast radiography: megacolon with adjoining narrow nondilated segments

Manometry:
- Normal bowel
  - normal peristaltic waves
  - hyperactivity
- Hypo-/aganglionic segments
  - uncoordinated contractions
  - no spontaneous relaxation
  - no filling adaptation
  - rectal stretching reflex abnormal (no inhibition of the internal sphincter with contraction of the rectal musculature)
  - increased myogenic tone

Histology/histochemistry of deep mucous membrane biopsy:
1. Demonstration of ganglion cells: lactate dehydrogenase (LDH) reaction +
   succinate dehydrogenase reaction +

1. Evidence for acetylcholinesterase
   → Normal: poorly demonstrated
   → Abnormal: raised acetylcholinesterase activity
   Interpretation: as a result of absent intramural ganglion cells, excessive terminal ramification of the cholinergic preganglionic fibers, i.e. increased enzyme content.

Types of congenital megacolon

Total colon aganglionosis

Segmental colon aganglionosis (Hirschsprung's disease)

Colon hypoganglionosis: ganglion cell-count per segment limited by 1/10; can be found combined with Hirschsprung's disease

Immature ganglion cells: abnormally small number of ganglion cells present from jejunum to rectum

Hypogenesis of the myenteric plexus: ganglion cell numbers in ileum and colon reduced to 1/3

Neural dysplasia of colon: increased acetylcholinesterase reaction, ganglion cell count in the plexus normal/increased

GASTROENTEROLOGY/NUTRITION

Disease stages of mucoviscidosis (Shwachman score)

Grade	Points	General activity	Clinical findings	Nutritional	Radiological findings
Very good (86–100)	25	Full normal activity; plays ball, attends school regularly etc.	Normal; no cough; pulse and breathing regular; lungs free; good posture	Weight and height above the 25th percentile; stools formed, almost normal; well-developed muscle and tone	Lung fields clear
Good (71–85)	20	Reduced staying power; tired in evenings; school attendance good	Pulse and respiration normal; rarely coughs or clears throat; no clubbed fingers or toes; lungs free; minimal emphysema	Weight and height between 15th and 20th percentile; stools slightly altered; adequate muscul-ature and tone	Minimally accentuated markings of bronchi and vessels; beginning of emphysema
Mild (56–70)	15	Rests during day; tires easily on effort; school attendance adequate	Occasional cough, e.g. on getting up in the morning; slight emphysema; coarse breath sounds, rarely, localized rales; clubbed fingers +	Weight and height above 3rd percentile; stools in general bulky and hardly ; formed abdomen distended very slightly if at all; slack muscle tone, reduced musculature	Slight emphysema, with patchy atelectasis; increased bronchial and vessel outlines
Moderate (41–55)	10	Only home tuition possible; dyspnea on mild exertion; rests a good deal	Frequent cough, usually productive; retraction of thorax; moderate emphysema; thorax may be deformed; rales; clubbed fingers ++ to +++	Weight and height below 3rd percentile; bulky, fatty, foul-smelling stools; substantially reduced musculature; slightly to moderately distended abdomen	Moderately severe emphysema; spreading areas of atelectasis and scattered foci of infection; minimal bronchiectasis
Severe (40 or under)	5	Orthopnea, bed-ridden or sitting	Severe coughing attacks; tachypnea with tachycardia and extensive lung findings; sometimes right heart failure; clubbed fingers +++ to ++++	Markedly poor nutrition; grossly distended abdomen; rectal prolapse; voluminous foul, fatty, frequent stools	Extensive changes with signs of airway obstruction and infection; lobar atelectasis and bronchiectasis

MEMORIX PEDIATRICS

Hyperbilirubinemia

Characteristics of hereditary syndromes
(A = autosomal, D = dominant, R = recessive)

Syndrome Characteristics	Crigler–Najjar Type I	Crigler–Najjar Type II	Meulengracht–Gilbert	Rotor	Dubin–Johnson
Dominant bilirubin form	Indirect (unconjugated)	Indirect (unconjugated)	Indirect	Conjugated	Conjugated
Serum bilirubin (mg/dl)	20–27	10–15	1–2	2–6	2–6
Bile acids in serum	n	n	n	n	n
Bilirubin-UDP-glycuronyl-transferase activity	0	Trace	ca. 50%	100%	100%
Conjugates in bile: Monoglycuronide Diglycuronide	0 0	95% 5%	40% 60%	20% 80%	20% 80%
Other glycuronide defects	+	+	–	–	–
Site of defect	Microsomes	Microsomes	Microsomes Plasma membrane	Cytosol	Canalicular secretion
Pathology	Kernicterus	(Kernicterus)	–	–	Dark brown liver pigmentation
Mode of inheritance	AR	AD/AR	AD	AR	AR
Diagnosis: bromsulfophthalein	n	n	(n)	Pathological	Pathological
Improved with phenobarbital	0	+	+		
Coproporphyrin urinary excretion pattern				Pathological	Pathological

Biliary atresia

Portoenterostomy (after Kasai)

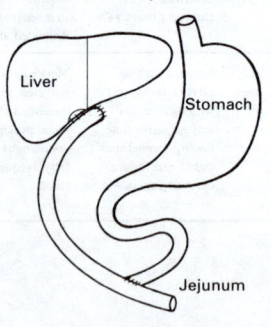

GASTROENTEROLOGY/NUTRITION

Cholelithiasis in childhood and adolescence

Site:
- Gallbladder
- Cystic duct
- Bile duct
- Intrahepatic

Combined
- Cholesterol stones
- Pigment stones
- Calcium bilirubinate (black)
- Calcium palmitate (brown)

Causation

Increased secretion of bilirubin (pigment stones):
- Hereditary hemolytic anemia
- Hereditary hyperbilirubinemia syndrome (hepatic)

Disorder of the enterohepatic circulation of the bile acids:
- Pancreatic insufficiency
- Mucoviscidosis
- Crohn's disease
- Short-bowel syndrome

Deficient secretory stimulus: Total parenteral nutrition

Metabolic diseases:
- Wilson's disease
- Metachromatic leukodystrophy

Bile duct anomalies:
- Primary anomalies
- Postcholangitic stenoses

Treatment:
- Shock-wave lithotripsy
- Ursodeoxycholic acid ⎫
- Chenodeoxycholic acid ⎭ — Stone dissolution

MEMORIX PEDIATRICS

Differential diagnosis of vomiting

Vomited secretions and other contents	Origin	Causes
Sour smell (litmus paper → red)	Stomach	See table below
+ foam	Esophagus, stomach	Ingestion of detergent
+ mucus	Esophagus, stomach	Bronchitis, gastritis
+ blood	Nose, pharynx → jejunum	All causes of hemorrhage
+ bile	Mid-duodenum	High ileal obstruction below Vater's papilla, ileus of upper ileum
+ feces	Jejunum, ileum	Ileus of lower ileum

Causes

Infections

Diagnostic program:
Blood count, CRP, ESR, urine
CSF, bilirubin
γGT/GPT/GOT
Microbiological diagnosis
Sonography/scintigraphy
Excretion urography

Gastritis
Peptic ulcer
Enteritis, appendicitis
Peritonitis
Hepatitis
Cholangitis, cholelithiasis
Pancreatitis
Pyelonephritis, ureteric stone
Meningitis
Pharyngitis, tonsillitis
Pertussis, bronchitis

Impaired passage
Abnormal propulsion

Diagnostic program:
Stomach tube, retained contents
Radiology, sonography
Blood gases, electrolytes (serum)
pH, endoscopy

Esophageal atresia/stenosis
Tracheoesophageal fistula
Achalasia
Hiatus hernia
Brachyesophagus
Gastroesophageal reflux
Foreign body
Pyloric stenosis
Anular pancreas
Duodenal atresia/stenosis
All forms of ileus
Hirschsprung's disease
Anal atresia/stenosis
Postabdominal operations

GASTROENTEROLOGY/NUTRITION

Metabolic disorders

Diagnostic program:
Blood gases, blood glucose, electrolytes
Creatinine, urea, ammonia
Lactate, ketone bodies (urine, serum)
17-hydroxyprogesterone
Uric acid (serum)

Metabolic acidosis in neonates
Enzyme defects of intermediary metabolism
Adrenogenital syndrome with salt loss
Hypoglycemia
Uremia
Reye's syndrome
Hyperuricemia

Psychological causes

Habitual vomiting
Anorexia nervosa
Aerophagy

Poisoning

Diagnostic program:
Fetor, mucosal inspection
Endoscopy
Screen for poisons (gastric secretion, urine)

Plant ingestion (laburnum)
Aflatoxin
Alkaloids
Colchicine
Alcohol
Botulinus toxin
Hydrocarbons
Alkalis/acids
Zinc chloride

Central cause

Migraine
Sunstroke
Raised intracranial pressure
Leukemic invasion of the meningococci
Trauma
Subdural hemorrhage

Vestibular cause

Labyrinthine stimulation (flying, rotation, seasickness)
Labyrinthitis
Herpes zoster oticus
Cholesteatoma
Ménière's disease

Therapeutic effect

Pediatric ipecacuanha emetic
Antitumor chemotherapy

Rough formula for length of nasogastric/orogastric tubes:

Tube length (nasal) = $0.252 \times$ body height (cm) + 5 $\Big\}$ infants/
Tube length (oral) = $0.226 \times$ body height (cm) + 6.7 $\Big\}$ adolescents

Indigestion/malabsorption: function tests

> Composition of the disaccharides:
> cellobiose = glucose + glucose
> lactose = galactose + glucose
> maltose = glucose + glucose
> saccharose (sucrose) = glucose + fructose
> trehalose = glucose + glucose

Indigestion/malabsorption

① **Screening of nonabsorbed carbohydrate:** feces – pH $\leq$ 5.5
Limitation: the pH is dependent on amount ingested, the transit time and the degree of intestinal bacterial colonization.

② **Screening for nonabsorbed sugar (reducing substances)**
Procedure: one part feces + two parts water; 15 drops of the mixture with one tablet of Clinitest placed in the reagent glass. Compare the color with the standard color chart after one minute.
Result: negative <0.25%; positive >0.5%.
Further investigation of glucose with the glucose oxidase test strip (as with blood sugar).
If negative results (saccharose, trehalose do not reduce), hydrolytic split: one part feces + two parts 0.1 normal HCl to be boiled for one min, then Clinitest as above.
Limitation: the result will be false-negative if all the sugars are bacteriologically broken down; false-positive due to bile pigments.

① and ② are always combined.

③ **Disaccharide loading test (oral)**
Procedure: morning fasting
insert indwelling needle, measure pretest glucose level 10% disaccharide solution in tea (2 g/kg or 50 g/m², maximum 100 g) by mouth or tube check blood sugar after 15, 30, 45, 60, 90, 120 min.
Result: normal = a rise in blood sugar >20 mg/dl (>1.1 mmol/l) in the first hour.
If result abnormal, repeat test with one of the two sugars of the disaccharide (1 g/kg) to exclude a monosaccharide absorption disorder.

④ **H₂ breath test**
Procedure: overnight fasting; give the disaccharide as with the oral loading test within the following 3–4 h, every 30 min; aspirate 3–5 ml of expired air, via tube or mask, in the second half of the expiratory phase, and analyze chromatographically.
If loading with a milk meal, the measurement phase must be extended to eight hours.
Results: An H_2 rise >22 ppm (parts per million, i.e. μmol/l) occurs with malabsorption.
With high 30-minute value, suspect bacterial colonization of the upper ileum.

> NB: More important than the measured values is the occurrence or worsening of the signs and symptoms of indigestion and malabsorption

GASTROENTEROLOGY/NUTRITION

Pathogenic (enterovirulent) *Escherichia coli* (EVEC)

Action group	Mechanism of action	Site of action	Accompanying diseases
Enteropathogenic *E. coli* (EPEC)	Bacterial adherence + toxic destruction of the ciliated epithelium	Lower ileum	Infantile diarrhea (dyspepsia)
Enterohemorrhagic *E. coli* (EHEC)	Ciliated epithelium and endothelial damage, verotoxin	Colon, endothelial vessels	Hemorrhagic colitis, hemolytic-uremic syndrome
Enterotoxic *E. coli* (ETEC)	Enterotoxins	Upper ileum	Cholera-like travel diarrhea
Enteroinvasive *E. coli* (EIEC)	Invasion + destruction of intestinal epithelial cells	Colon	Diarrhea

Diagnosis of dehydration

Classification by grades of severity (clinical signs)

Symptoms \ Grade	Dehydration Slight	Moderate	Severe
Weight loss. infants other children	≤5% ≤3%	5–10% 3–6%	10–15% 6–9%
Skin turgor Skin color Mucosa	n/↓ Pale Moist/dry	↓↓ Pale-gray Dry	↓↓↓ (marked folds, wrinkled) Gray, marbled Chapped
Fontanelle	Level/slight depression	Depressed	Deeply depressed
Pulse rate	n	↑	↑↑
Urine production	n	Oliguria	Anuria

Types of dehydration (pathophysiological signs)

Type Loss ratio salt:H$_2$O	Isotonic salt = water	Hypotonic salt > water	Hypertonic salt < water
Laboratory criteria Osmolality (serum) mosmol/kg Osmolality (urine) Na (serum) mmol/l Hematocrit Urea-N (serum)	 281–297 ↑ 133–145 ↑ n, ↑	 <281 ↑ <133 ↑ ↑	 >297 ↑ >145 ↑ ↑
Symptoms: CNS Skin turgor Skin temperature Pulse rate/quality	 Apathy, lethargy ↓ Cold ↑/soft	 Stroke, unconsciousness ↓↓ (Marbled) cold ↑↑↑/amplitude ↓↓	 Stroke, irritability Doughy Warm ↓/n
Causes	Diarrhea + vomiting	Salt-loss syndrome: sweating in mucoviscidosis cholera	Diabetes insipidus (renal, central), diarrhea, fluid deficiency

GASTROENTEROLOGY/NUTRITION

Oral rehydration

(Recommendations of the Ges. für Pädiatrische Gastroenterologie und Ernährung (1992).)
ORS = oral rehydration solution.

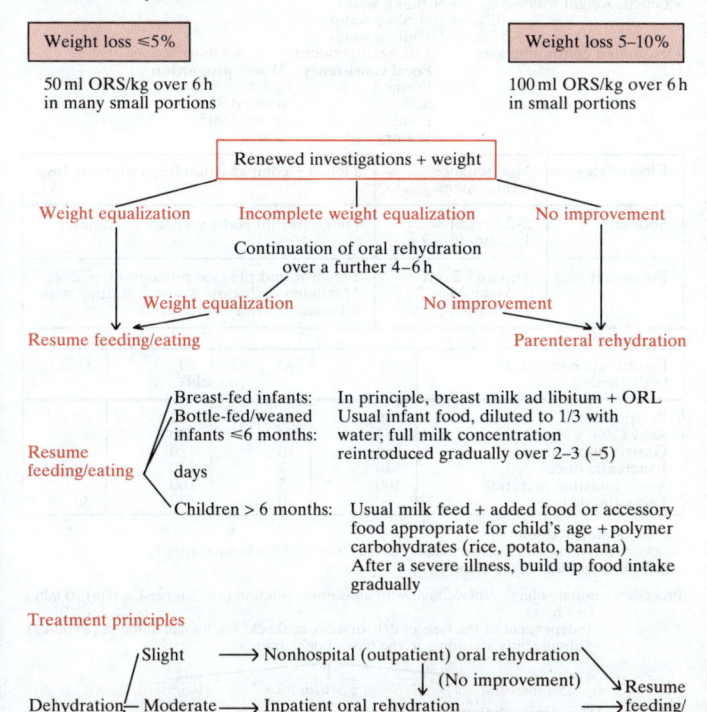

Weight loss ≤5%	Weight loss 5–10%
50 ml ORS/kg over 6 h in many small portions	100 ml ORS/kg over 6 h in small portions

Renewed investigations + weight

- Weight equalization → Resume feeding/eating
- Incomplete weight equalization → Continuation of oral rehydration over a further 4–6 h
  - Weight equalization → Resume feeding/eating
  - No improvement → Parenteral rehydration
- No improvement → Parenteral rehydration

Resume feeding/eating

- Breast-fed infants: In principle, breast milk ad libitum + ORL
- Bottle-fed/weaned infants ≤6 months: Usual infant food, diluted to 1/3 with water; full milk concentration reintroduced gradually over 2–3 (–5) days
- Children > 6 months: Usual milk feed + added food or accessory food appropriate for child's age + polymer carbohydrates (rice, potato, banana). After a severe illness, build up food intake gradually

Treatment principles

Dehydration
- Slight → Nonhospital (outpatient) oral rehydration
  - (No improvement) ↓
- Moderate → Inpatient oral rehydration
  - (No improvement) ↓
- Severe → Inpatient parenteral rehydration

→ Resume feeding/eating

Parenteral rehydration

Parenteral rehydration (amount per 24 h):
= basic water requirement
+ deficit: weight loss ~5% → 50 ml/kg water
~10% → 100 ml/kg water
~15% → 150 ml/kg water
+ estimated continuing loss

Estimated amounts in acute diarrhea

Fecal consistency	Water proportion
Formed	<80%
Soft	around 85%
Fluid	around 90%
Watery	>90%

Electrolytes	Maintenance requirement	Deficit + compensation for continuing loss
Sodium	2–3 mmol/l ≤ 2 y 1–2 mmol/l > 2 y	$(140 - [serum\ Na]^+) \times kg \times 0.2 = mmol/l$
Potassium	1 mmol/l 2–7 d 2–3 mmol/l ≤ 2 y 1–2 mmol/l > 2 y	Serum K and pH (see nomogram, p. 294) Maximum daily dose 8 mmol; starting with 0.1 mmol if urine is produced

Electrolyte content in body fluids	Na^+	K^+	Cl^-	HCO_3^-
	(mmol/l)			
Perspiration	30	10	30	
Saliva	15	30	30	
Gastric juice	50	10	120	
Pancreatic juice	140	7	120	30
Small intestine secretion	100	5	100	
Feces (liquid)	70	40	70	30

Choice of prepared solutions:
Acidosis: solutions with organic anions (lactate, acetate, bicarbonate, citrate).
Alkalosis: solutions high in chloride.

Procedure: initial volume replacement with an isotonic solution (e.g. Ringer-Lactate) 20 ml/kg in 1 h.
Independent of the type of dehydration, in shock: 5% human albumin (20 ml/kg).
Subsequently according to the type of dehydration:

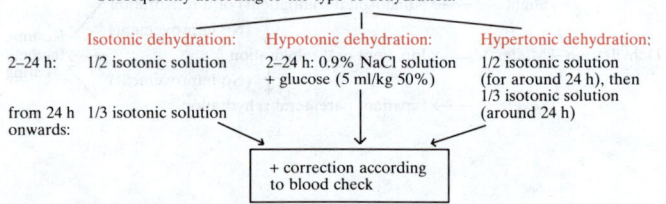

	Isotonic dehydration:	Hypotonic dehydration:	Hypertonic dehydration:
2–24 h:	1/2 isotonic solution	2–24 h: 0.9% NaCl solution + glucose (5 ml/kg 50%)	1/2 isotonic solution (for around 24 h), then 1/3 isotonic solution (around 24 h)
from 24 h onwards:	1/3 isotonic solution		

+ correction according to blood check

pH < 7.15/bicarbonate < 12 mmol/l → buffering $(15 - actual\ bicarbonate) \times kg \times 0.6 = ml$ of 8.4% bicarbonate solution.

GASTROENTEROLOGY/NUTRITION

Nutrition in the first year of life
(Modified from Schöch, Chahda and Kersting (1988).)

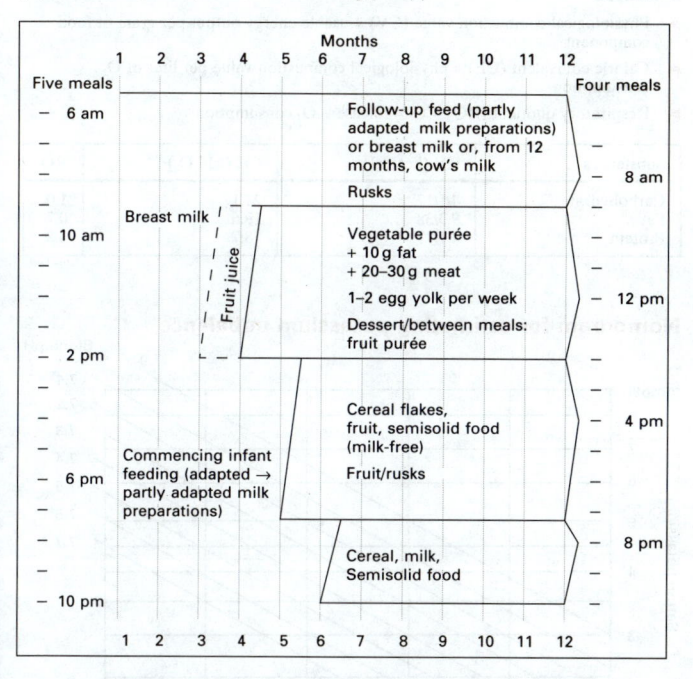

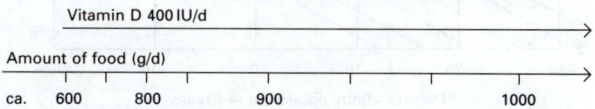

Five meals	Months 1–12		Four meals
6 am	Breast milk	Follow-up feed (partly adapted milk preparations) or breast milk or, from 12 months, cow's milk / Rusks	8 am
10 am	Breast milk / Fruit juice	Vegetable purée + 10 g fat + 20–30 g meat / 1–2 egg yolk per week / Dessert/between meals: fruit purée	12 pm
2 pm			
6 pm	Commencing infant feeding (adapted → partly adapted milk preparations)	Cereal flakes, fruit, semisolid food (milk-free) / Fruit/rusks	4 pm
10 pm		Cereal, milk, Semisolid food	8 pm

Vitamin D 400 IU/d →

Amount of food (g/d)

ca. 600   800   900   1000

MEMORIX PEDIATRICS

Nutritional energy

Definitions:

- ▶ Physiological combustion value (CV) = usable energy output per gram of food component
- ▶ Caloric equivalent (CE) = physiological combustion value per liter of O_2 consumption
- ▶ Respiratory quotient (RQ) = CO_2 release ÷ O_2 consumption

Substances	CV (kcal/kJ)	CE (kJ/l O_2)	RQ
Carbohydrate	4.1/17	21.1	1.0
Fat	9.3/38	19.6	0.7
Protein	4.1/17	18.7	0.8

Nomogram for estimating potassium imbalance

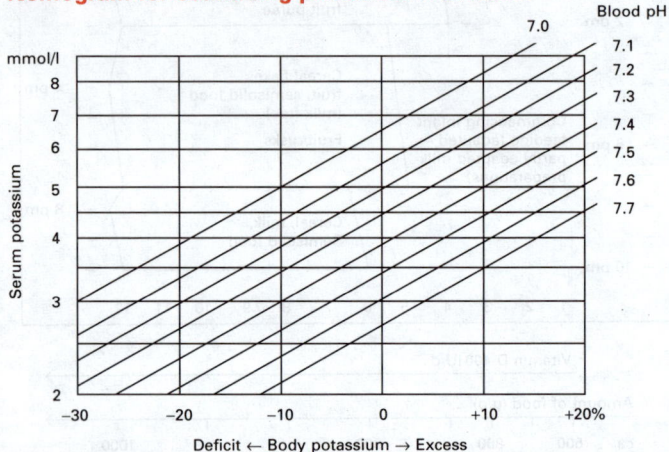

GASTROENTEROLOGY/NUTRITION

Parenteral nutrition
Basic water requirement
Age-independent calculation: 1.5 ml/kcal (0.4 ml/kJ)/d
1500 ml/m² body surface area (BSA)/d

Age-related volumes
(Recommendations of the German Society for Nutrition, 1986)

Age	ml/kg/d
1 d	50–70
2 d	70–90
3 d	80–100
4 d	100–120
5 d	100–130
1 y	100–140
2 y	80–120
3–5 y	80–100
6–10 y	60–80
11–14 y	50–70

Age-related 'rule of six' (ml/kg/d)

<6 kg	100 ml
<16 kg	80 ml
<36 kg	60 ml
<56 kg	50 ml
>56 kg	40 ml

Additional water requirements Fever: +5 ml/kg/d for every °C above 37.5°C rectal temperature

Hyperventilation, mechanical ventilation: +10 ml/kg/d

Basic requirement – electrolytes
(Recommendations of the German Society for Nutrition, 1986)

	mmol/kg/d
Sodium	3–5
Potassium	1–3
Calcium	0.1–1–3*
Magnesium	0.1–0.7
Chloride	3–5
Phosphate	0.5–1–2.5*

*Growth requirement for prematures

Food and energy requirement per kg per day

	Energy (kcal)	Glucose (g)	Fat (g)	Amino acids (g)
1st y	60–100	8–15	2–3	1.5–2.5
2nd y	70–90	12–15	2–3	1.5
3–5 y	60–70	12	1–2	1.5
6–10 y	50–60	10	1–2	1.0
10–14 y	50	8	1	1.0

MEMORIX PEDIATRICS

Survey of vitamin requirements

Vitamin	Prematures	0–6 months	6–12 months	2–11 y	>11 y
A	450	420	400	400–700	700
B_1 (mg)	0.7	0.3	0.5	0.7–1.2	1.1–1.4
B_2 (mg)	0.9	0.4	0.6	0.8–1.4	1.3–1.6
B_3 (mg)	11	6	8	9–16	15–18
B_6 (mg)	0.65	0.3	0.6	0.9–1.6	1.8
B_{12} (µg)	0.65	0.5	1.5	2–3	3
C (mg)	30	35	35	45	50
D (IU)	500	400	400	400	200
E (mg)	4.6	3–4	4–5	5–7	7
K (µg/kg)	15	15	15	15–30	10
Folic acid (µg)	90	30	45	100–300	400
Biotin (µg)	4	20	20	20–120	120
Pantothenic acid (mg)	2	2	2	2–4	5

Directions for the addition of trace elements (µmol/d): iron: 1–2
zinc: 1–2–4.6 (prematures)

Side-effects

Problem	Possible causes	Other findings	Measures
Cholestasis	1. Amino acid overload	Ammonia ↑, metabolic acidosis	Lower supply of amino acids
	2. Lipid supply	Triglyceride ↑, intravasal coagulation ↑	Reduce lipid supply
Hyperglycemia	Blood sugar, 150 mg/dl	Osmolality ↑ (serum, urine)	Reduce sugar supply
Hypoglycemia	Blood sugar 50–60 mg/dl	Serum: ketone bodies ↑ Urine: acetone ↑	Increase sugar supply
Alkaline phosphatase	Deficiency of vitamin D, calcium, phosphate		Substitution
Thin skin, cracks	Zinc deficiency	Serum zinc ↓	Supply ↑

Ready-made milk feeds

Definition	Initial infant feed	Infant milk feeds	Later feeds	Later milk
Age indication	From birth onwards	From birth onwards	>4 months	>4 months
Protein source	Cows' milk or soya protein	Cows' milk only	Cows' milk or soya	Cows' milk only

Adaptation: protein content < 2.5 g/100 kcal, whey protein : casein ≥ 1

GASTROENTEROLOGY/NUTRITION

Breast milk: nutrition in prematures

Composition	Mature human breast milk	ESPGAN recommendations
Energy (kcal/100 ml)	67	65–85
Protein (g/100 kcal)	1.33	2.25–3.1
Whey : casein (%/%)	77:28	
Fat (g/100 kcal)	5.15	4.6–6.6
MUFA (% fat)	15	
MCT (% fat)	5.9	40
Linolic acid (% kcal)	5.5	4.5
Carnitine (µmol/100 kcal)		≥7.5
Linolenic acid (mg/100 kcal)	89	55
Carbohydrate (g/100 kcal)	11.0	7–14
Lactose (g/100 kcal)	10.1	3.2–12
Other carbohydrates (g/100 kcal)	0.9	
Protein : fat : carbohydrate (%/kcal)	7:48:45	
Minerals and trace elements Calcium (mg/100 kcal)	46	70–140
Phosphorus (mg/100 kcal)	22	50–90
Ca : P	2.1	1.4–2.0
Magnesium (mg/100 kcal)	5.5	6–12
Sodium (mg/100 kcal)	22	23–53
Potassium (mg/100 kcal)	78	90–152
Chloride (mg/kcal)	63	57–89
Zinc (µg/100 kcal)	363	550–1100
Iron (µg/100 kcal)	99	1500 from 8 weeks old
Copper (µg/100 kcal)	57	90–120
Iodine (µg/100 kcal)	12	10–65
Manganese (µg/100 kcal)	3	2.1–7.5

MUFA = multiple unsaturated fatty acids; MCT = medium-chain triglycerides.

Breast milk: nutrition in prematures (continued)

Composition	Mature human breast milk	Recommendations of ESPGAN
Vitamins (additional) A (µg/100 kcal)	79	90–150
D (IU/100 kcal)	6	800–1600 IU/d
E (IU/100 kcal)	0.8	0.6
E (IU/g linolic acid)	1.4	0.9
K (µg/100 kcal)	2.2	4–15
B_1 (µg/100 kcal)	22	20
B_2 (µg/100 kcal)	55	60
Niacin (µg/100 kcal)	254	800
Pantothenic acid (µg/100 kcal)	313	330
B_6 (µg/100 kcal)	15	35
Biotin (µg/100 kcal)	1.0	1.5
Folic acid (µg/100 kcal)	6.4	6.0
B_{12} (µg/kcal)	0.04	0.15
C (mg/100 kcal)	7	7
Feeding recommendations: kcal/kg/d	130	130
ml/kg/d	200	150–200
Protein (g/kg/d)	1.78	2.9–4

MUFA = multiple unsaturated fatty acids; MCT = medium-chain triglycerides.

GASTROENTEROLOGY/NUTRITION

Special nutrition in metabolic defects

Diet adjustments

Indicated in:	Changes to diet: – to be reduced + to be increased
Maple-syrup disease	Isoleucine –/leucine –/valine –
Fructose intolerance	Fructose –
Galactosemia	Lactose –
Urea cycle enzyme defect	Essential amino acids +
Histidinemia	Histine –
Homocystinuria	Methionine –/cystine +
Hyperlysinemia	Lysine –
Isovaleric acidemia	Leucine –
Leucine sensitive hypoglycemia	Leucine –
Methylmalone aciduria	Isoleucine –/methionine –/threonine –/valine –
Phenylketonuria	Phenylalanine –
Proprionic acidemia	Phenylalanine –
Tyrosinemia	Phenylalanine –/tyrosine –

MEMORIX PEDIATRICS

Fever types
Examples
Continuous (amplitude <1°C): typhoid, viral pneumonia
Remittent: not diagnostic
Intermittent: sepsis, malignancy
Periodic: viral infections, e.g. measles, polio (biphasic), malaria
Undulating: Hodgkin's disease, brucellosis
End of fever: by lysis, by crisis

Fevers with no obvious initial cause
- Rare infections
- Autoimmune diseases
- Malignancy
- Medication

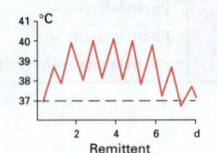

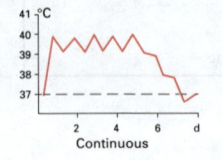

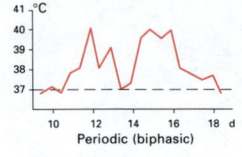

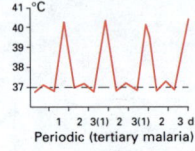

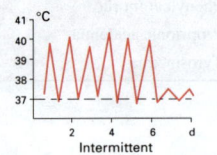

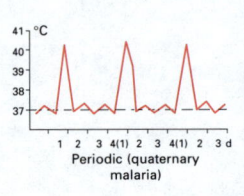

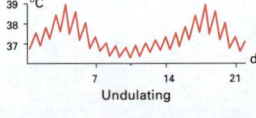

INFECTIONS/IMMUNOLOGY/RHEUMATOLOGY

Bacteriology
Structure of the bacterial cell

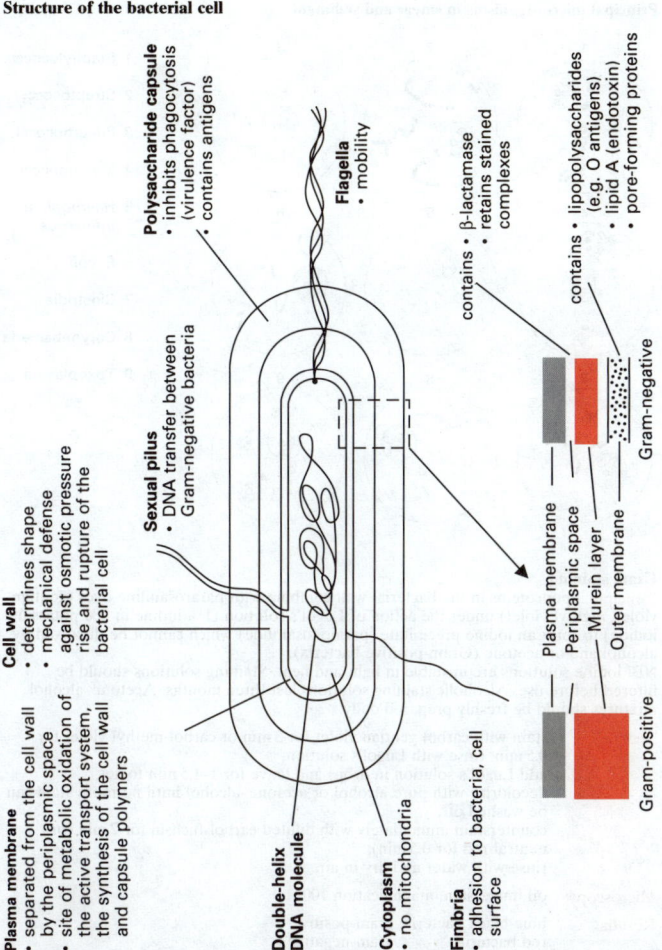

Polysaccharide capsule
- inhibits phagocytosis (virulence factor)
- contains antigens

Flagella
- mobility

contains
- β-lactamase
- retains stained complexes

contains
- lipopolysaccharides (e.g. O antigens)
- lipid A (endotoxin)
- pore-forming proteins

- Plasma membrane
- Periplasmic space
- Murein layer
- Outer membrane

Gram-negative

Gram-positive

Sexual pilus
- DNA transfer between Gram-negative bacteria

Cell wall
- determines shape
- mechanical defense against osmotic pressure rise and rupture of the bacterial cell

Plasma membrane
- separated from the cell wall by the periplasmic space
- site of metabolic oxidation of the active transport system, the synthesis of the cell wall and capsule polymers

Double-helix DNA molecule

Cytoplasm
- no mitochondria

Fimbria
- adhesion to bacteria, cell surface

MEMORIX PEDIATRICS

Diagnostic bacterial microscopy
Principal microorganisms in smear and sediment

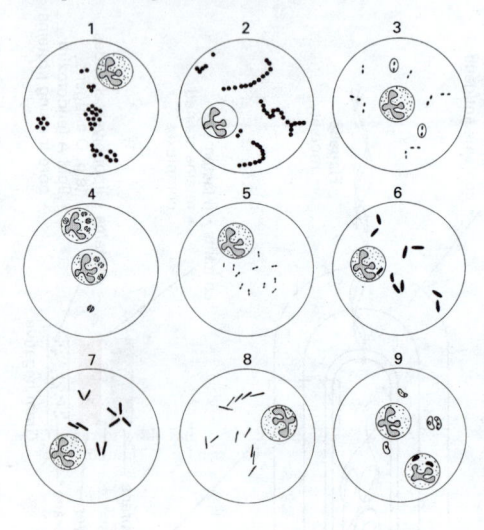

1 Staphylococci

2 Streptococci

3 Pneumococci

4 Meningococci

5 *Haemophilus influenzae*

6 *E. coli*

7 Clostridia

8 Corynebacteria

9 Toxoplasma

Gram staining

Principle: lipoproteins in the bacterial wall combine with pararosaniline dyes (gentian violet, methyl violet) under the action of Lugol's solution (1% iodine in 2% potassium iodide) to form an iodine precipitate (paraiodosaniline) which cannot be dissolved by alcohol and/or acetone (Gram-positive bacteria).
NB: iodine solutions are unstable in light and heat. Staining solutions should be filtered before use. Alcoholic staining solutions last three months. Acetone–alcohol mixtures should be freshly prepared daily.

Technique: stain with carbol-gentian violet for 3 min or carbol-methyl violet for 0.5 min; rinse with Lugol's solution;
add Lugol's solution in drops and leave for 1–1.5 min to act;
decolorize with pure alcohol or acetone–alcohol until no more stain can be washed off;
counterstain immediately with diluted carbol-fuchsin for 2 min (or neutral-red for 0.5 min);
rinse with water and dry in air.

Microscopy: oil immersion, magnification 100:1.

Results: blue-black bacteria: gram-positive
red bacteria: gram-negative.

INFECTIONS/IMMUNOLOGY/RHEUMATOLOGY

Differentiation of human pathogenic organisms by Gram staining

Gram-positive
Staphylococci
Streptococci
Pneumococci
Listeria
Corynebacterium diphtheriae
Mycobacteria
Fungi
Yeasts

Gram-negative
Meningococci
Haemophilus influenzae
Escherichia coli
Moraxella catarrhalis
Salmonella
Shigella
Campylobacter
Gonococci
Proteus
Pseudomonas

Ziehl–Neelsen staining

Principle: hydrophobic elements in the cell wall form a complex with carbol-fuchsin which cannot be completely removed either by acid or alcohol.

Technique: allow film to air dry and quickly fix over a flame.
Cover with concentrated carbol-fuchsin solution and leave for 5 min.
Intermittently pass through the flame and heat until vaporization starts.
Do not dry completely.
Rinse in running water.
Add decolorizing solution (HCl-alcohol) in drops and allow to run off, then dip into the decolorizing solution and agitate for 2–4 min until no more red stain is washed off.
Rinse with running water.
Counterstain with diluted methylene blue solution for 15–25 sec, depending on the thickness of the slide.
Rinse with running water, dry in air.

Result: acid-fast mycobacteria stain red, others stain blue.

Meningitis: diagnosis of cerebrospinal fluid

Cell count
The diluting solution (acetic acid plus methyl violet) is drawn up from an hour-glass bowl into a leukocyte pipette to mark 1. From a second bowl, fresh cerebrospinal fluid (CSF) is drawn up to mark 2. The contents of the ampulla of the pipette are mixed by rotating, the contents of the capillary part of the pipette are discarded, and a Fuchs–Rosenthal chamber filled with some drops. The leukocyte count in the chamber (volume 3.2 µl) divided by 3 = the CSF count (rounded off to whole numbers).

Upper limit of normal: neonates (first week)   20/cells/µl
                       all children over 1 month 5/cells/µl

Further cell differentiation from the CSF sediment (allow the preparation to dry in air, then stain with Giemsa or Pappenheim's stain).

Interpretation of findings
Note the time of the subarachnoid space puncture in relation to the time course of the inflammation. The cell count is only suitable for diagnosis and to check on progress, not for etiological differentiation.

Phase of inflammation	Duration	Cell picture (main cell type)	Type of inflammation
1 Granulocytic	Hours to 1 day >1 day	Neutrophils >60%	Meningitis of every etiology bacterial meningitis
2 Lymphocytic	Hours to weeks 1–2 weeks	Lymphocytes (>80%) (>50%)	Serous meningitis (viral) Uncomplicated bacterial meningitis
3 Monocytic	>2 weeks	Monocytes + lymphocytes	'Reparative stage'

Note: • *Listeria*, myobacteria and *Salmonella* cause a mixed picture of all inflammatory cells.
• In immune deficiency, changes occur in the cellular reaction (mostly minus or compensatory), depending on the system affected.

INFECTION/IMMUNOLOGY/RHEUMATOLOGY

Treatment of bacterial meningitis

(Recommendations of der Arbeitsgemeinschaft "Meningitis" der Paul-Ehrlich-Gesellschaft e.V. (supplemented))

Organism	Antibiotic treatment*		In penicillin allergy
	First choice	Alternative (sensitivity confirmed)	
Unknown Hemophilus influenzae	Cefotaxime or ceftriaxone	Chloramphenicol or ampicillin	
Neisseria meningitidis Streptococcus pneumoniae	Penicillin G	Cefotaxime or ceftriaxone or chloramphenicol	Chloramphenicol
Group B streptococci	Penicillin G	Cefotaxime or ceftriaxone	
E. coli	Cefotaxime or ceftriaxone	Combined with tobramycin or gentamicin	
Listeria monocytogenes	Ampicillin	Combined with gentamicin or tobramycin	

* Additional treatment with dexamethasone (0.15 mg/kg four times a day, beginning with the antibiotic treatment, for four days).

Duration of treatment of meningitis: normalization time for C-reactive protein (CRP) plus three days
– beyond the neonatal period for at least seven days
– neonates and infants two to three weeks

Note: three to four days after treatment is finished, repeat CRP check in order to spot the beginning of a relapse. No CRP monitoring is possible under corticosteroid treatment.

Treatment of meningitis – daily dosage

Penicillin G	$6 \times 50\,000$ IU/kg
Ampicillin	$4 \times 75–100$ mg/kg
Ceftriaxone	initially 1×100 mg/kg, then 1×75 mg/kg
Cefotaxime	4×50 mg/kg
Chloramphenicol[1,2]	4×25 mg/kg
Gentamicin[1,3]	2–3 times 2–2.5 mg/kg
Tobramycin[1,3]	2–3 times 2–2.5 mg/kg

[1] Check serum concentration.
[2] Check blood picture and reticulocyte count twice a week.
[3] Check renal function and adjust dosage accordingly.

MEMORIX PEDIATRICS

Tuberculosis: contacts, diagnosis and treatment

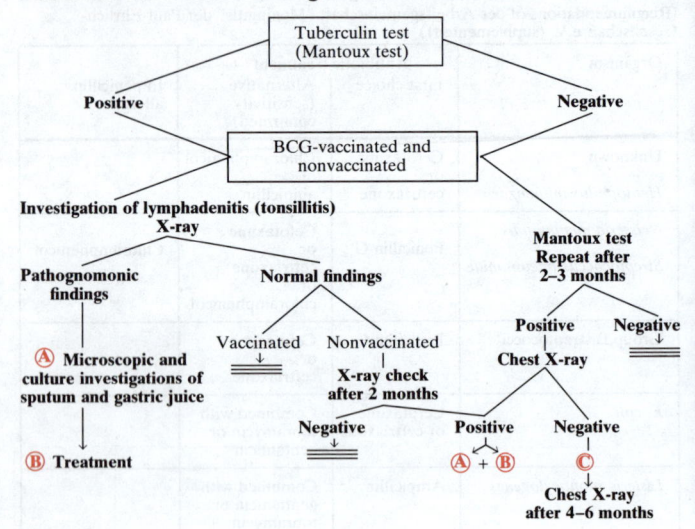

```
                    Tuberculin test
                    (Mantoux test)
          Positive                    Negative
                 BCG-vaccinated and
                   nonvaccinated

Investigation of lymphadenitis (tonsillitis)
            X-ray
                                                 Mantoux test
                                                 Repeat after
                                                 2–3 months
Pathognomonic       Normal findings
  findings
                                              Positive    Negative
                  Vaccinated  Nonvaccinated      ↓
Ⓐ Microscopic and                             Chest X-ray
culture investigations of
sputum and gastric juice    X-ray check
                            after 2 months
                                          Negative  Positive  Negative
Ⓑ Treatment                    Negative           Ⓐ + Ⓑ       Ⓒ
                                                            Chest X-ray
                                                           after 4–6 months
```

Ⓑ Treatment of organ tuberculosis and/or tuberculous meningitis

Initial stage (two to three months): Isoniazid (INH) + rifampicin + pyrazinamide + (streptomycin in extensive infection or INH resistance) daily, plus vitamin B_6.
Ethambutol is an alternative to pyrazinamide.
Corticoids for the first four weeks in meningitis and marked granulations.

Stabilizing stage (4–10 months): INH + rifampicin daily plus vitamin B_6.

Ⓒ Preventive chemotherapy (after conversion negative → positive in Mantoux test):

INH + vitamin B_6 for three months.

Chemoprophylaxis (for unaffected people who have been exposed to infectious patients

INH + vitamin B_6 according to the exposure.

INFECTION/IMMUNOLOGY/RHEUMATOLOGY

Toxoplasmosis

Diagnostic tests

1 Qualitative: **Screening tests**

  Direct agglutination test (DA)
  Indirect immunofluorescence test (IIFT)
  Sabin–Feldman test (SFT)

2 Quantitative: **Toxoplasma-IgM-antibodies**

  Enzyme immunoassay (EIA-IgM)
  Immunosorbent agglutination assay (ISAGA)

  Clarification tests

  IIFT quantitative } (titer stages 1:16, 1:64, etc.)
  SFT quantitative

Three-step diagnosis (recommendations of the BGA-Kommission "Toxoplasmose und Schwangerschaft"):

  Antibody test ⟶ IgM-antibody test ⟶ Clarification test

Serodiagnosis of prenatal infection

Investigation point postpartum* (precautionary)	Test used EIA-IgM or ISAGA	Result IIFT or SFT	Interpretation Prenatal infection: + yes, – no	Comments†
1st day maternal and child's blood	Positive ⟶ Negative ⟶	≥ 1:4096 ≥ 1:256 1:1024	+ + – ?	+ +
4–6 weeks	Positive ⟶ Negative ⟶	≥ 1:4096 ≤ 1:256 1:1024	+ + – ?	+ +
3–4 months	Positive ⟶ Negative ⟶	≥ 1:4096 ≥ 1:256 1:1024	+ + – ?	+ +
5–6 months	Positive ⟶ Negative	≥ 1:1024 ≥ 1:1024 ≤ 1:256	+ + + –	+ + +

* The various times are meant as progress or starting points.
† Titer checks with IIFT or SFT.

Diagnosis of postnatal toxoplasmosis infection

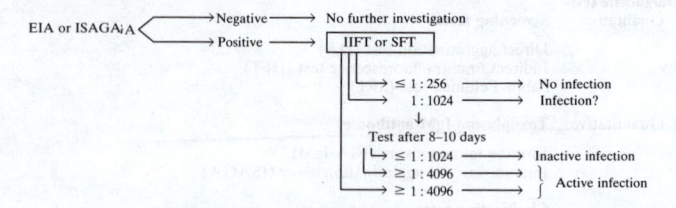

```
EIA or ISAGA₁A  →  Negative  →  No further investigation
                →  Positive  →  IIFT or SFT
                                    ↓
                                    → ≤ 1 : 256   →  No infection
                                    → 1 : 1024    →  Infection?
                                         ↓
                                    Test after 8–10 days
                                    → ≤ 1 : 1024  →  Inactive infection
                                    → ≥ 1 : 4096  →  ⎫
                                    → ≥ 1 : 4096  →  ⎬ Active infection
```

Identification of parasites in blood

Technique

Blood film
– Put small drops of blood from finger tip or ear lobe at the edge of a microscope slide and place on another slide at an angle of 45°. After contact of the blood with the second slide, move the first slide flat over the second one without pressure.

– Allow the preparation to air dry, then fix in water-free methanol, air dry again and put under microscope.

Thicker drops
– Put large drops of blood directly on to a microscope slide. Then transfer to another slide with a glass rod or edge of a slide and spread it over an area of ca. 1.5 cm².

– Leave the preparation lying horizontally to dry for about 2 h at room temperature (do not fix with heat or alcohol).

– Removal of hemoglobin:
  a) with Giemsa stain
  b) for 5–10 min, place the slide with the covered side down in a vessel containing distilled water, with one slide edge on the vessel wall. Finally stain with Giemsa without fixing.

INFECTION/IMMUNOLOGY/RHEUMATOLOGY

Syphilis: serodiagnosis of infection with treponemes pathogenic in humans

Antibody tests:
      Cardiolipin reaction (complement fixation reaction (CFR) or venereal disease research laboratory test (VDRL))
      FTA AT (fluorescence *Treponema* antibody absorption test)
      TPHA (*Treponema pallidum* hemagglutinin assay)

Quantitative antibody differentiation: IgM in the immunofluorescence test or ELISA
                                                  IgG in the enzyme immunoassay.

Diagnostic procedure

TPHA ⟶ ± ⟶ FTA AT ⟶ ± ⟶ cardiolipin reaction ⟶ IgM

Test patterns and interpretation

TPHA	FTA AT	Tests Cardiolipin test	IgM	IgG	Interpretation	Comments
–	–	–			No infection	Up to ca. two weeks before
++++	++++	++++	++++		Infection	Treatment necessary
+	+	–	+		Infection	Treatment necessary plus serology checks
++++	++++	(+)	+		Reinfection (primary infection some time previously)	IgG suppressed IgM synthesis
+++	++++	++	++	++++	Infection healed	'serum scar'
+++	++++	++	(+)	++++		
+	+	–	–	+		
+	–					
–	++	–			Nonspecific findings	

MEMORIX PEDIATRICS

Notification of infectious diseases
Obligatory notification
(differs between countries)

Disease	Causative organisms	Notifiable if: suspected	Notifiable if: disease	Notifiable if: excreting	Death	Special rules
Meningitis	all		×		×	
Encephalitis	all		×		×	
Cytomegalovirus	CMV		×*		×*	*only congenital
Early summer meningo-encephalitis (ESME)	Flavivirus		×		×	
Yellow fever	Flavivirus		×		×	
Japanese encephalitis B	Flavivirus		×		×	
Hemorrhagic fever	Hantavirus Puumala virus	×	×		×	
Hepatitis A	Picornavirus		×		×	
Hepatitis B	Hepadnavirus		×		×	
Hepatitis C	Togavirus (?)		×		×	
Hepatitis D	RNA-virus		×		×	
Hepatitis E	?		×*		×	
Herpes simplex	human herpesvirus 1		×*			*only in meningo-encephalitis
Genital herpes	Human herpesvirus 2		×*			
Influenza						
Measles	Paramyxovirus		×*		×	*only in public health institutions
Mumps	Paramyxovirus		×*¹		×*	*only meningitis ¹ increased incidence in residential homes, kindergartens and hospitals
Smallpox	Orthopoxvirus	×	×		×	
Polio	Enterovirus	×	×		×	
Rubella	Rubivirus		×*		×*	*only embryopathy
Rabies	Rhabdovirus	×	×		×	
Varicella zoster	human herpesvirus 3		×*		×	+ only encephalitis
Borreliosis (relapsing fevers)	Borrelia	×	×		×	not Lyme disease
Botulism	Clostridium botulinum	×	×		×	
Brucellosis (Mediterranean fever)	Brucella melitensis		×			
Cholera	Vibrio cholerae	×	×			quarantine
Diphtheria	Corynebacterium diphtheriae		×			

INFECTION/IMMUNOLOGY/RHEUMATOLOGY

Notification of infectious diseases (continued)

Disease	Causative organism	Notifiable if: suspected	Notifiable if: disease	Notifiable if: excreting	Death	Special rules
Typhus	*Rickettsia prowazeki*	x	x		x	
Gas gangrene	*Clostridium perfringens*		x		x	
Leprosy	*Myobacterium leprae*	x	x		x	
Listerosis	*Listeria monocytogenes*		x*		x*	*only if congenital
Syphilis	*Treponema pallidum*		x+[1]		*	*if congenital, otherwise anonymous
Anthrax	*Bacillus anthracis*	x	x		x	
Ornithosis	*Chlamydia psittaci*	x	x		x	
Paratyphoid A, B, C, (and other salmonella infections)	*Salmonella paratyphi* and others	x	x	x	x	
Pertussis	*Bordetella pertussis*		x*		x	
Plague	*Yersinia pestis*	x	x*		x	*wide quarantine
Puerperal sepsis						
Q fever	*Coxiella burneti*		x			
Glanders	*Pseudomonas mallei*				x	
Scarlet fever	*Streptococcus* group A		x*		x	*only in public institutions
Shigella (dysentery)	*Shigella*	x		x	x	
Tetanus	*Clostridium tetani*		x		x	
Trachoma	*Chlamydia trachomatis*		x		x	
Tuberculosis	*Mycobacterium bovis tuberculosis avium*		x		x	
Tularemia	*Bacterium tularense*	x	x		x	
Typhoid	*Salmonella typhi*	x	x	x	x	
Malaria	*Plasmodia*		x*		x	*(+ relapse)
Toxoplasmosis	*Toxoplasma gondii*		x*		x*	*only congenital
Trichinosis	*Trichinella spiralis*		x		x	

MEMORIX PEDIATRICS

Immunization schedule

Age	Disease; immunization against	Schedule
2 months	*Haemophilus influenzae* (type B) (Hib) Diphtheria–tetanus–pertussis (DTP) Polio Tuberculosis (BCG) (in special circumstances)	Injection Injection Oral Injection
3 months	Hib DTP Polio	Injection Injection Oral
4 months	Hib DTP Polio	Injection Injection Oral
12–15 months	Measles–mumps–rubella (MMR)	Injection
3–5 years	Tetanus–diphtheria (Td)	Injection
School entry	Polio	Oral
10–14 years	Rubella (girls only)	Injection
15–18 years	Tetanus Polio Tuberculosis (BCG)	Injection Oral Injection

INFECTION/IMMUNOLOGY/RHEUMATOLOGY

Indications for immunization

Disease immunization against	Indications/target group	Application
Tuberculosis	Exposed tuberculin-negative children and adults without evidence of immune defect	BCG vaccine strictly intracutaneous. Neonates and infants up to 6 weeks old without testing Tuberculin testing: *1. Before immunization, multiple test (10 IU/PRD), if Mantoux puncture test negative (100 IU/PRD) *2. >3 months after immunization, as for preimmunization. If negative, repeat immunization if possible
Pneumococci	At-risk patients with chronic organic disease, functional asplenia, before splenectomy	1 injection s.c., i.m. for children ≥2 y; below this age only on strong indications
Hepatitis A	People taking holidays in epidemic areas, medical personnel (pediatrics), personnel in day nurseries, kitchen staff, laundry workers drug addicts	3 injections (i.m., upper arm) Schedule: 0, 1 month, 6–12 months
Hepatitis B	Preexposure: people in close contact with HBsAg-positive subjects at high risk of infection; patients with raised risk of infection: frequent blood transfusions, dialysis, heart-lung machine; patients in institutions (behavioral or psychological disorders); medical personnel, paramedics, police	Basic immunization as recommended by manufacturers Anti-HBs check required >8 weeks after the basic immunization
	Postexposure: neonates of HBsAg-positive mothers; medical personnel in injuries with hepatitis B-containing items	Instant combined prophylaxis: vaccine + contralateral hepatitis B immunoglobulin i.m. (at least 200 IU)
Early summer meningoencephalitis encephalitis (ESME)	Children and adults in endemic areas	Basic immunization: second injection 1–3 months after the first, third injection 9–12 months after the second. Booster after 3 years
Influenza	Children and adults with chronic organic disease (heart, airways, anemias, metabolic or renal diseases, immunosuppression) People at increased risk of infection	Annual immunization (late summer, autumn) Vaccine with current antigen combination
Varicella	The immunosuppressed, susceptible children and adults, seronegative prepregnant women	1 injection s.c., possibly repeat later

313

Incomplete immunization

Disease; immunization against	Problem/indication	Measures
Tetanus	No injury: – Complete basic immunization – Incomplete basic immunization After injury (exposure): – complete basic immunization • insignificant superficial injury • all other injuries – incomplete basic immunization • at least two toxoid injections in the past 10 years • immunized twice + injury >24 h before Only immunized once Unsure if immunized Not immunized Extensive burns	Booster with Td, if last immunization ≥10 years previously, complete with DT; complete with Td in children >8 years old No treatment or booster (Td) if last immunization ≥10 years earlier Booster (Td) if last immunization ≥5 years before Booster (Td) } Combined immunization: 250 IU antitoxin +75 IU tetanus toxoid; second injection (toxoid only) after 4 weeks; first booster (toxoid) after 6–12 months Combined immunization with 2 × 250 IU and then antitoxin, each injection 36 h apart
Diphtheria	After complete basic immunization Incomplete basic immunization Incubation	Booster every 10 years (Td) until age 40 Completion: children >8 years, immunization dose = 75 IU toxoid (D) children <8 years and adults, immunization dose = 5 IU toxoid (d) Completion if possible with DT, or Td Basic immunization if not immunized Booster if last immunization >3 years before
Polio	No immunization Incomplete basic immunization Immunization of a child or an adult in a community or residential home Travel to endemic areas	Basic immunization 1 immunization dose (trivalent) orally Basic immunization or booster for inhabitants if last dose >10 years before (booster = 1 oral dose) Booster

INFECTION/IMMUNOLOGY/RHEUMATOLOGY

Immunization in pregnancy
Measures if exposure during pregnancy and negative or uncertain history of immunization

General:
- history of infection and immunization of mother and older children
- arrange medical examination of the affected contacts
- if necessary, determine the antibody status of the mother.

Special prophylaxis:
Rules:
- no immunization with live vaccine during pregnancy (exceptions below)
- if possible avoid active immunization during pregnancy (inflamatory-autonomic effect on the mother)
- active immunization given by mistake is no indication for termination of pregnancy.

Procedure

Disease	Active immunization (D = dead vaccine; L = live vaccine)	Passive immunization (St-Ig = standard immunoglobulin; H-Ig = immunoglobulin with high titer for specific antibodies)	Special circumstances
Rubella		H-Ig	
Measles		St-Ig 0.1 ml/kg	
Mumps		St-Ig 0.1 ml/kg	
Varicella zoster		H-Ig	If necessary, treat the affected mother with acyclovir
Polio	L/D		Killed vaccine only for booster before pregnancy
Hepatitis A		St-Ig 0.1 ml/kg	
Hepatitis B		H-Ig	
ESME		H-Ig	
Influenza		St-Ig	Only if antibody deficiency
Rabies	D		
Yellow fever	L		Only in endemic areas
Tetanus	D		Should be done as active or combined immunization
Diphtheria	D (d)		Treat nonimmunized cases with antitoxic serum and penicillin G
Pertussis			Chemoprophylaxis with erythromycin
Tuberculosis	L		BCG immunization only on the strictest indications
Typhoid	L		Only if at high risk in epidemic areas
Cholera	D		Only in epidemic areas

MEMORIX PEDIATRICS

Immunization: special indications

Immunization in immune deficiency

- If immune deficiency is suspected, postpone immunization and define deficiency precisely.
- Use only passive immunization in contact cases.
- Use active immunization only if patient is in good general condition and in the absence of active inflammatory processes.

Type of immune deficiency	Active immunization possible
Primary (congenital) Pure granulocyte function defect Intracellular bactericidal disorder (granulocytes, monocytes)	1. Diphtheria, tetanus, pertussis, pneumococci, *Haemophilus influenzae* type b, meningococci, cholera polio (parenteral, Salk vaccine), hepatitis B, ESME, rabies, influenza (killed vaccine) 2. Varicella, mumps, rubella (live vaccine) Active immunization is contraindicated against: tuberculosis (BCG), measles, polio (oral, Sabin vaccine), typhoid orally
Functional defects of T-cells and B-cells and all combinations	1. Immunization with killed vaccine is possible, but check the effectiveness of immunization by measuring the antibody titer and decide on an individual basis whether a booster is necessary 2. Varicella, mumps, rubella Immunization is contraindicated against: tuberculosis (BCG), measles, polio oral (Sabin vaccine), typhoid orally
Secondary (acquired) HIV infection: Children, adolescents and children of HIV-infected mothers in the asymptomatic stage of the disease	Diphtheria, tetanus, measles, mumps, rubella according to the immunization schedule Polio (Salk vaccine): three times at intervals of six to eight weeks, booster after 6–12 months Indications: hepatitis B, influenza, pertussis – as in the non-infected
Symptomatic HIV infection	No immunization with live vaccine

Immunosuppression (ionizing radiation, drugs)	Preconditions for immunization:
	  – no chemotherapy induction phase
	  – interrupt any chemotherapy for one week before and after the immunization
	  – lymphocyte count $\geq 1200/\mu l$
	  – positive skin reaction (type IV, tuberculin type) to PPD (tuberculin), candida and other 'recall antigens'
	Diphtheria, tetanus, polio (Salk vaccine), hepatitis B, varicella
	
	Contraindications to immunization as for primary immunodeficiency

Note: healthy children living with immunocompromised persons should be immunized with polio vaccine (Salk) (attenuated viruses in the oral vaccine can mutate in the immunized person and re-attain their neurovirulence).

INFECTION/IMMUNOLOGY/RHEUMATOLOGY

Schedule for rabies immunization

Vaccine: HDC (human diploid cell culture) vaccine

Schedule	Indication	Procedure
Prophylactic immunization	Frequent trips to endemic rabies areas; animal with rabies (infected cadaver): make sure no contact with saliva, no skin damage before or after contact If immediate or postexposure immunization has begun, but investigations reveal the animal to have been healthy, continue with prophylactic immunization	1 immunization dose on days 0, 28, 56 and after 1 year or 1 dose on days 0, 7 and 21 and after 1 year
Postexposure immunization	Rabies suspected animal (cadaver): salivary contact, skin damage Animal shows rage: type of exposure unclear (no injury) After renewed exposure, if complete immunization > 5 years ago	1 immunization dose on days 0, 3, 7, 14, 30 and 90
Postexposure combined immunization	Animal (cadaver) suspected of rabies, enraged or wild animal (and unavailable for examination): treat as for salivary contact of skin/mucosa, bite injury	20 IU/kg human rabies immunoglobulin + schedule of postexposure immunization

For all schedules: 1 booster every 2–5 years
Reexposure immunization (mild cases/severe cases):
   complete immunization < 1 year previously → 1 immunization dose on day 0/days 0 and 3
   complete immunization 1–5 years previously → 1 immunization dose on days 0 and 3/days 0, 3 and 7		

Local wound treatment after exposure to rabies
(After WHO (1984).)

First aid: Wash and rinse the wound with water and detergent or soapy water. Wash away soap thoroughly. Then treat the wound with 40–70% alcohol, tincture of iodine or 0.1% quaternary ammonium solution.

Wound treatment: After cleansing, spray rabies immunoglobulin into the depth of the wound and infiltrate the surroundings. Postpone suture of the wound. Give prophylaxis against tetanus and infection.

Vaccine data

(Summarized from manufacturers' information and Spiess (1987).)

Vaccine	Abbreviation	Characteristics	Application	Combined vaccines
Dead vaccine				
Bacteria				
Tetanus	T	} Toxoid	i.m.	} DT, Td, DPT
Diphtheria	D, d		i.m.	
Pertussis	P	} Inactivated bacteria	i.m.	
Cholera	–		i.m.	
Haemophilus influenzae	Hib	}	i.m.	} With capsular protein, meningococci B or toxoid D, T.
Meningococci A, C	–	} Capsular polysaccharide	i.m.	
Pneumococcus	–		i.m.	
Viruses				
Hepatitis B	HB	HBsAg by gene technology	i.m.	
Early summer meningoencephalitis		} With formaldehyde-inactivated viruses	i.m.	
Polio	(Salk)		i.m.	–
Influenza			i.m.	
Rabies		With betapropriolactone-inactivated viruses	i.m.	
Live vaccine				
Bacteria				
Bacillus Calmette-Guérin	BCG	Attenuated by culture bovine mycobacteria	i.c.	
Typhoid	–	*Salmonella typhi* with enzyme defect mutant	oral	
Viruses				
Measles	–	} Attenuated by culture viruses	s.c.	} MMR
Mumps	–		s.c.	
Rubella	–		s.c.	
Polio	(Sabin)	Avirulent polio viruses	oral	–
Yellow fever	–	Attenuated viruses	s.s	
Varicella	–	Attenuated viruses	s.c.	

INFECTION/IMMUNOLOGY/RHEUMATOLOGY

Recommendations for hepatitis B prophylaxis after exposure
(After DVV (1986).)

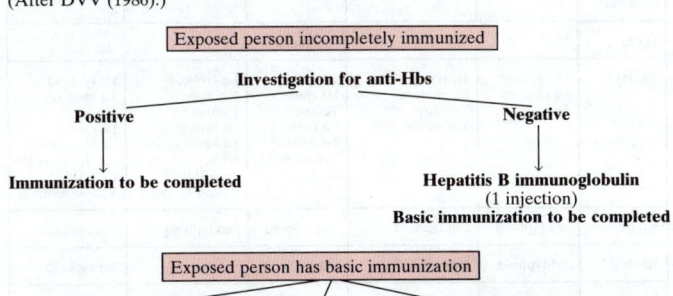

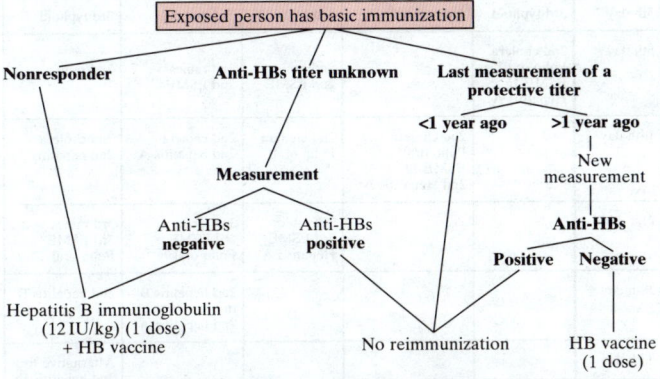

Exposed person incompletely immunized

Investigation for anti-Hbs

- **Positive** → Immunization to be completed
- **Negative** → **Hepatitis B immunoglobulin** (1 injection) **Basic immunization to be completed**

Exposed person has basic immunization

- **Nonresponder** → Hepatitis B immunoglobulin (12 IU/kg) (1 dose) + HB vaccine
- **Anti-HBs titer unknown** → **Measurement**
  - Anti-HBs negative → Hepatitis B immunoglobulin (12 IU/kg) (1 dose) + HB vaccine
  - Anti-HBs positive → No reimmunization
- **Last measurement of a protective titer**
  - <1 year ago → No reimmunization
  - >1 year ago → New measurement → **Anti-HBs**
    - Positive → No reimmunization
    - Negative → HB vaccine (1 dose)

After active immunization check titer (protective anti-HBs titer: >10 IU/l).

MEMORIX PEDIATRICS

Schedule for travelers' immunization

Time until departure	8 days	2 weeks	3 weeks	4 weeks	5 weeks
Date	Immunizations				
1st day	1st typhoid 1st cholera Tetanus*	1st typhoid 1st cholera Tetanus* Yellow fever	1st typhoid 1st cholera Tetanus* 1st rabies 1st ESME[§] Yellow fever	1st typhoid 1st cholera Tetanus* 1st rabies 1st hepatitis A 1st hepatitis B 1st ESME[§] Yellow fever	1st typhoid 1st cholera Tetanus* 1st rabies 1st Hepatitis A 1st Hepatitis B 1st ESME[§] Yellow fever
3rd day	2nd typhoid	2nd typhoid	2nd typhoid	2nd typhoid	2nd typhoid
5th day	3rd typhoid	3rd typhoid	3rd typhoid	3rd typhoid	3rd typhoid
8th day	2nd cholera Polio oral* ESME-Ig Hepatitis A[†]		2nd rabies 2nd ESME	2nd rabies 2nd ESME	2nd rabies
14th day		2nd cholera Polio oral* ESME-Ig 2nd Hepatitis A[†]	2nd cholera Polio oral*	2nd cholera 2nd hepatitis A[†]	2nd cholera 2nd hepatitis A[†]
21st day			3rd rabies 3rd ESME Hepatitis A[†]	3rd rabies 3rd ESME Polio oral	3rd rabies 3rd ESME Polio oral
28th day				2nd hepatitis B or 2nd hepatitis A[†]	2nd hepatitis B
35th day					Alternative to 2nd hepatitis B: hepatitis A[†]

* = booster; [†] = immunoglobulins if no active immunization possible; [‡] = complete basic immunization achieved only with 3rd injection after 6 months; ESME-Ig = immunoglobulin; [§] = rapid immunization schedule.

INFECTION/IMMUNOLOGY/RHEUMATOLOGY

Immunization in allergy or suspected allergy/combined immunization

Vaccine	Allergen	Alternative measures
Measles–mumps		1. **Intracutaneous test** with diluted material according to the degree of presumed allergy. Begin with 1/100. Result negative → immunization.
Yellow fever	Chicken egg albumin	2. **Fractionated immunization** if result positive. Degree and quantity of fractions according to the grade of the immediate reaction. Injection intervals 15–20 min.
ESME		In general, begin with 0.05 cm^3, doubling the next doses (do not vary the total dosage).
Rabies		Inoculation with HDC rabies vaccination.
Influenza		1. Allergy testing. 2. Immunization with split vaccines.

Intervals between different immunizations

Rules: 1. No specific interval is required when using dead material (inactivated organisms).

2. With living material (attenuated, still possibly multiplying organisms) there should be an interval of ≥ four weeks, provided that the immunization reaction is completed and has faded without complications.
   Measles, mumps and rubella immunizations can be given simultaneously, but not after an interval of days to four weeks.

   Exceptions: after yellow fever immunization, a live vaccine can be given after two weeks.

   Interval between oral immunization against:

$$\text{Typhoid} \xleftarrow[14 \text{ days}]{3 \text{ days}} \text{Polio}$$

3. Vaccines of live and dead organisms can be given at the same time if they are not directed against the same disease.

4. Between immunoglobulin administration and parenterally applied living vaccine there should be an interval of at least three months.

   Exceptions: oral immunization against polio and typhoid (build-up of intestine-associated immunity).

5. Further intervals in live immunization:
   ≥ three weeks after steroid treatment
   ≥ six months after splenectomy
   two weeks before or after an operation.

MEMORIX PEDIATRICS

Course of serology in acute (red) and chronic (gray) hepatitis B

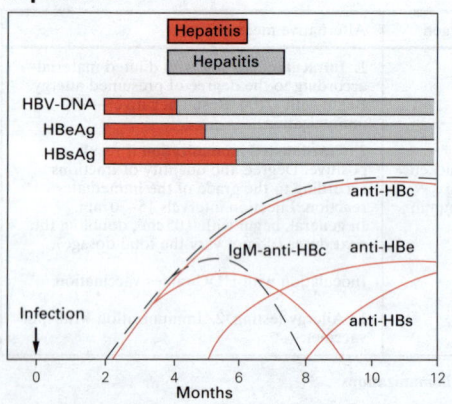

Controlled hepatitis B immunization

Engerix B vaccine (SmithKline Beecham)
Immunization with hepatitis B vaccine (e.g. Engerix B, SmithKline Beecham)

	1st dose	2nd dose	3rd dose	Booster
Basic immunization	Birth	1 month	6 months	5 years
Fast-track immunization	Birth	1 month	2 months	1 year

8 weeks after measurement of the anti-HBs titer		
Check results	Measurements	Further checks
Anti-HBs titer (IU/l) ⓐ <10 ⓑ 10–100 ⓒ 100–1000 ⓓ 1000–10 000 ⓔ >10 000	Repeat immunization immediately Check after 2–3 months Check after 1 year Check after 2.5 years Check after 5 years	Check after 4 weeks proceed to ⓐ or ⓑ or ⓒ or ⓓ or ⓔ

Note: If after proper basic immunization and two further ones no anti-HBs antibodies are demonstrable, the subject is probably a non-responder. Further injections are not indicated. Give HBV immunoglobulin after exposure.

INFECTION/IMMUNOLOGY/RHEUMATOLOGY

Diagnostic components of the hepatitis B virus

Surface: Antigens → Antibodies
- HBsAG → Anti-HBs-Ab
- Pre-S1-Ag → Ant-pre-S1-Ab
- Pre-S2-Ag → Anti-Pre-S2-Ab

Core:
- HBcAg → Ant-HBc-Ab
- HBeAg → Anti-HBe-Ab

Additional: double-stranded DNA, DNA polymerase, reverse transcriptase, protein bound to DNA (HBx-antigen?)

Antigen–antibody pattern for the assessment of hepatitis B infectivity

Infectivity	Positive (Findings)	Negative
None	Ant-HBs-Ab	
None	Anti-HBs-Ab Anti-HBc-Ab Anti-HBe-Ab	HBsAg
Low	HBsAg Anti-HBc-Ab Anti-HBe-Ab	
High	HBsAg HBe-Ag Anti-HBc-Ab	
Very high	HBs-Ag HBV-DNA Anti-HBc-Ab	

Course of serology in hepatitis A

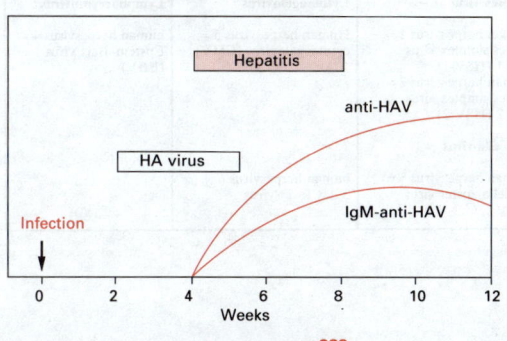

Early summer meningoencephalitis (ESME)
Treatment after tick-bite in an endemic area

Time interval after the bite \ Immune status	No immunization	1st immunization ≤ 14 days before the bite	1st immunization > 14 days before the bite	2nd immunization before the bite
≤ 48 h	ESME immunoglobulin 0.1 ml/kg		2nd partial immunization	Only in immunodeficiency: active/passive immunization
48–96 h	0.2 ml/kg ESME immunoglobulin			
≥ 96 h	No passive immunization 2nd partial immunization 4 weeks after the 1st immunization Nonimmunized healthy subject has basic immunization after incubation period			3rd partial immunization 9–12 months after the 2nd

Classification of herpes viruses

Family	Herpesviridae		
Subfamily	Alpha herpesvirus	Beta herpesviridae	Gamma herpesvirus
Characteristics	Rapid growth, short reproductive cycle, rapid propogation of the infection in culture, high cytolytic potential, frequent persistence in ganglion cells	Slow-growing, relatively longer reproduction cycle, cytomegaly, less cytolysis than alpha herpesvirus, persists in salivary glands, kidneys, lymphoreticular lymph cells	Tropism to T or B lymphocytes, replication in the T or B cell range
Genus	Simplex virus	Cytomegalovirus	Lymphocryptovirus
in human host	Human herpesvirus 1 = herpes simplex virus type 1 (HSV-1) Human herpesvirus 2 = herpes simplex virus type 2 (HSV-2)	Human herpesvirus 5 = cytomegalovirus (CMV)	human herpesvirus 4 = Epstein–Barr virus (EBV)
Genus	Varicella virus	?	
in human host	Human herpesvirus 3 = varicella-zoster virus (VZV)	human herpesvirus 6 = 3-day fever virus	

INFECTION/IMMUNOLOGY/RHEUMATOLOGY

Diagnostic survey of the commonest viral diseases
(After Wiegand (1992).)

How to obtain specimens:
Type of specimen, transport medium and investigative method (e.g. nucleic acid + PCR) to be discussed with viral laboratory.

Nasopharyngeal sample:
– if adequate secretion present, take specimen by direct aspiration, or
– instill drops of 0.9% NaCl, about 0.5–1 ml, into each nostril, the head bent forward and the nasal contents caught in a sterile glass, or
– ca. 10 ml NaCl (0.9%) to be gargled and then spat into sterile container.

Urine specimen: midstream specimen.

Blood specimen: whole blood (5 ml) for serology, heparinized (10 IU/ml) for viral isolation.

Pustule: aspirate contents.

Preserve all cell-holding specimens (blood, CSF, biopsies) at −70 °C.

Disease/symptom	Viruses in question	Investigations indicated
Arthralgia	Rubella Hepatitis B Parvovirus B19	Serum Serum Serum
Airways infection	Influenza Parainfluenza types 1–4 Respiratory syncytial virus (RSV) Rhinoviruses Adenoviruses Coronaviruses	Nasopharyngeal secretion, serum Nasopharyngeal secretion, serum Nasopharyngeal secretion, serum Nasopharyngeal secretion, swab Nasopharyngeal secretion, serum Nasopharyngeal secretion, serum
Neonates	Varicella-zoster (VZV) Enteroviruses Measles Cytomegalovirus (CMV)* Epstein–Barr virus (EBV)* Herpes simplex (HSV)*	Nasopharyngeal secretion Feces Serum Serum Serum Nasopharyngeal secretion
Embryopathies (malformations, diagnosis in the neonatal period)	Rubella CMV Hepatitis B* VZV* Parvovirus B19	Urine, serum Urine, serum Serum, (liver biopsy) Urine, serum Serum
Exanthemata	Measles Rubella EBV VZV Human herpes virus 6 (HHV 6) HSV Coxsackievirus A16 and others Enteroviruses	Serum, nasopharyngeal secretion Serum, nasopharyngeal secretion Serum Serum Serum Serum, pustular content Nasopharyngeal secretion, serum, feces Nasopharyngeal secretion, serum

* Rare organisms or rarely investigated.

MEMORIX PEDIATRICS

Disease/Symptom	Viruses in question	Investigations indicated
Encephalitis, serous meningitis (brain biopsy not indicated)	Measles	Serum, CSF
	Mumps	Serum, CSF
	Rubella	Serum, CSF
	Enterovirus	Nasopharyngeal secretion, feces, CSF, serum
	ESME	Serum
	HIV	Serum
	Lymphocytic choriomeningitis	Serum
Gastroenteritis	Rotaviruses	Feces, serum
	Adenoviruses (types 40, 41)	Feces, serum
	Norwalk	Feces
	Enteroviruses*	Feces, serum
	Calicivirus	Feces
	Astrovirus	Feces
Hepatitis	Hepatitis A	Feces, serum
	Hepatitis B	Serum, biopsy
	Hepatitis C	Serum
	Epstein–Barr (EBV)	Serum
	Cytomegalovirus (CMV)	Serum
Conjunctivitis (keratitis)	Adenoviruses (types 8, 19, 37)	Serum, swab
	Coxsackievius A24	Serum, swab
	Enterovirus 70	Serum, swab
Lymphadenitis	EBV	Serum
	CMV	Urine, serum
	HIV	Serum
	Human herpesvirus 6 (HHV 6)	Serum
Myocarditis	Coxsackievirus B	Feces, nasopharyngeal secretion, serum
	Influenza	Nasopharyngeal secretion, serum
	Coxsackievirus A*	Nasopharyngeal secretion, feces, serum
	ECHO*†	Nasopharyngeal secretion, feces, serum
	Adenoviruses*	Nasopharyngeal secretion, feces, serum
	CMV*	Serum
Pancreatitis	Mumps	Serum
	Coxsackievirus B	Nasopharyngeal secretion, feces, serum
Stomatitis	Herpes simplex (HSV)	Nasopharyngeal secretion, serum
	Coxsackievirus A	Nasopharyngeal secretion, feces, serum

* Rare organisms or rarely investigated.
† ECHO = enterocytopathogenic human orphan virus.

INFECTION/IMMUNOLOGY/RHEUMATOLOGY

Human enteroviral diseases
(Modified from Melnick (1982).)

Symptoms/Disease	Enteroviruses	Types
Serous meningitis	Polio Coxsackievirus A Coxsackievirus B ECHO Enterovirus	1–3 2, 4, 7, 9, 10, 23 1–6 1–11, 13–23, 25, 27, 28, 30, 31 71
Encephalitis	Polio Coxsackievirus B ECHO Enterovirus	1–3 1–5 2, 6, 9, 19 (3, 4, 7, 11, 14, 18, 22?) 71
Paralysis	Polio Coxsackievirus A ECHO	1–3 7, 9 2, 4, 6, 9, 11, 30 (1, 7, 13, 14, 16, 18, 31?)
Conjunctivitis (acute, hemorrhagic)	Coxsackievirus A Enterovirus	24 70
Fever + influenza, 'colds', summer flu	Polio Coxsackievirus A Coxsackievirus B	1–3 21, 24 and others 1–6
Herpangina, pharyngitis + lymphadenitis	Coxsackievirus A Coxsackievirus A	2–6, 8, 10 10
Respiratory tract infection + pneumonia	Coxsackievirus A Coxsackievirus B ECHO Enterovirus	9, 16 4, 5 4, 9, 11, 20, 25 (1–3, 6–8, 16, 19, 22?) 68
Pleurodynia (+ Bornholm's disease)	Coxsackievirus B ECHO	1–5 1, 6, 9
Myocarditis, pericarditis	Coxsackievirus B ECHO	1–5 1, 6, 9, 19
Hepatitis	Hepatitis A (= enterovirus 72) Coxsackievirus A Coxsackievirus B ECHO	 4, 9 5 4, 9
Pancreatitis	Coxsackievirus B	1, 2, 4
Diabetes mellitus	Coxsackievirus B	4

MEMORIX PEDIATRICS

Symptoms/Disease	Enteroviruses	Types
Diarrhea	Coxsackievirus A ECHO	18, 20–24 No fixed association
Exanthema	ECHO	2, 4, 6, 9, 11, 16, 18 (1, 3, 5, 7, 12, 14, 19, 20?)
Exanthema, macular	Coxsackievirus A Coxsackievirus B	2, 4, 9, 16, 23 1, 3, 5
Exanthema, vesicular	Coxsackievirus A	4–6, 9, 10, 16
Foot-and-mouth disease	Coxsackievirus A Enterovirus	5, 10, 16 71

328

INFECTION/IMMUNOLOGY/RHEUMATOLOGY

Malaria prophylaxis/recommendations

Measures: exposure prophylaxis – chemoprophylaxis – chemoprophylaxis + standby therapy (administration of a therapeutically effective medication in a feverish illness in an endemic area)

Prophylaxis by stage

Stage of organism	Plasmodia			
	P. vivax (tertian malaria)	P. ovale (tertian malaria)	P. malariae (quartan malaria)	P. falciparum (tropical malaria)
Sporozoites (from mosquito) ↓		Proguanil	Proguanil	Proguanil
Hypnozoites (in the liver) ↓	Primaquine	Primaquine		
Schizonts (in the liver) ↓		Proguanil	Proguanil	Proguanil
Merozoites (in blood) ↓	Chloroquine Quinine Mefloquine Halofantrine	Chloroquine Quinine Halofantrine	Chloroquine Quinine Halofantrine	Chloroquine Quinine Mefloquine Halofantrine Tetracycline
Gametocytes (in blood)	Chloroquine Quinine Pyrimethamine	Pyrimethamine	Pyrimethamine	Chloroquine Quinine Pyrimethamine

Recommendations for prophylaxis modified according to risk
(After Leichsenring, Bussman and Bremer (1991))

E = exposure prophylaxis; P = chemoprophylaxis; s = standby treatment

Regions with little risk of infection, no resistance to chloroquine:
  Very little risk: E + s (chloroquine)
  Higher risk: E + P (chloroquine)

Regions with medium risk of infection, possible resistance to chloroquine:
  E + P (chloroquine, possibly + proguanil) + s

High risk areas (resistance to varisos medications):
Duration of stay < 1 month and body weight > 15 kg: E + P (mefloquine)
Duration of stay > 1 month or body weight < 15 kg: E + P (chloroquine + proguanil) + s

Dosage:
Chloroquine   5 mg/kg/week orally
Proguanil   3 mg/kg/day orally
Mefloquine   15–19 kg: 1/4 tablet/week ⎫
             20–30 kg: 1/2 tablet/week ⎬ Weeks 1–4, then fortnightly doses
             31–45 kg: 3/4 tablet/week ⎪
             >45 kg: 1 tablet/week   ⎭

Begin chemoprophylaxis one week before arriving at the malarial region.
Terminate the prophylaxis four weeks after leaving the area.
In pregnancy use chloroquine and/or proguanil.
The medication passes into breast milk in very small amounts, giving no protection for the infant.

Kawasaki's syndrome

Diagnostic signs

A Fever, without other obvious cause, lasting five days

B Bilateral conjunctival hyperemia
Mucosal inflammation, strawberry tongue, dry and red lips
Distal limbs: edema, palmar and plantar erythema, scaling (2–3 weeks)
Trunk: polymorphic rash
Cervical (lateral) lymph node enlargement

C Exclude (differential diagnosis) other infections:
measles, streptococcal infection, leptospirosis, *Rickettsia*

Diagnosis possible in the presence of:

A + B + C
A + 4 of B + C
A + 3 of B + sonographic verification of a coronary aneurysm

Treatment

Medication	Dosage	Treatment duration
Acetylsalicylic acid (aspirin)	60–100–130 mg/kg/d orally Serum level 20–25 mg/dl	1–2 weeks
	50 mg/kg/d	3 weeks
	3–5 mg/kg/d	from 3 weeks
Gammaglobulin	2 g/kg infusion over 10 h or 0.4 g/kg/d i.v.	5 days
Steroids (if no fall in temperature after 3 days)	2 mg/kg/d orally	3–4 weeks

Morphological staging in Kawasaki's syndrome

Stage I 1–2 weeks	Perivasculitis, vasculitis (arterioles, small arteries and veins), intimal inflammation of medium and large arteries.
Stage II 2–4 weeks	Regression of inflammation in the smallest vessels, vasculitis in the medium-sized arteries, development of aneurysms, stenoses, thrombi (particularly in coronary arteries).
Stage III 4–7 weeks	Smallest vessels as in stage II, granulating inflammation in medium-sized arteries.
Stage IV from 7 weeks	Scarring stage: aneurysms, stenoses from scar contraction and intimal hypertrophy, development of thrombi in medium-sized arteries, no acute inflammation, persistence of healing of lesions.

INFECTIONS/IMMUNOLOGY/RHEUMATOLOGY

Sequence of immunological findings after HIV infection (children >6 months)

(Modified from Stiehm and Wara (1991).)

Note: After perinatal HIV infection, the disease progresses more rapidly than in juveniles or adults.

Criterion	Stages/findings (n = normal, age-dependent normal values)			
	Asymptomatic		Symptomatic	
	Early	Late	Early	Late
HIV antibodies*	+	+	+	+
Absolute Lymphocyte count	n >1500/µl	n >1500/µl	↓ 150–1000/µl	↓ <1000/µl
CD4 cells (absolute)	n > 1200/µl	1200–800/µl	800–400/µl	<400/µl
CD8 cells (absolute)	n > 800/µl	n	n/↓	<200/µl
Helper:suppressor = CD4:CD8 ratio	n (>2.0)	1.0–0.75	0.75–0.5	<0.5
B lymphocytes	n	↑ (>15%)	↑	
Immunoglobulins (IgG + IgA + IgM)	n 600–1500 mg/dl	↑ >1800 mg/dl	↑	
Antibody formation against neoantigens	n	Defect	Defect + ↓	0
Antibody formation against repeated antigen contact (recall antigens)	n	n	n to ↓	↓ to 0
NK (natural killer) cytotoxicity	n	n	↓	↓

*Some neonates and prematures have no HIV antibodies if there is an association with a hypogammaglobulinemia.

MEMORIX PEDIATRICS

HIV infection: definitions

(After the Centers for Disease Control Criteria (1987) and the recommendations of the German Federal AIDS Center (BGA).)

Definition of HIV infection in children >15 months (perinatal infection)
Reason for age limit: prenatally transferred maternal antibodies can persist until the 15th month of life.

Infection is present if:

1. The virus is demonstrable in blood or tissues.

   or

2. Antibodies are present (screening test [enzyme immunoassay] + positive confirmatory test [e.g. Western blot]).
   plus   Signs of cellular and humoral immune defects
          (gammaglobulin ↑ + lymphocyte count ↓, or
          CD4 cells (T4 helper) ↓ or CD4:CD8 ratio ↓).
   plus   Finding of infection symptomatic of HIV (→CDC classification PII).

   or

3. A disease pointing to AIDS (see below) is diagnosed.

   or

4. Antibodies are identified in serum (positive screening and confirmatory tests), but the mother was not infected during the pregnancy.

Definition of HIV infection in children >15 months to ≤13 years (vertical = perinatal infection, horizontal = later infection)
(Adolescents >13 years are subject to the adult classification.)

An HIV infection is established by:
1. Identification of HIV in blood or tissues.
2. Identification of antibodies.
3. Confirmed diagnosis of a disease pointing to AIDS.

(CDC = Centers for Disease Control, Atlanta, USA; BGA = Federal Health Office.)

INFECTIONS/IMMUNOLOGY/RHEUMATOLOGY

HIV infection: Centers for Disease Control classification
(Children ≤13 years old)

Class (P-pediatric)	Features	Further diagnostic measures
P0 (suspected infection)	Children ≤15 months: Exposure against infected mother with antibody cover: neither proof of virus antigen nor symptoms	Check: Changes in antibody titer Development Infections Immunological parameters
PI (asymptomatic infection)	Definition of HIV infection is met	
Subclass A	Normal immunological function	
Subclass B	One or more abnormal immunological functions associated with HIV infection (hypergammaglobulinemia, T4 (CD4) lymphopenia, T4:T8 ratio ↓, absolute lymphopenia)	Exclude other causes (e.g. genetic immune defects, pharmacogenic immune suppression, Hodgkin's disease, ALL*, CML†, non-Hodgkin's lymphoma, except primary cerebral lymphoma)
Subclass C	Children with incomplete immunological testing	Complete investigation
PII (symptomatic infection)	Appropriate definition of HIV infection plus signs/symptoms of an infectious disease Depending on the symptoms, patients can belong to more than one subclass	Causes other than HIV infection must be excluded
Subclass A	≥2 nonspecific findings that persist for ≥2 months: fever, dystrophy, weight-loss >10%, hepatomegaly, splenomegaly, generalized lymphadenopathy, persistent or recurrent parotitis (≥2 episodes within 2 months), diarrhea (≥2 thin stools/d)	Ascertain immune status; microbiological and virological differential diagnosis
Subclass B	Encephalopathy: (1) arrest or reduction of mental and/or motor development; (2) progressive cerebral motor disorders with 2 or more symptoms (paresis, ataxia, pathological reflexes, abnormal muscle tone); (3) abnormal CNS growth in MRI or CT scans	Exclude neurometabolic and other hereditary metabolic defects

* ALL = acute lymphocytic leukemia.
† CML = chronic myelogenous leukemia.

CDC classification of HIV infection (children ≤13 years old, continued)

Class (P-pediatric)	Features	Further diagnostic measures
PII		
Subclass C	Interstitial lymphoid pneumonia (either histologically proven or persisting for ≥2 months despite antibiotics)	Subclasses C and D. Diagnostic tests clarify individual findings (e.g. X-rays), exclude a genetically determined immune defect, identify infection by serological, cultural, cytological and histological investigation. If toxoplasmosis in the first 3 months, include the mother in the serological testing
Subclass D	Secondary infectious diseases due to HIV-conditioned immunodeficiency	
	Category D1: *Pneumocystis carinii* pneumonia, chronic cryptosporidiosis, toxoplasmosis (onset beyond the 1st month of life), extraintestinal strongyloidiasis, chronic isosporiasis, disseminated coccidioidomycosis, candidiasis (bronchopulmonary, esophageal), extrapulmonary cryptococcosis, disseminated histoplasmosis, nocardiosis, other disseminated mycobacterial infections, cytomegalovirus or herpes simplex virus infection after the first month of life, progressive multifocal leukoencephalopathy	
	Category D2: ≥2 bacterial infections in 2 years (sepsis, meningitis, pneumonia, osteomyelitis, organ abscess, joint empyema)	Exceptions are otitis media and superficial skin and mucosal abscesses
	Category D3: oral candidiasis for ≥2 months, ≥2 oral herpes attacks per year, herpes zoster in several dermatomes	
Subclass E	Secondary malignancies: Category E1: Kaposi's sarcoma, primary cerebral lymphoma, non-Hodgkin's lymphoma of B-cell type	Exclude T-cell lymphoma
	Category E2: high grade lymphoma	
Subclass F	Other diseases as possible sequelae of an HIV infection: hepatitis, carditis or cardiomyopathy, glomerulonephritis, autoimmune hemolytic anemia, thrombocytopenia, chronic dermatitis	Look for autoantibodies, immune complexes

Notes: class PII (subclasses A–E) includes diseases pointing to AIDS (CDC case definition for pediatric AIDS). Perinatally infected children can show AIDS-associated symptoms before their parents. On proof of antibodies in a child, the parents should be included in the investigative process.

INFECTIONS/IMMUNOLOGY/RHEUMATOLOGY

Biological properties of the immunoglobulins

Characteristics	IgA1	IgA2	IgG1	IgG2	IgG3	IgG4	IgM	IgE	IgD
Reaction with Fc-receptor to: Neutrophils			+		++				
Basophils (+ mast cells)								+++	
Lymphocytes			++	?	++	?			
Macrophages	+	+	+		++				
Thrombocytes			+	+	+	+			
Complement-binding: 'classic pathway'			+++	+	+++		+++		
'alternative pathway'	+	+	+	+	+	+	?	+	+
Placental transfer			+	+	+	+			
Presence of secretion	+	+++					+	+	

Allergies: Types of allergic reactions
(After Gell and Coombs (1963).)

Type of reaction	Reagents* Immunopathology	Reaction site	Cardinal symptoms	Clinical picture
Type I Anaphylactic reaction immediate reaction after s/min	AB: specific, homocytotropic IgE = reagents = precipitating AB 0 complement binding Cells: basophil, mast cells Mediators: histamine, serotonin, heparin, leukotrienes (C_4, D_4, E_4) prostaglandins	Surface of mast cells and basophils	Blister, urticaria, edema, shock	Anaphylactic shock, allergic rhinitis/conjunctivitis, bronchial asthma, eczema
Type II Cytotoxic reaction	AB: specific IgG (IgM) mediate – phagocytosis of target cells via granulocytes, macrophages – cytolysis by large lymphocytes – cytolysis by complement	Surface of own and foreign cells	Exanthema, purpura and others	Blood transfusion reaction; drug-induced thrombocytopenia, hemolytic anemia, agranulocytosis; myasthenia gravis; Hashimoto's thyroiditis; Goodpasture's nephritis
Type III Arthus reaction, immune complex reaction, after 4–6 h	AB: IgG (IgM) bind complement, formation of small immune complexes	Edema + cell infiltration in vessel walls, glomeruli, synovia	Rosette formation	Allergic vasculitis (e.g. Henoch–Schönlein purpura), serum disease, glomerulonephritis, allergic alveolitis
Type IV cell-mediated reaction, later type, after 24–72 h	AB: none Cells: T-lymphocytes, macrophages, fewer granulocytes Precipitating factors: intracellularly surviving bacteria, parasites	Skin, perivascular connective tissue	Papules, granuloma	Contact eczema, graft versus host reaction, tuberculosis, leprosy, brucellosis, mycoses

* AB = antibodies.

INFECTIONS/IMMUNOLOGY/RHEUMATOLOGY

Immunodeficiency syndrome
Immune defects associated with other diseases

Disease	Immunoglobulin + antibodies (serum)	B cells	T cells	Presumed pathogenesis	Other symptoms	Mode of inheritance
Ataxia telangiectasia	IgA → or ↓ IgG → or ↓ IgE →	n	→	Maturation defect of T cells	Ataxia, telangiectases, α-fetoprotein ↑, lymphoreticular malignoma	AR
DiGeorge syndrome	n/↓	n	→	Thymus aplasia, T cell defect	Hypoparathyroidism, aortic arch and/or other cardiac defects	?
Partial albinism	↓ all isotypes	n	n/↓	?Natural killer cell defect	Cerebral atrophy	AR
Transcobalamine-2 deficiency	↓ all isotypes	n	n	Cell proliferation defect (Vit B_{12})	megaloblastic anemia, villar atrophy	AR
Wiskott-Aldrich syndrome	IgM ↓, IgA ↑, IgE ↑	n	n → ↓	Membrane defect of the hematopoietic stem cells	Eczema, thrombocytopenia, lymphoreticular malignoma	X

337

Primary immune defects: WHO classification

Term	Phenotype				
	Serum immunoglobulin + serum antibodies	Circulating B cells	Circulating T cells	Presumed pathogenesis	Mode of inheritance
A Preponderent antibody defects (antibody deficiency syndrome)					
X-chromosomal agammaglobulinemia	All isotypes ↓	Absent	n	Differentiation defect Pre-B → B cells	X
X-chromosomal agammaglobulinemia with severe growth hormone deficiency	All isotypes ↓	Absent or very little	n	Differentiation defect	X
Autosomal recessive congenital agammaglobulinemia	All isotypes ↓	↓	n	Differentiation defect	AR
Ig deficiency with high IgM (hyper-IgM syndrome)	IgM ↑, IgD ↑/n, other Ig ↓	n (IgM-, IgD- forming lymphocytes)	n	Switch defect in specific B cell maturation	X, AR, AD
IgA deficiency 1.	IgA ↓, IgA2 ↓ ± IgG2, IgG3, IgG4	n	n	Defect in terminal B cell differentiation	?AR, ?AD, increased incidence in families with CVID (common variable immunodeficiency)
2.	IgA1 or IgA2 ↓	n	n	Partial deletion 14q32	AR
Selective Ig deficiency	One or more isotypes ↓, others normal	n?	n	Terminal Ig-isotype differentiation defect	?
κ-chain defect	κ-chain of Ig ↓, AB reaction ↓/n	κ+ –B– ↓	n	In part, punctate mutation 2p11	?
Immunodeficiency syndrome (IDS) with thymoma	All isotypes	Absent or ↓	Variable	?	?
Transitory hypogammaglobulinemia of early childhood	↓ IgG, ↓ IgA	n	T helper cells ↓	Retarded maturation of helper cell function	Increased incidence in families with IDS

INFECTIONS/IMMUNOLOGY/RHEUMATOLOGY

Term	Phenotype				
	Serum immunoglobulin + serum antibodies	Circulating B cells	Circulating T cells	Presumed pathogenesis	Mode of inheritance
B Combined variable immunodeficiency (CVID)					
CVID with predominant B cell defect	Variable, several isotypes ↓	n/↓	n	Differentiation defect T helper cell function ↓	AR AD
CVID with predominant T cell defect	Variable, several isotypes ↓	n	n/↓	?Differentiation disorder in thymus, T-suppressor function ↑	AR
CVID with autoantibodies against T or B cells	Variable ↓	↓	↓	No differentiation	?
C Severe combined immunodeficiency (SCID)					
Reticular dysgenesis	↓	↓	↓	Differentiation disorder of T and B cells	AR
T or B cells reduced	↓	↓	↓	⎫ Maturation ⎬ disorder ⎭	AR/X
T cells ↓ B cells normal	↓	n	↓		AR
Bare lymphocyte syndrome	↓	↓	↓	No HLA determinants on T and B cells	AR
D Other combined immune defect syndromes					
Immune defect after Epstein–Barr infection	After infection ↓	After infection ↓	n	? (+ aplastic anemia)	AR/X
Adenosine deaminase defect (ADA)	↓	↓	↓	Metabolic lymphocyte damage (+ dysosteogenesis)	AR
Purine-nucleoside phosphorylase deficiency (PNP)	n → ↓	n	n → ↓	Metabolic T-cell damage (+ anemia, retardation)	AR

Complement defects and associated diseases

Complement defect	Relapsing infectious diseases	Rheumatic diseases
C1q		Membranoproliferative glomerulonephritis, congenital poikilodermia
C1r		Glomeruonephritis, lupus erythematosus-like (LE-like syndrome)
C1s		LE-like syndrome, vasculitis, arthritis
C1 inactivator		Hereditary angioneurotic edema
C2, C4		Forms of LE, vasculitis, polymyositis, glomerulonephritis
C3, C3b inhibitor	Otitis media, pneumonia, sepsis, meningitis	Glomerulonephritis, LE-like syndrome, vasculitis
C5	Meningococci, gonococci	Systemic lupus erythematosus (SLE)
C6	*Neisseria*	SLE, rheumatoid arthritis
C7	*Neisseria*	Vasculitis
C8	*Neisseria*	SLE
C9	*Neisseria*	

INFECTIONS/IMMUNOLOGY/RHEUMATOLOGY

Complement activation (schematic)

Symbols: P = properdin; D = C3-proactivator-convertase; B = C3-proactivator; I = C3b/
C4b- inactivator; H = β_1-H-globulin.

- Addition of the symbols denotes binding of the individual components to the cell surface in cooperative distance from one another.
- a,b = effective fragments after limited proteolysis.
- i = inactive components.
- If a component/complex is enzymatically active, this is denoted by a horizontal line: $\overline{\text{(C4b2a)}}$. C1 = C1q + C1r + C1s ∿∿∿ split-off polypeptide; red = inhibitors.

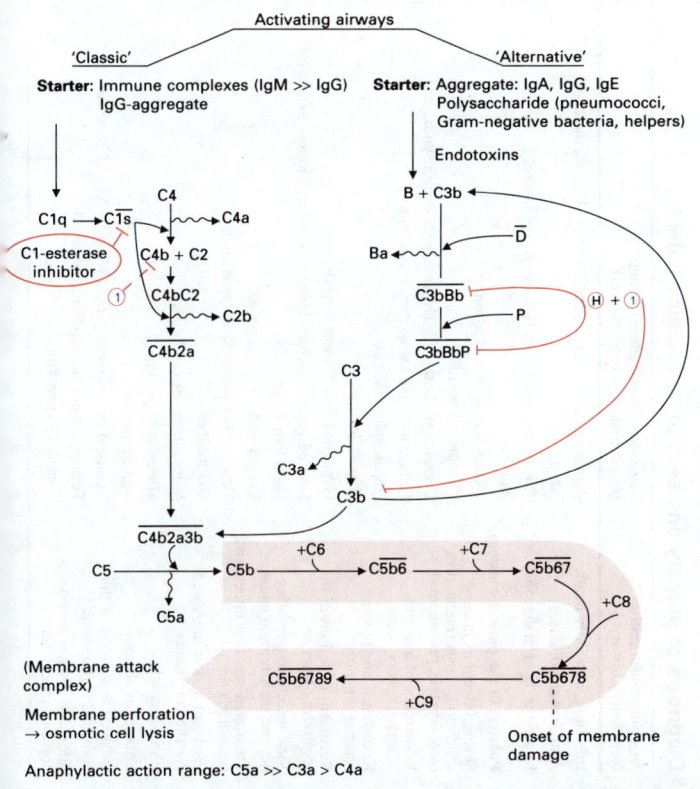

Activating airways

'Classic' | 'Alternative'

Starter: Immune complexes (IgM ≫ IgG)
IgG-aggregate

Starter: Aggregate: IgA, IgG, IgE
Polysaccharide (pneumococci, Gram-negative bacteria, helpers)
Endotoxins

C1q → $\overline{\text{C1s}}$
C1-esterase inhibitor
C4 → C4a
$\overline{\text{C4b + C2}}$
C4bC2 → C2b
$\overline{\text{C4b2a}}$

B + C3b
$\overline{\text{D}}$
Ba
$\overline{\text{C3bBb}}$
P
$\overline{\text{C3bBbP}}$
H + ①

C3
C3a
C3b

$\overline{\text{C4b2a3b}}$

C5 → C5b → $\overline{\text{C5b6}}$ → $\overline{\text{C5b67}}$
C5a
+C6   +C7
+C8

(Membrane attack complex)

$\overline{\text{C5b6789}}$ ← +C9 ← $\overline{\text{C5b678}}$

Membrane perforation
→ osmotic cell lysis

Onset of membrane damage

Anaphylactic action range: C5a ≫ C3a > C4a

341

Diagnosis of primary and secondary immune defects

Suggestive information from family history	Suggestive investigative findings (single and/or in combination)	Suspicious laboratory findings
Infections with early death	Albinism (oculocutaneous), (Chédiak–Higashi disease)	Persistent elevation of erythrocyte sedimentation rate and C-reactive protein
Autoimmune diseases	Alopecia	
Infections, later malignancy	Aortic arch anomalies (DiGeorge syndrome)	Low erythrocyte sedimentation rate despite severe infection
Pointers in the patient's history	Anemia	
Severe infections in early childhood, sepsis (meningitis, osteomyelitis, pneumonia)	Ataxia (Louis–Bar syndrome)	Persistent lymphopenia (absolute count ≤ 1500/µl)
	Chronic dermatitis	
Recurrence of a severe infection (every year)	Eczema (Wiskott–Aldrich syndrome, Hiob's syndrome)	Leukocytosis
	Failure to thrive (Shwachman syndrome)	Neutropenia
Recurrence due to same (micro) organism	Hepatosplenomegaly	Rise in all serum immunoglobulin concentrations
	Hypertelorism	
Recurrent infections of the respiratory tract	Hypogonadism (Blooms' syndrome)	Single immunoglobulins or all immunoglobulins diminished or absent
	Stunted growth (Schwachman syndrome, Blooms' syndrome)	
Viral infections persisting beyond their normal course	Head hair hypoplasia	Anemia
Treatment-resistant infections (sinusitis, otitis)	Lymph nodes ('nil palpable')	Calcium in serum (↓)/ parathormone (↓)
	Melena (Wiskott–Aldrich syndrome)	
Frequent and/or untreated diarrhea in infancy	Deformities	
	Mucocutaneous candidiasis	
Chronic colitis	Muscular hypotonia	
Cutaneous abscess	Nail dystrophy	
Delayed separation of the umbilical cord remnant	Neonatal thrombocytopenia (Wiskott–Aldrich syndrome)	
	Telangiectasias (Louis–Bar syndrome)	
Infectious disease in spite of previous inoculation	Tonsillar hypoplasia	

INFECTIONS/IMMUNOLOGY/RHEUMATOLOGY

Immune defect: step-by-step diagnosis

Basic program
Blood picture + morphology
Thrombocyte count
ESR, CRP*
Bone-marrow in peripheral cytopenia
Immunoglobulins A, E, G, M
Serum electrophoresis
Thymus size (sonography/X-rays)
Microbiological investigation
Urine, feces, swabs (throat, conjunctiva, skin), aspiration (abscess, empyema)
Organ investigation according to history and findings: exclusion of other diseases (e.g. disordered mucociliary clearance, bronchial maldevelopment, urinary tract disease, functional diarrhea)

Immunological diagnostic program

System	Screening	Further investigations
Granulocytes	Absolute count, morphology	NBT test* Chemofluorescence Adherence Chemotaxis In vitro migration Phagocytosis Enzyme activity: cytochrome-b-oxidase glucose-6-phosphate-dehydrogenase myeloperoxidase glutathione synthetase, glutathione reductase deficiency Cell wall proteins: adherence proteins CD-11/CD-18 glycoprotein
Monocytes	Absolute count (n = 300–1100/µl)	Surface marker Cytokine production Antigen presentation (autologous cell proliferation
T lymphocytes	Absolute count (n = 155–2500/µl) Mérieux multitest (recall antigens)	Surface marker Subpopulations (CD 4, CD 8) quantitatively (CD cluster designation) In-vitro stimulation (antigens, mitogens) Cytokine production Cytotoxicity test
B lyphocytes	Absolute count (n = 100–300/µl) Isoagglutinins (blood group) Immunoglobulin sublcasses (IgG 1, 2, 3, 4) Vaccine antibodies	Surface marker Immunoglobulin synthesis after stimulation (Pokeweed mitogen)
Natural killer cells	Absolute count (n = 70–200/µl)	Cytotoxicity test
Complement	Total hemolytic activity for classic and alternative routes C3, C4 quantitatively	Individual components (immunochemical, functional
Enzyme	See T and B cells	Adenosine deaminase deficiency (enzyme activity in the erythrocytes)
	See T cells	Purine-nucleoside phosphorylase deficiency (enzyme activity in erythrocytes)
	B cells, granulocytes, blood picture	Transcobalamin-II deficiency (enzyme activity in fibroblast culture)
		Multiple carboxylase deficiency
HLA antigens		Look for lymphocytes, monocytes

* ESR = erythrocyte sedimentation rate; CRP = C-reactive protein; NBT test = nitroblue tetrazolium test.

MEMORIX PEDIATRICS

Cell–cell interactions: synopsis of cytokines

	Cytokines	Target cell or tissue	Direct/indirect functions
Monocyte, macrophage	IL-1 (α, β)	Bone marrow (BM) stroma cells, endothelium, fibroblasts	Liberation of GM-CSF, G-CSF, M-CSF
		T cells	IL-3 → BM proliferation
		Granulocytes (IL-1a)	Secretion of IL-2 (T cell proliferation)
		Endothelium	Phagocytosis ↑, mobility ↑, metabolism ↑
			Permeability ↑ (with TNF)
		Liver	Fever, catabolism
			Induction of acute-phase proteins
	IL-6	Liver	
		T cells, NK cells	Activation
		B cells	Ig synthesis
		BM stem cells	Megakaryocytopoiesis ↑
		AP	ACTH ↑
	IL-8	Neutrophils	Chemotaxis
	G-CSF	BM myelopoesis	Neutrophil proliferation and function ↑
	M-CSF	BM monocytopoiesis	Monocyte proliferation and function ↑
	TNF-α	Tumor cells	Necrosis
		Endothelium, vessels	Granulocyte adhesion ↑, endotoxic shock
		Granulocytes, monocytes, B cells	Activation
		Liver	Acute-phase protein ↑
			Fever, catabolism
T lymphocyte	IFN-α	Infected cells	Antiviral action
	IL-2	T cells	Proliferation + differentiation of T cells and B cells, cytotoxic activity of T and NK cells ↑, secretory and other cytotokines ↑
		B cells	
		NK cells	
	IL-3	BM stem cells	Myelo- and erythropoiesis ↑
	IL-4	T cells (cytotoxic)	Proliferation ↑
		B cells	Production of IgG$_1$, IgE ↑
	IL-5	B cells	Production of IgA, IgM ↑
		Eosinophils	Function ↑
	IL-6	B cells	Differentiation + Ig production ↑
		Liver	Acute-phase protein ↑
	IL-7	T cells, B cells	Proliferation
	IL-8	Neutrophils	Chemotaxis ↑
	GM-CSF	BM	Myelopoiesis ↑, activation of monocytes, neutrophils, eosinophils
	TNF-β	B cells, monocytes, granulocytes	Activation
		Tumor cells	Necrosis
	INF-γ	B cells, monocytes, granulocytes	Activation

IL = interleukin; G-, M-, GM-CSF = interleukin, monocyte/macrophage colony stimulating factor; TNF = tumor necrosis factor; IFN = interferon; BM = bone marrow; NK = natural killer; AP = anterior pituitary; ACTH = adrenocorticotropic hormone.

INFECTIONS/IMMUNOLOGY/RHEUMATOLOGY

Synopsis of juvenile chronic arthritis (JCA) (Still's disease)

(Onset: < age 16 years; duration of symptoms: three months)

Type of course	♀:♂	Age of onset (years)	Joints affected	Other manifestations	ANA	RF	HLA type	Complications/ prognosis
Systemic JCA (Still's disease) (15%)	4:5	5	60% polyarticular 40% oligoarticular Beginning discretely, all joints may become involved	Intermittent, high fever synchronous with maculopapular rash. Inflammation of reticuloendothelial system, serositis, leukocytosis, thrombocytosis, microcytic anemia	–	–		Deformed growth of affected joints (25%) Amyloidosis, infections Mortality 2%
Pauciarticular JCA Type I (50%)	7:1	2	≤4 joints, 3/4 monarticular Large joints, mostly asymmetrical, at onset 50% in knee joint	Chronic uveitis (up to 80%)	+ (60–80%)	–	A2, DR5 (40%)	Contractures, secondary hyperostosis, cataracts, glaucoma, amaurosis (17%)
Pauciarticular JCA Type II (spondylo- arthritis) 15%	1:10	10	Large joints of lower limbs, mostly asymmetrical	Sacroileitis, calcaneitis, first metatarsophalangeal joint, enthesiopathy, plantar fasciitis, tendon sheath inflammation, acute iridocyclitis attacks	Rarely + at onset	–	B 27 (90%) Positive family history: 60%	Iridocyclitis/ ankylosing spondylitis (Bechterew's disease), destructive hip-joint arthritis
Polyarticular JCA Seronegative type (10%)	8:1	Peak: 3, whole childhood	≥5 joints Mostly all joints, symmetrically also cervical spine, maxillary joints, proximal interphalangeal and metacarpophalangeal joints	Subfebrile temperatures, malaise, tendovaginitis of the flexors, rheumatoid nodules	+ (25%)	–		Deformed growth
Polyarticular JCA Seropositive type (10%)	6:1	>12	As for seronegative type	Subfebrile temperature, rheumatoid nodules, tendovaginitis of the extensors	+ (50–70%)	+	DR4 (70%)	Chronic destructive arthritis, later adult PCP, 50% invalidity after 40 years

ANA = antinuclear antibody; RF = rheumatoid factor; HLA type = human lymphocytic antigen; PCP = primary chronic polyarthritis.

American Rheumatism Association criteria for classification of chronic rheumatoid arthritis
(After Arnett (1990).)

Criterion	Definition
1 Morning stiffness	In and around the joints, lasting at least 1 h until complete relief.
2 Arhtritis in three or more joints,	History of effusion in at least three joints or swelling of the soft tissues. Joints affected are: proximal interphalangeal joints (PIP), metacarpophalangeal joints (MCP), metatarsophalangeal joints (MTP), elbow, hand, knee and ankle joints.
3 Arthritis in the joints of the hand	Swelling of at least one joint (see criterion 2) of one hand, MCP and/or PIP joint.
4 Symmetrical arthritis	Bilateral in MCP, MTP or PIP.
5 Rheumatoid nodules	Subcutaneously over joint extensor surface, adjacent to the joint or over a bony projection
6 Rheumatoid factor in serum	Raised titer. (The laboratory test must give a positive result in <5% of control cases.)
7 Radiological changes	Erosions or demineralization in the affected hand and finger joints (p-a film).

Evaluation: Criteria 1–4 must have been present for at least six weeks. Rheumatoid arthritis is present if at least four of the seven criteria are present.

Jones criteria for the diagnosis of rheumatic fever
(After American Heart Association, Council or Rheumatic Fever and Congenital Heart Disease (1984).)

Main criteria	Additional criteria
Carditis: Change in heart murmurs or new dilated cardiomyopathy Pericarditis	Fever Arthralgia History of rheumatic fever
Polyarthritis (migratory) Sydenham's (minor) chorea Erythema marginatum Rheumatoid nodules (subacute)	ESR ↑, CRP ↑ Rising antistreptolysin titer ECG: P-R interval prolonged

Diagnosis:	Probable	with two main criteria or one main and two additional criteria.
	Doubtful	if there is no pointer to a previous (two to five weeks) streptococcus A infection, i.e. history of scarlet fever, rising antistreptolysin titer, positive throat swab.

ESR = erythrocyte sedimentation rate; CRP = C-reactive protein.

INFECTIONS/IMMUNOLOGY/RHEUMATOLOGY

Selection of antibiotics

(After Simon and Stille (1989).)
1 = 1st choice; 2 = 2nd choice; 3 = effective, substitute only in special cases; 4 = ineffective.

Organism	Penicillin G	Ampicillin, amoxycillin	Azlocillin	Piperacillin	Flucloxacillin	Cefazolin	Cefuroxime	Cefoxitin	Cefotaxime	Cefaclor	Imipenem	Gentamicin, tobramycin	Amikacin	Ofloxacin, ciprofloxacin	Doxycycline	Co-trimoxazole	Erythromycin	Clindamycin	Vancomycin
Bacteroides melaninogenicus	1	3	3	3	4	4	3	2	3	4	1	4	4	3	2	3	3	1	4
Bacteroides fragilis	4	4	2	2	4	4	4	2	4	4	1	4	4	3	3	3	3	1	4
Chlamydia trachomatis	4	4	4	4	4	4	4	4	4	4	4	4	4	3	1	2	1	4	4
Chlamydia psittaci	4	4	4	4	4	4	4	4	4	4	4	4	4	3	1	4	3	4	4
Clostridium	1	3	3	3	4	3	3	3	3	3	4	4	4	3	2	4	2	3	2
E. coli	4	2	3	1	4	2	1	1	1	2	1	2	2	2	3	1	4	4	4
Enterobacter aerogenes	4	4	4	3	4	3	2	2	1	3	1	2	1	1	3	2	4	4	4
Enterobacter cloacae	4	4	4	4	4	4	4	4	1	4	1	2	1	1	3	3	4	4	4
Enterococcus	3	1	2	2	4	3	3	4	3	3	2	4	4	3	2	3	2	4	2
Gonococcus	3	3	3	3	4	3	1	1	1	3	1	3	3	1	3	3	3	4	4
Haemophilus influenzae	4	2	2	2	4	3	1	3	1	2	2	3	3	1	2	3	3	4	4
Klebsiella pneumoniae	4	4	4	4	4	3	1	1	1	3	1	2	1	1	2	2	3	4	4
Legionella pneumophila	4	4	4	4	4	4	4	4	3	4	3	4	4	3	3	4	1	4	4
Listeria	3	1	3	2	4	2	4	4	4	4	2	3	3	2	3	3	1	3	3
Meningococcus	1	3	3	3	4	3	2	3	2	3	2	3	3	2	3	3	3	4	4

MEMORIX PEDIATRICS

Selection of antibiotics (continued)

1 = 1st choice; 2 = 2nd choice; 3 = effective, substitute only in special cases; 4 = ineffective.

Organism	Penicillin G	Ampicillin, amoxycillin	Azlocillin	Piperacillin	Flucloxacillin	Cefazolin	Cefuroxime	Cefoxitin	Cefotaxime	Cefaclor	Imipenem	Gentamicin, tobramycin	Amikacin	Ofloxacin, ciprofloxacin	Doxycycline	Co-trimoxazole	Erythromycin	Clindamycin	Vancomycin
Moraxella	3	3	3	3	3	3	2	3	2	3	2	3	3	2	1	2	2	4	4
Mycoplasma pneumoniae	4	4	4	4	4	4	4	4	4	4	4	4	4	3	1	4	2	4	4
Pneumococcus	1	3	3	3	3	3	2	3	3	2	2	4	4	3	3	3	2	2	2
Proteus vulgaris	4	4	2	1	4	3	2	1	2	4	1	4	1	1	3	1	4	4	4
Proteus mirabilis	4	1	1	1	4	2	2	1	3	3	1	4	1	1	3	1	4	4	4
Pseudomonas aeruginosa	4	4	1	1	4	4	4	4	3	4	2	2	1	1	4	4	4	4	4
Salmonella typhi	4	3	3	4	4	3	4	4	1	3	3	4	4	1	3	1	4	4	4
Salmonella typhimurium	4	2	3	3	4	3	3	3	2	2	2	4	4	1	4	1	4	4	4
Serratia marcescens	4	4	4	3	4	4	4	3	3	4	1	2	1	2	2	3	4	4	4
Shigella	4	1	3	3	4	3	3	3	2	3	2	3	4	1	4	1	4	4	4
Staph. epidermidis	4	4	4	4	2	2	2	2	2	3	2	3	3	2	2	4	4	4	4
Staphylococcus aureus	2	3	3	3	1	1	1	3	3	3	2	3	3	3	3	3	3	3	1
Streptococcus A, B	1	3	3	3	3	3	2	2	2	3	2	4	4	4	2	4	2	2	3
Treponema pallidum	1	3	3	3	3	2	2	3	3	3	3	3	3	3	3	3	3	4	4
Yersinia enterocolitica	4	4	3	4	3	3	3	3	3	4	2	3	3	1	2	1	4	4	4

INFECTIONS/IMMUNOLOGY/RHEUMATOLOGY

Antibiotics against rarer organisms
(After Simon and Stolle (1989).)
1 = 1st choice; 2 = moderate action; 3 = effectiveness uncertain; 4 = ineffective;
? = action unknown.

Organism	Penicillin G	Ampicillin	Cefazolin	Cefoxitin	Cefotaxime	Imipenem	Gentamicin	Doxycycline	Chloramphenicol	Erythromycin	Clindamycin	Ofloxactin, ciprofloxactin	Co-trimoxazole
Acinetobacter	4	4	4	4	3	2	2	3	4	4	4	1	4
Actinomyces israelii	1	2	2	2	2	2	4	2	3	2	2	3	2
Aeromonas hydrophila	4	4	4	2	2	2	2	2	4	4	2	2	2
Bacillus anthracis	1	2	2	2	2	2	2	2	2	2	2	2	2
Bordetella pertussis	4	2	4	4	4	?	4	1	2	1	4	2	2
Borrelia burgdorferi	1	2	2	2	2	2	?	2	2	2	4	4	4
Borrelia recurrentis	2	2	2	2	2	2	?	1	2	2	4	4	4
Brucella	4	4	4	4	4	?	2	1	2	4	4	2	2
Campylobacter jejuni	4	2	4	4	3	2	2	2	2	1	4	2	4
Citrobacter	4	4	4	4	3	2	1	2	2	4	4	2	1
Corynebacterium diphtheriae	1	2	2	2	2	2	4	2	2	2	2	2	2
Erysipelothrix rhusiopathiae	1	2	2	2	2	2	4	2	2	2	2	2	2
Francisella tularensis	4	4	4	4	?	?	1	1	2	4	4	?	4
Fusobacterium	1	2	2	2	2	2	4	2	2	2	1	2	2
Haemophilus ducreyi	4	2	2	2	2	?	?	2	2	2	4	2	1
Leptospira	1	2	2	2	2	?	?	1	2	?	?	?	4
Nocardia asteroides	4	4	4	2	2	4	2	4	2	4	2	?	1
Pasteurella multocida	1	2	2	2	2	2	2	2	2	2	?	2	2
Pseudomonas cepacia	4	4	4	4	4	4	4	4	2	4	4	3	2
Pseudomonas mallei	4	4	4	4	?	?	2	1	2	4	4	2	2
Pseudomonas maltophilia	4	4	4	4	4	4	4	2	2	4	4	3	2
Pseudomonas pseudomallei	4	4	4	4	?	2	4	2	2	4	4	?	2
Rickettsia	4	4	4	4	4	4	4	1	1	2	4	2	4

MEMORIX PEDIATRICS

Antibiotic treatment

Antibiotic	Daily dose (mg/kg)	Number of single doses	Mode of administration
Aminoglycosides			
Amikacine	10–15	2	i.v., i.m.
Gentamicin	4–7.5	2–3	i.v., i.m.
Netilmicin	4–5	2–3	i.v., i.m.
Tobramycin	4–7.5	2–3	i.v., i.m.
Aztreonam	45–120	3–4	i.v.
Cephalosporins			
Cefaclor	30–50	3–4	p.o.
Cefadroxil	20–40	2	p.o.
Cefalexin	80–100	3–4	p.o.
Cefamandole	100–150	3–4	i.v., i.m.
Cefazolin	50–100	2–3	i.v., i.m.
Cefixime	8–12	2	p.o.
Cefotaxime	50–100–150	3	i.v., i.m.
Cefoxitin	50–100	3	i.v., i.m.
Cefradine	80–100	2–3	p.o., i.v.
Ceftazidime	50–100	2–3	i.v., i.m.
Ceftizoxime	50–100	2–3	i.v., i.m.
Ceftriaxone	50–80	1–2	i.v., i.m.
Cefuroxime	50–100	3–4	i.v., i.m.
Chloramphenicol	25–50–80–100	4	p.o., i.v.
Clindamycin	10–20	3–4	p.o., i.v.
Co-trimoxazole	5(–20)T*/ 25(–100)S†	3–4	p.o., i.v.
Fusidic acid	20	3	i.v., p.o., local
Glycopeptides			
Teicoplanin	Initially 6, thereafter 3–6	1	i.v.
Vancomycin	20–30–40	2–3	i.v.
Imipenem	50–80–100	2	i.v.
Macrolides			
Clarithromycin	15	2–3	p.o.
Erythromycin	30–50	2–4	p.o., i.v.

p.o. = by mouth; * = trimethoprim; † = sulfamethoxazole.

INFECTION/IMMUNOLOGY/RHEUMATOLOGY

Antibiotic	Daily dose (mg/kg)	Number of single doses	Mode of administration
Spiramycin	12.5–25	4	p.o.
Metronidazole	20–30	2–3	i.v., p.o.
Nitrofurantoin	4	2	p.o.
Penicillins			
Benzylpenicillin	200 000–600 000 U	4–6	i.v.
Benzylpenicillin	10^6–1.5×10^6 U	1	i.m.
Oral penicillins			
Penicillin V	30–60	4–6	p.o.
Flucloxacillin	20–80	2–3	p.o.
	50–100	4	i.v.
Acylaminopenicillins			
Azlocillin	200–300	4	i.v.
Piperacillin	100–300	4	i.v.
Aminobenzylpenicillins			
Ampicillin	60–100	3–4	p.o.
	100–300	3–4	i.v.
Amoxycillin	50–100	3	p.o.
Bacampicillin	20	2–3	p.o.
Combinations			
Amoxicillin + clavulanic acid	37.5	3	p.o.
Ticarcillin + clavulanic acid	20		i.v.
	80–260	2–3	i.v.
Rifampicin	10–15	1–2	p.o., i.v.
Sulfonamides			
Sulfadiazine	100	1	p.o.
Sulfasalazine	30–40–60	3	p.o., Enema

p.o. = by mouth.

MEMORIX PEDIATRICS

Antibiotic	Daily dose (mg/kg)	Number of single doses	Mode of administration
Tetracyclines			
Doxycycline	First dose 4, then 4	2	p.o.
Minocycline	First dose 4, then 4	2	p.o., i.v.
Antituberculous drugs			
Ethambutol	20–25	1	p.o., i.v.
Isoniazid	5–10	1	p.o.
Pyrazinamide	30–40	1	p.o.
Streptomycin	10–20–30	3	i.v., i.m.
Antiviral drugs			
Acyclovir	15–30	3	i.v., p.o.
Zidovudine	60	6	p.o.
Foscarnet	60–120	3/1	i.v.
Ganciclovir	5–10	2/1	i.v.
Ribavirin	6 g in 300 ml nebulized over 12–18 h		Aerosol
Antifungal drugs			
Amphotericin B	0.1–0.3–1.0	1	i.v.
	10	2–4	Inhalation
	400–800 mg	2–4	p.o., local
Clotrimazole			Local
Fluconazole	1–2 (surface mycosis)	1	i.v., p.o.
	3–6 (systemic mycosis)	1	i.v.
Flucytosine	150	4	i.v.
Ketaconazole	2.5–5	1	p.o.
Miconazole	20	4	p.o.
Nystatin	$2–8 \times 10^5$ IE	4	p.o.

p.o. = by mouth.

HEMATOLOGY/HEMOSTASIS/ONCOLOGY

Schema of the coagulation system

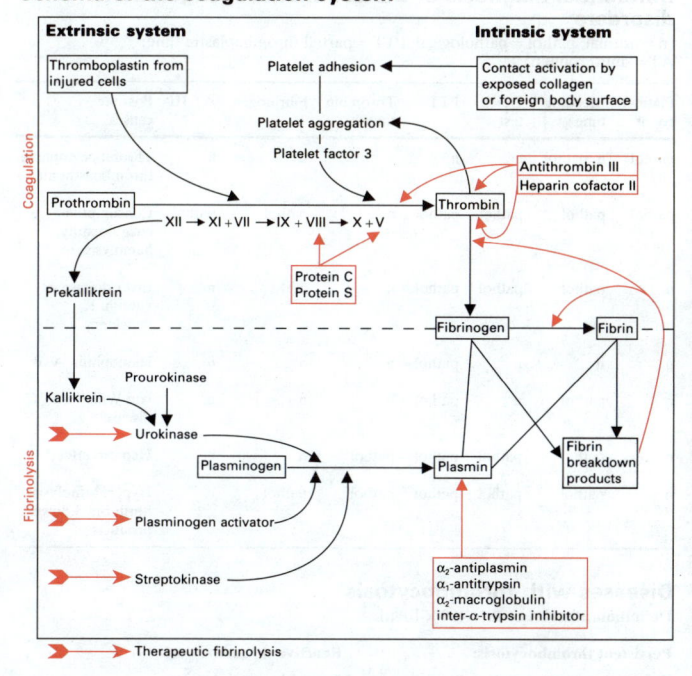

Extrinsic system | **Intrinsic system**

Coagulation:
- Thromboplastin from injured cells
- Platelet adhesion ← Contact activation by exposed collagen or foreign body surface
- Platelet aggregation
- Platelet factor 3
- Prothrombin
- XII → XI + VII → IX + VIII → X + V
- Thrombin
- Antithrombin III
- Heparin cofactor II
- Protein C / Protein S
- Prekallikrein
- Fibrinogen → Fibrin

Fibrinolysis:
- Kallikrein
- Prourokinase
- Urokinase
- Plasminogen
- Plasminogen activator
- Streptokinase
- Plasmin
- Fibrin breakdown products
- α_2-antiplasmin
- α_1-antitrypsin
- α_2-macroglobulin
- inter-α-trypsin inhibitor

→ Therapeutic fibrinolysis

MEMORIX PEDIATRICS

Differential diagnosis of the commonest coagulation disorders

(n = normal; pathol = pathological; PTT = partial thromboplastin time; AT = antithrombin)

Platelet count	Bleeding time	Quick test	PTT	Thrombin time	Fibrinogen	AT III	Possible causes
pathol	n, pathol	n	n	n	n	n	Thrombocytopenia, thromboasthenia
pathol	pathol	pathol	pathol	n	pathol	pathol	Consumptive coagulopathy, hemolysis
n	pathol	pathol	pathol	n	n	n	Liver disease, vitamin K deficiency
n	n	n	pathol	n	n	n	Hemophilia A, B
n	pathol	n	pathol	n	n	n	von Willebrand's disease
n	pathol	pathol	pathol	pathol	n	n	Heparin effect
n	pathol	pathol	pathol	pathol	pathol	n	Hyperfibrinolysis, fibrin breakdown products

Diseases with thrombocytosis

Definition: Platelet count >450 × 10^3/μl

Persistent thrombocytosis:

Essential thrombocythemia
Polycythemia vera
Sideroblastic anemia
5q syndrome
Infantile cortical hyperostosis
Myeloproliferation

Reactive thrombocytosis

Acute/chronic infection
Autoimmune diseases
Functional asplenia
After splenectomy
Postoperative
Posthemorrhagic
After thrombocytopenia
Iron deficiency
Vitamin E deficiency
Hemoglobinopathies
Chronic hemolytic anemia
Neoplasia
Medication (Vinca alkaloids)
Prematurity (? cause)

HEMATOLOGY/HEMOSTASIS/ONCOLOGY

Synopsis of von Willebrand's disease

Characteristics \ Type	I	IIa	IIb	III
Frequency (%)	ca. 80	ca. 6	ca. 4	ca. 10
Mode of inheritance	AD	AD	AD	AR
Bleeding time	↑, n	↑	↑	↑↑↑
von Willebrand factor (VWF)	↓	↓	↓	↓↓↓, ∅
Factor VIII: C	↓	n, ↓	n, ↓	↓↓↓
Ristocetin factor	↓, n	↓, ∅	↓, n	∅
Ristocetin-induced platelet aggregation	↓, n	∅	↑	∅
Polymers:				
plasma	n	Medium + large	large ∅	∅
platelets	n	∅	All available	∅
Treatment:				
Factor VIII concentrate	+	+	+	+
or				
Desmopressin 0.4 µg/kg/d	+	+	–	–

AD = autosomal dominant; AR = autosomal recessive; ∅ = absent.

Causes of thrombophilia

* = Hereditary; + = acquired.

Antithrombin III deficiency* (+ nephrotic syndrome)

Protein C deficiency*

Protein S deficiency*

Plasminogen deficiency* (+ nephrotic syndrome)

Homocystinuria*

Paroxysmal nocturnal hemoglobinuria+

MEMORIX PEDIATRICS

Diagnosis of anemia: erythrocyte forms in blood smears

Normal form	
Anisocytosis	Anemias
Poikilocytosis	Severe anemias
	Hemolytic anemia with macro- or microangiopathy, e.g. hemolytic uremic syndrome (HUS)
	Hereditary pyropoikilocytosis
	Hereditary elliptocytosis of neonates
Anulocytes	Hyperchromic anemia
Microspherocytes	Hereditary spherocytosis
Elliptocytes	Hereditary elliptocytosis, thalassemia, megaloblastic anemia
Sickle cells	Sickle cell anemia
Target cells	Hypochromic anemia, β thalassemias, hemoglobin C disease

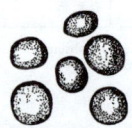

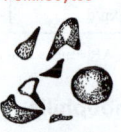

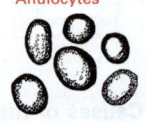

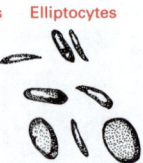

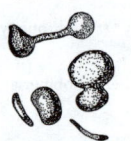

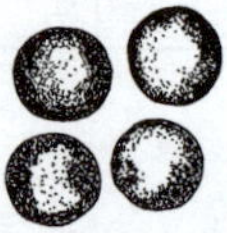

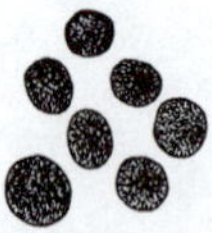

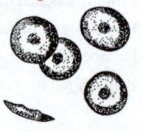

HEMATOLOGY/HEMOSTASIS/ONCOLOGY

Microscopy of erythrocytes: Staining variants

Type	Staining characteristics, unstained	Occurs in
Anisochromia	Differing staining of the erythrocytes (different Hb contents)	Anemias, after transfusion in hypochromic anemia
Hypochromasia	Pale erythrocytes (Hb production reduced), + variations in shape (mostly microcytosis)	Iron deficiency, thalassemia, sideroblastic anemia
Polychromasia	Intense staining of individual cells (base stains)	Increased erythropoiesis (regeneration)
Basophilia stippling	Strong staining, blue-black spots (RNA + ribonucleoprotein residue)	Regeneration of erythropoiesis (normal to $4/10^4$ erythrocytes)
Cabot rings (nuclear remnants)	Violet ring-shaped bodies in the erythrocytes	Erythropoiesis
Heinz bodies	Blue, eccentrically placed spheres (denatured/precipitated Hb)	Toxic hemolytic anemia, hemoglobinopathies
Howell–Jolly bodies	Stain red with Giemsa (nuclear residues as single spots)	Erythropoiesis after splenectomy, functional hyposplenia
Reticulocytes	Bluish-gray network after staining with cresyl blue brilliant (ribonucleoprotein, ribosome aggregate)	Measure of normal erythropoiesis

MEMORIX PEDIATRICS

Definitions of automatic blood cell analysis

MCV   mean (red cell) corpuscular volume (μm^3, fl)

RDW   red cell distribution width (scatter of red cell volumes)

$$RDW-CV = \frac{\text{standard deviation}}{\text{mean value of RDW}} \times 100 \, (\%)$$

Normal value of RDW: 11.5–14.5%, the greater the percentage, the more marked the anisocytosis

MCH   mean corpuscular hemoglobin (Hb_E) (pg)

$$\text{Calculation}: \frac{\text{Hb concentration}}{\text{erythrocyte count}}$$

MCHC   mean corpuscular hemoglobin concentration

$$\text{Calculation}: \frac{\text{Hb} \, (g/dl)}{\text{hematocrit}}$$

MPV   mean platelet volume (fl)

Biological errors that may be the cause of primarily reduced measurements

Parameter	Variation in result	
	Upwards (false positive)	Downwards (false negative)
Erythrocyte count	High leukocytosis Platelet aggregation	Marked microcytosis (+ fragmentation) Agglutination (counted as leukocytes) Hemolysis
Leukocyte count	Platelet aggregation (antibodies) Normoblasts	Agglutination of the leukocytes
Platelet count	Hemolysis (red cell ghosts) Cytoplasm fragments (leukemias) Microcytosis Cryoglobulinemia Lipid infusion	Platelet aggregation (antibodies) Macrothrombocytosis Platelet adhesion to leukocytes
Hb	*In vivo* hemolysis Hyperbilirubinemia Hyperlipidemia	
MCV	Agglutination (antibodies) Hyperglycemia (erythrocyte osmolality ↑)	

HEMATOLOGY/HEMOSTASIS/ONCOLOGY

Morphological differentiation of the anemias

Type	Blood values	Bone marrow (BM) findings	Disease (examples)
Normocytic, normochromic	Hb ↓, MCV n, MCH n, MCHC n	Quantitatively variable Erythropoiesis ↓ Hypo- or aproliferative anemias	Erythroblastopenias (congenital, acquired) Panmyelopathies (congenital, acquired) Hemolytic anemias Chronic kidney/liver failure Acute bleeding before regeneration
Macrocytic, normochromic	Hb ↓, MCV ↑, MCH n	Megaloblastic BM	Normal in neonates Vitamin B_{12} deficiency
		Normoblastic BM	Folic acid deficiency Orotic aciduria Hypothyroidism Liver diseases Anemias with raised regeneration
Microcytic, hypochromic	Hb ↓, MCV ↓, MCH ↓, MCHC ↓	Variable Hb production disorder	Iron deficiency Sideroblastic anemia Chronic infection Thalassemias Hemoglobinopathies (unstable Hb)

MEMORIX PEDIATRICS

Pathophysiological differentiation of the anemias

Insufficient erythropoiesis (renal failure)

- Erythropoietin deficiency (kidney failure)
- Erythroblastopenia
  congenital: Diamond–Blackfan syndrome
  acquired: infections
- Panmyelopathy
  congenital: Fanconi's anemia Estren–Damashek type, Zinsser–Cole–Engman syndrome
  acquired: infectious, toxic
- Aplastic crisis in chronic hemolytic anemia
- Displacement: leukemias, neuroblastoma, histiocytosis, myelofibrosis, osteopetrosis

Inefficient erythropoiesis (maturation disorder)

- Primary dyserythropoietic anemia
- Disordered nuclear formation
  Vitamin B_{12}/folic acid deficiency
  Hemoglobin formation disorder
  Thalassemias
  Iron deficiency anemia
  Sideroblastic anemia
  Sideroachrestic anemia
  Copper deficiency anemia

Increased erythrocyte breakdown in RES

- Hemolytic anemias:
  Enzyme and/or membrane defects
  Variants in shape of hemoglobin and erythrocytes
  Allo-autoimmune hemolysis

Increased erythrocyte loss

- Acute/chronic bleeding

RES = reticuloendothelial system

HEMATOLOGY/HEMOSTASIS/ONCOLOGY

Hemoglobin development

Phase	Hemoglobin	Polypeptides
Early embryonic	Gower 1	$\zeta_2 \epsilon_2$
	Gower 1	$\alpha_2 \epsilon_2$
	Portland	$\zeta_2 \gamma_2$
Fetal	Hb F	$\alpha_2 \gamma_2$
Birth	Hb F around 80%	
	Hb A around 20%	
	Hb A_2 <0.5%	
Postnatal	Hb A	$\alpha_2 \beta_2$
	Hb A_2	$\alpha_2 \delta_2$

Hemoglobin structure variants

Qualitative ↓

Variations in the primary structure of the polypeptide chains α, β, γ, δ

- Interchange of 1 amino acid
- Interchange of 2 amino acids (2 different nucleotide bases)
- Deletion of 1–5 amino acids in sequence
- Cross-over of nonhomologous nucleotide sequences in the genes of the β, γ and δ chains; fusion hemoglobins
- Lengthening of the α or β chains

Nomenclature: Hb polypeptide, position of amino acid exchange in the primary sequence, position in segments A–H of the helix, symbol of the amino acids.
Example: Hb S:β6 (A3) Glu → Val

Quantitative ↓

Disorders of polypeptide chain synthesis
α chain → α thalassemia
β chain → β thalassemia

Gene deletion (mostly α thalassemias)
Defects of transcription, of RNA processing, of translation (mostly β thalassemias)

	α thalassemias	β thalassemias
Defect	α chain	β chain
Excess	β chain → $β_4$	α chain → Hb A_2
	γ chain → $γ_4$	→ Hb F

Nomenclature α^+, β^+ = chain production suppressed
α^-, β^- = no chain synthesis

↓

Functional results

Hb precipitation in the erythrocytes*
(Heinz bodies)

O_2 transport ↓ or ↑

*Reduced globin causes hypochromia
*Excess globin shortens lifespan of erythrocytes
→ hemolysis + anemia

Tendency to aggregation of the erythrocytes with variations in shape (e.g. Hb C, Hb S)

Exchange transfusions

Selection of donor blood
Rules: The donor's erythrocytes must not react with alloantibodies (of the mother) in the child.
Donor plasma must not contain antibodies against the child's erythrocytes.

Blood groups		Donor's blood group	
Mother	Child	ABO system	Subgroups
A	B	O, poor in anti-B lysin	
A	AB	O	
B	A	A_2 or O, poor in anti-A lysin	
B	AB	O, poor in anti-AB lysin	Like the child's
O	A	A_2 or O, poor in anti-A lysin	
O	B	O, poor in anti-B lysin	
rh (d)	**Rh (D)**	Blood group compatible with the maternal isoagglutinins, usually group O. After a prenatal blood transfusion, a postnatal exchange transfusion must always be with **O rh-negative erythrocytes in AB plasma**	**rh (ccddee)**

How to constitute combined donor blood: O erythrocytes with the recipient's subgroup, washed once and resuspended in isoagglutinin-free AB plasma. Hematocrit (HC) around 60%.

Calculation of amount of blood required:

$$\text{Exchange volume (ml)} = \text{circulating blood volume (ml)} \times \frac{HC_{actual} - HC_{required}}{HC_{actual}}$$

Circulating blood volume (ml) ca. 1/10 bodyweight (g)

Effectiveness:

single → exchange volume → exchange of 63%
double → exchange volume → exchange of 87%   } of the child's blood volume
treble → exchange volume → exchange of 95%

Alternative to blood exchange in Rh incompatibility:
Condition: bilirubin level below exchange limit.
Treatment: immunoglobulin (IgG, 500 mg/kg i.v. over 2 h). If anemia, erythrocyte concentrate (O rh-negative, washed erythrocytes).

Polycythemia
Partial exchange transfusion for reduction of the HC:
Calculation of the exchange volume:

$$ml = \text{blood volume} \times \frac{HC_{actual} - HC_{required}}{HC_{actual}} = 80\,ml \times kg \times \frac{HC_{actual} - 0.55}{HC_{actual}}$$

Procedure: calculated blood volume removed in 10 ml units and replaced by 10 ml plasma (FFP).

HEMATOLOGY/HEMOSTASIS/ONCOLOGY

Blood transfusion: reactions

Calculation of the volume to be transferred (ml):

ca. 6 ml/kg of whole blood (= 3 ml erythrocytes) raises the Hb concentration by 1 g/dl

Whole blood: ml = ($Hb_{required}$ − Hb_{actual}) × kg × 3 or
ml = ($HC_{required}$ − HC_{actual}) × kg × 2
maximum 15–20 ml/kg (single transfusion)

Erythrocyte concentrate: ml = ($Hb_{required}$ − Hb_{actual}) × kg × 6 or
ml = ($HC_{required}$ − HC_{actual}) × kg
maximum 10–15 ml/kg (single transfusion)

Fresh plasma: maximum 20 ml/kg (single transfusion)

Granulocyte concentrate: target dose 10^{10} neutrophils
2 drops/kg/min. If compatible, after 30 min, 4 drops/kg/min

Platelet concentrate: 12×10^9 fresh platelets in 10 ml plasma per kg, more in consumption

Transfusion reactions

Type	Occurrence (C = concentrates)	Possible causes (AB = antibodies)	Treatment (always stop the transfusion), prophylaxis
Fever (after 30–120 min)	Whole blood Granulocyte C Thrombocyte C Erythrocyte C (contaminated)	AB against donor cells, escape of pyrogens from recipient's leukocytes	Antipyretics
Urticaria	Plasma-containing stored fluid	Donor antigens + specific IgE of the recipient	Antihistamines
Anaphylaxis	IgA-containing stored blood	Anti-IgA AB in IgA defect	Adrenaline, corticosteroids
Lung infiltration (fever, cough)	Antileukocytic erythrocyte C	Agglutination of recipient's leukocytes	Corticosteroids
Hemolysis			
Nonimmunological	Damaged stored blood	Hemolysis after transfusion	Symptomatic
Immunological			
Acute, intravascular (hypotension)	ABO-incompatible stored blood, particularly in group O recipients	Complement activation by IgM (anti-A, anti-B)	Symptomatic
Acute, extravascular (fever)	Incompatibility with Rh, Kell, Duffy, Kidd	IgG antibodies, erythrocyte destruction	Corticosteroids, high dosage IgG (?)
Delayed (anemia, jaundice, fever after 2–10 d)	Blood group incompatibility with low AB titers	Patient already sensitized	–

MEMORIX PEDIATRICS

Transfusion reactions (continued)

Type	Occurrence (C = concentrates)	Possible causes (AB = antibodies)	Treatment (always stop the transfusion), prophylaxis
Graft versus host disease (fever, maculopapular erythema, diarrhea, vomiting, hepatomegaly, pancytopenia)	Lymphocyte-containing or contaminated preparation (killer cells)	Congenital/acquired immune defect in the lymphomonocytic system	Symptomatic, prophylaxis: irridiation of transfusate
Hypervolemia (cardiac failure, pulmonary edema, headache)	Plasma containing preparation	Volume overloading	Furosemide administer O_2, venesection
Pulmonary embolus	Old reserve	Microemboli from cell detritus	Prophylaxis: filter
Hemosiderosis	Frequent blood transfusions	Iron accumulation	Prophylaxis: desferoxamine

Diagnosis of leukemia

Checklist of diagnostic tests in acute leukemias

Complete blood picture, reticulocytes, platelets

Bone marrow puncture (cytology, cytochemistry, blast immunology, chromosomal analysis, DNA content)

Lumbar puncture (CSF, cell sediment after centrifugation)

Coagulation state (Quick test, partial thromboplastin time, thrombin time, fibrinogen, antithrombin III)

Blood group, HLA-typing (patient, siblings, parents)

Urine

Blood chemistry (uric acid, urea, creatinine, gammaglutamyl transpeptidase, SGOT*, SGPT*, alkaline phosphatase, alpha amylase, immunoglobulins, electrolytes including calcium and magnesium)

Radiological investigation (chest X-ray in two planes, cranial computed tomography)

Abdomonal sonography (liver, spleen, kidneys, enlarged lymph nodes)

ECG, echocardiogram

Electroencephalogram

Ophthalmoscopic investigation

Microbiological investigation (throat swab, *Candida* and *Aspergillus* titers; viruses: hepatitis B, herpes simplex, cytomegalovirus, varicella, Epstein–Barr, measles)

*SGOT = serum glutamic-oxaloacetic transaminase (aspartate aminotransferase); SGPT = serum glutamic-pyruvic transaminase (alanine aminotransferase).

HEMATOLOGY/HEMOSTASIS/ONCOLOGY

FAB (French-American-British) classification of the acute leukemias

(After Bennet, Catovsky and Daniel (1981).)

Cytological characteristics	L1*	L2*	L3*
Cell size	Mainly small cells	Heterogeneous large cells	Homogeneous large cells
Nuclear chromatin	Always homogeneous	Always heterogeneous, variable	Homogeneous, finely stippled
Nuclear structure	Evenly round, occasionally constricted or indented	Irregular, notching or cleft frequent	Evenly oval to round
Nucleoli	Unrecognizable, small and inconspicuous, more vesicular	One or more, frequently large and variable	One or more clearly identifiable
Cytoplasm:			
– border	Thin to hardly recognizable	Broad	Moderately broad
– basophilia	Small to moderate rarely intense	Variable, intense in some cells	Very intense
– vacuole count	Variable	Variable	Usually numerous
Cell morphology frequent in:	(common) ALL[†] T cell ALL[†]	T ALL[†] ± E rosette formation	B cell ALL[†] AUL[‡]

* L1, common type in children; L2, commoner in adults; L3, occurring in both children and adults.
[†] ALL = acute lymphocytic leukemia.
[‡] AUL = acute undifferentiated leukemia.

FAB classification of ANLL

(After Bennet *et al.* (1985).)
ANLL = acute nonlymphocytic leukemia.

Classification	Morphological	Cytochemical Peroxidase	Cytochemical Esterase	PAS	Immunological HLA–DR	Immunological CDw13	Immunological CD11b	CD14	CD15
AML Acute myeloblastic leukemia without maturation (M1)	Large nongranular cells, one or more discrete nucleoli, variably azure granules and Auer rods. Like L2. ≥90% of the white cells are blasts	+ ≥3%	(+)	–/(+)	+	+	–/+	–	–
Acute myeloblastic leukemia with maturation (M2)	Maturation to the promyelocyte stage. In the bone marrow, >90% are blasts, ≥10% of the whites are promyelocytes and mature granulocytes, <20% belong to the monocyte group. Cells have Auer rods and azure granules	++	(+) >85%	–	+/–	+/–	+	–	Inconstant
(Hypergranular) APL Acute promyelocytic leukemia (M3)	Nuclear shape and size variable, granules pink-red, ≥30% blasts and intensely granular cells (promyelocytes). Auer rods in a few granulated cells in groups. Variations: abnormal microgranular promyelocytes	++	+ >85%	+	–	+/–	+	–	+
AMMOL Acute myelomonocytic leukemia (M4)	Blasts as in AML 2 ≥ 30%. ≥ 30% myeloblasts, myelocytes and granulocytes. <80% of the white cells are monoblasts, promonocytes and monocytes. Variants as in M3 plus eosinophilia	++	+ >20%	–/+	+	+	+	+	+
AMOL Acute monocytic leukemia (M5)	>30% of the cells are blasts. Few differentiated variants with many monoblasts, further variants with more monocytes. Histochemical features: presence of NaF-inhibiting naphthol-as-acetate esterase	–/+	++	+	+	+	Inconstant	+	–

+/– = changing findings.

HEMATOLOGY/HEMOSTASIS/ONCOLOGY

Classification		Criteria							
	Morphological	Cytochemical			Immunological				
		Peroxidase	Esterase	PAS	HLA–DR	CDw13	CD11b	CD14	CD15
AEL Erythroleukemia (Di Guglielmo's syndrome) (M6)	≥50% erythroblasts; nuclei multilobed, many nucleoli; Almost always, transition to M1, M2 or M4	+	+	+	–	–	–	–	–
AMegL Acute megakarioblastic leukemia (M7)	≥30% leukemic cells with positive peroxidase reaction in the platelets	–	+	+	Immunochemical evidence of glycoproteins Ib, IIb, or IIIa				

+/– = changing findings.

Classification of the histiocytoses in childhood

Class I	Class II	Class III

Disease:

| Langerhans cells granulomatosis (histiocytosis X) | Infection-associated hemophagocytic syndrome (IAHS) | Malignant histiocytosis Acute monocytic leukemia |
| | Familial erythrophagocytic lymphohistiocytosis (FEL) | Histiocytic large cell lymphoma |

Cellular characteristics:

| Langerhans cells microscopically deelply indented nuclei and Birbeck's granules, S-100 and CD 1 surface antigens, eosinophilic granulocytes in some cells, occasional multinuclear giant cells | Apparently normal macrophages with clear erythrophagocytosis in the whole reticuloendothelial system | Focal or generalized malignant cell proliferation of macrophages and monocytes |

Presumed pathogenesis:

| Langerhans cells with normal antigen activity, partially uncontrolled immunological stimulation | Secondary histiocytic reaction after binding of foreign antigen on the erythrocytes: erythrophagocytosis | Neoplasia: clonal autosomal proliferation |

MEMORIX PEDIATRICS

Schema of lymphocytopoiesis and phenotypical classification of the leukemias (children, juveniles)

(Modified from Foon and Todd (1986).)

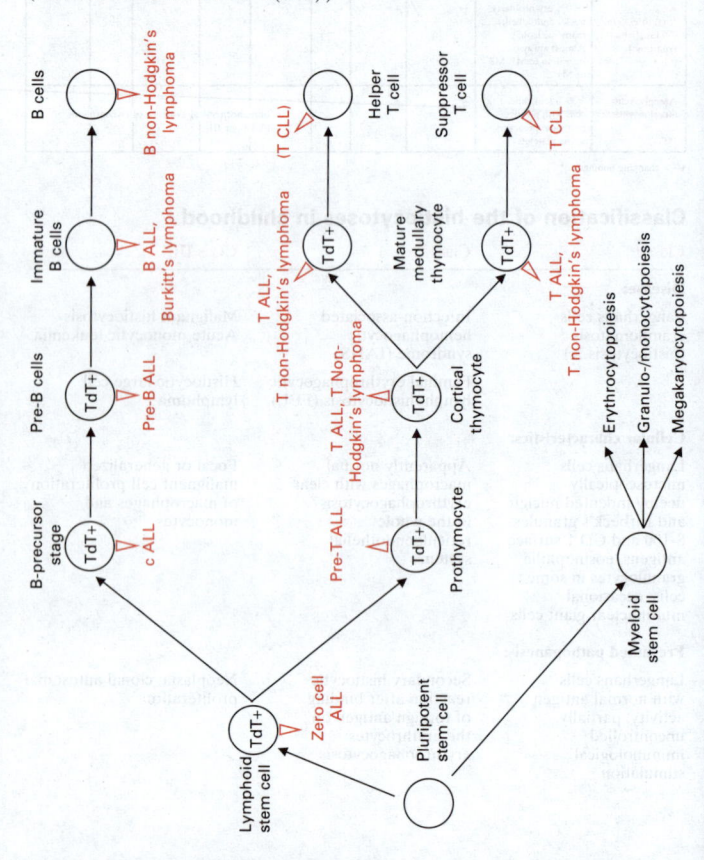

C ALL = common acute lymphoblastic leukemia; T CLL = chronic T lymphocytic leukemia; rare in children and juveniles.
TdT = terminal deoxynucleotidyl-transferase.

HEMATOLOGY/HEMOSTASIS/ONCOLOGY

Schema for hematopoiesis and classification of acute nonlymphocytic leukemias (ANLL) according to the FAB classification

(After Foon and Todd (1986).)

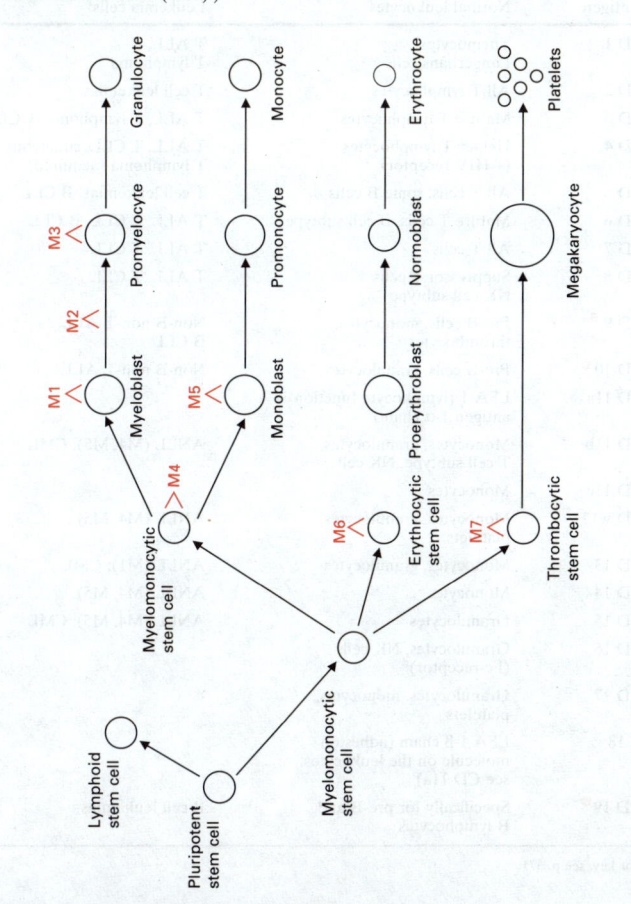

MEMORIX PEDIATRICS

CD antigens on normal and neoplastic leukocytes

(CD cluster of differentiation)

Antigen	Normal leukocytes	Leukemia cells
CD 1+	Thymocytes, Langerhans cells	T ALL, T lymphoma
CD 2+	All T lymphocytes	T cell leukemias
CD 3+	Mature T lymphocytes	T ALL, T lymphoma, T CLL
CD 4+	Helper T lymphocytes (+ HIV receptor)	T ALL, T CLL, cutaneous T lymphoma (acquired)
CD 5	All T cells, some B cells	T cell leukemias, B CLL
CD 6	Mature T cells, B cell subtype	T ALL, T CLL, B CLL
CD 7+	All T cells	T ALL, T CLL
CD 8+	Suppressor T cells, NK cell subtype	T ALL, T CLL
CD 9●	Pre-B cells, monocytes, thrombocytes	Non-B non-T ALL, B CLL
CD 10●	Pre-B cells, granulocytes	Non-B non-T ALL
CD 11a	LFA 1 (lymphocyte function antigen 1-α chain)	
CD 11b	Monocytes, granulocytes, T cell subtype, NK cells	ANLL (M4, M5); CML
CD 11c	Monocytes	
CD w12	Monocytes, granulocytes, platelets	ANLL (M4, M5)
CD 13	Monocytes, granulocytes	ANLL (M1); CML
CD 14	Monocytes	ANLL (M4, M5)
CD 15	Granulocytes	ANLL (M4, M5); CML
CD 16	Granulocytes, NK cells (Fc-receptor)	
CD 17	Granulocytes, monocytes, platelets	
C 18	LFA 1-β chain (adhesion molecule on the leukocytes, see CD 11a)	
CD 19●	Specifically for pre-B and B lymphocytes	B cell leukemias

For key, see p. 371.

HEMATOLOGY/HEMOSTASIS/ONCOLOGY

Antigen	Normal leukocytes	Leukemia cells
CD 20 ●	Specific for B cells	B cell leukemia
CD 21 ●	Early B cells (Epstein–Barr virus receptor) C3d complement receptor	B cell leukemia
CD 22	B cells	B cell leukemia
CD 23	B cell subtype	
CD 24	B cells, granulocytes	non-B non-T ALL
CD 25	Interleukin-2 receptor	HTLV-1 infective T ALL

ALL = acute lymphoblastic leukemia; CLL = chronic lymphocytic leukemia; ANLL = acute nonlymphocytic leukemia; M1, M4, M5 = FAB classification; + = differentiation antigens of the T lymphocytes; ● = differentiation antigens of the B lymphocytes.

Common antigen pattern of ALL:
Ia+, CD 9+, CD 10+, CD 19+, CD 20−, surface immunoglobulin−(SIg−)
Ia+, CD 9−, CD 10+, CD 19+, CD 20+, SIg−

TNM classification
(After Union Internationale Contre le Cancer (1989).)

Clinical categories

T Extent of the primary tumor
N Absence/presence/extent of regional lymph node metastases
M Absence/presence of distant metastases

Pathological categories: pT, pN, pM

C factor (certainty factor): grading of confirmatory methods of diagnosis.

C1: Inspection, palpation, endoscopy, standard radiography.

C2: Sonography, special radiography, computed tomography, magnetic resonance imaging, endoscopy, biopsy, cytology.

C3: Surgical exploration, targeted biopsy and cytology.

C4: Information about tumor growth from surgical tumor excision and histological examination.

C5: Autopsy.

The C factor should be shown separately for T, N and M, e.g. T4 C2, N2 C2, M1 C2.
The pathological categories pT, pN, and pM correspond to C4.

TN classification of the neuroblastomas

TX	Primary tumor not gradable
T0	No primary tumor
T1	Single tumor <5 cm (maximal diameter)
T2	Single tumor 5–10 cm (maximal diameter)
T3	Single tumor >10 cm (maximal diameter)
T4	Primary multicentric tumors (e.g. thorax and abdomen)
NX	Regional lymph nodes not gradable
N0	No regional lymph node metastases
N1	Regional lymph node metastases

Lymph node regions: cervical region (cervical and supraclavicular lymph nodes), thoracic region (intrathoracic and infraclavicular lymph nodes), abdominal and pelvic region (subdiaphragmatic, intraabdominal and pelvic lymph nodes, including nodes of the external iliac vessels), other regions

pTN classification of the neuroblastomas

pTX	Ungradable primary tumor
pT0	No primary tumor
pT1	Complete tumor excision, borders microscopically tumor-free
pT2	Not applicable
pT3	Residual tumor
pT3a	Microscopic residual tumor
pT3b	Macroscopic residual tumor and obviously incomplete excision
pT3c	Surgical exploration, no tumor resection
pT4	Multicentric tumor
pNX	Regional lymph nodes ungradable
pN0	No regional lymph node metastases
pN1	Regional lymph node metastases
pN1a	Completely resected
pN1b	Incompletely resected

HEMATOLOGY/HEMOSTASIS/ONCOLOGY

TN classification of nephroblastoma (Wilms' tumor)

TX	Primary tumor cannot be assessed
T0	No primary tumor found
T1	Unilateral tumor, radiographic area ≤80 cm^2 (area of the tumor shadow = maximal length × maximal width including kidney)
T2	Unilateral tumor >80 cm^2 (tumor + kidney)
T3	Unilateral tumor, ruptured before treatment
T4	Bilateral tumor
NX	Regional lymph nodes not gradable
N0	No regional lymph node metastases
N1	Regional lymph node metastases

pTN classification of nephroblastoma (Wilms' tumor)

pTx	Same as TX
pT0	Same as T0
pT1	Intrarenal tumor, complete tumor capsule, completely resected, histologically tumor-free surrounding tissue
pT2	Tumor also growing outside the capsule or the renal parenchyma (microscopic tumor adhesion, infiltration or thrombus in the renal vessels, renal pelvis and/or ureter)
pT3	Same as pT2, incomplete excision or rupture (pre- or intraoperatively)
pT3a	Residual tumor confirmed microscopically to the tumor bed
pT3b	Macroscopically residual tumor, tumor seeds, ascites with tumor cells
pT3c	Surgical exploration, no resection
pT4	Bilateral tumors
pNX	Same as NX
pN0	Same as N0
pN1	Regional lymph node metastases
pN1a	Completely resected
pN1b	Incompletely removed

TN classification of soft tissue sarcoma

TX Primary tumor ungradable
T0 No obvious primary tumor
T1 Primary tumor limited to the originating tissue or organ
  T1a Tumor <5 cm (maximal diameter)
  T1b Tumor >5 cm (maximal diameter)
T2 Tumour growing into adjacent organ or tissues and/or malignant seeding
  T2a <5 cm (maximal diameter)
  T2b >5 cm (maximal diameter)

NX Regional lymph nodes not gradable
N0 No regional lymph node metastases
N1 Regional lymph node metastases

Abbreviations for primary tumor localization: Orbits (ORB), head and neck (HEA), thorax + organ + diaphragm + thoracic wall (THO), abdomen + organ + abdominal wall (ABD), pelvis + organ + enclosing walls (PEL), limbs (LIM), other (OTH). Lymph node regions are: head and neck (cervical and supraclavicular), abdominal and pelvic (subdiaphragmatic, intra-abdominal and ilioinguinal), upper limbs (ipsilateral epitrochlear and axillary), lower limbs (ipsilateral popliteal and inguinal). Contralateral lymph node involvement is a distant metastasis.

pTN classification of soft tissue sarcoma

pTX Same as TX
pT0 Same as T0
pT1 Same as T1, complete excision, tissue borders microscopically tumor-free
pT2 Tumor growing outside its organ or tissue origin, complete excision, microscopically tumor-free borders
pT3 Same as pT2 but incomplete excision
  pT3a microscopically residual tumor
  pT3b macroscopically residual tumor or malignant infiltration in neighboring tissues
  pT3c Exploratory surgery, 'soft tissue sarcoma', no tumor resection

HEMATOLOGY/HEMOSTASIS/ONCOLOGY

Lymphoma

Kiel classification of highly malignant lymphoma

Category	Cell type Immunological	Morphological (FAB classification)
Lymphoblastic		
Convoluted cell type	T	L1/L2
Unclassified	pre-T, pre-B	
Burkitt type	B	L3
Immunoblastic	B, (T)	L3
Centroblastic	B	

Risk grouping of the B cell lymphomas

Group I   Primary completely excised lymphoma
          Stages I, IIR, III

Group II Regionally limited lymphoma, not or incompletely excised
          Small residual tumor or tumor mass
          Stage IIR, III

Group III Lymphoma with large tumor mass, disseminated, not resectable
          Stages II, IV
          (also B ALL)

Stages of Burkitt's lymphoma

Stage	Manifestation
I	One tumor in the facial area
II	Multiple tumors in the facial area
III	Mediastinal and/or abdominal tumors
IV	Intracranial tumor

MEMORIX PEDIATRICS

Stages of Hodgkin's disease

Stage	Manifestation
I IE	One lymph node region One extralymphatic organ
II IIE	≥2 lymph node regions above/below the diaphragm One or more lymph node regions on the same side of the diaphragm and focal in extralymphatic organs
III IIIE IIIS IIIES	Lymph node regions on both sides of the diaphragm III + focal in extralymphatic organs/tissues III + spleen III + IIIE + IIIS
IV	Disseminated + nonlymphatic organs

Stages of non-Hodgkin's lymphoma

Stage I	Single nodal/extranodal tumors without local extension Exception: mediastinal and/or abdominal and/or epidural localization
Stage II	Several nodal and/or extranodal tumors on the same side of the diaphragm with/without local extension Exception: mediastinal, extensive abdominal and/or epidural localization
Stage IIR (resected)	Abdominal tumor microscopically excised
Stage IINR (not resected)	Abdominal tumor macroscopically incompletely or not excised
Stage III	Tumors above and below the diaphragm; all thoracic (mediastinum, pleura, thymus), all epidural, all extensive abdominal tumors
Stage IV	Mixed primary involvement of the spinal cord, CNS and/or the skeleton (multifocal), independent of all other localizations

HEMATOLOGY/HEMOSTASIS/ONCOLOGY

Stages of the neuroblastomas

After the Pediatric Oncology Group

Stage

A   Tumor macroscopically radically removed, microscopically + tumor residues
Lymph nodes retained only in the tumor area or attached to the tumor
No liver metastases in cases of abdominal or pelvic tumors

B   Same as stage A
Tumor macroscopically not radically removed

C   Same as stage A or B
Intracavitary (thorax, abdomen) lymph nodes not attached to the tumor

D   Organs affected beyond those involved by intracavitary lymph node spread (e.g. liver, bone marrow, skin, extracavitary lymph nodes)

After Evans

Stage I   Tumor limited to an organ or structure

Stage II   Tumor has not grown in continuity across the midline
Ipsilateral regional lymph nodes may be affected

Stage III   Tumor has grown across the midline
Regional lymph nodes on both sides may be affected

Stage IV   Distant metastases, e.g. in bones, bone marrow, lymph nodes and other organs

Stage IVS   Same as Stage I or II
Distant metastases in bone marrow (no osteolysis), liver and/or skin

Neuroblastoma

Excretion pattern of catecholamines in 24 h urine
(After Gutjahr (1987).)

Catecholamine	Neuroblastoma	Pheochromocytoma
Adrenaline	Normal	+++
Metanephrine	Normal	+++
Noradrenaline	+	+++
Normetanephrine	++	+++
3,4-Dihydroxymandelic acid	++	++
3-Methoxy-4-hydroxyphenylglycol	+++	+++
Vanillylmandelic acid	+++	+++
Dopamine	+++	Normal
3-Methoxytyramine	+++	Normal
3,4-Dihydroxyphenylacetic acid	+++	Normal
Homovanillic acid	++	Normal
Dopa	+/++	Normal
3-Methoxytyrosine	+/++	Normal

+++ = Usually and/or strongly raised
 ++ = Often and/or moderately raised
  + = Occasionally and/or slightly raised

Staging of Wilms' tumor (nephroblastoma)

Stage I	Tumor limited to the kidney
Stage II	Tumor has penetrated the renal capsule, regional lymph nodes free or infiltrated
Stage III	Tumor extending beyond the hilar lymph nodes, tumor invasion into the inferior vena cava All biopsied tumors
Stage IV	Metastases in lungs, liver, bones or other organs
Stage V	Tumor growth in both kidneys

HEMATOLOGY/HEMOSTASIS/ONCOLOGY

Postoperative stages of Wilms' tumor

Stage I	Renal capsule not infiltrated or penetrated
Stage II	Tumor confirmed to the renal site, completely excised
Stage III	Residual tumor and/or local metastases not excised Biopsy or rupture of the tumor during the operation
Stage IV	Distant metastases
Stage V	Bilateral tumors

Stages of ovarian tumors (intraoperative classification)

Stage I	Tumor confined to the ovary
Stage II	Tumor spread to the pelvis
Stage III	Tumor invasion of small intestine and omentum Intraperitoneal metastases or retroperitoneal lymph node metastases
Stage IV	Tumor in other organs, including liver

Histopathological stages of testicular tumors

Stage I	Tumor confined to the testis
Stage IIA	Single retroperitoneal metastasis up to 2 cm in diameter
Stage IIB	Single metastasis up to 5 cm in diameter or several retroperitoneal metastases
Stage IIC	Retroperitoneal metastases only partially excised and/or large palpable abdominal tumors
Stage III	Generalized metastases

MEMORIX PEDIATRICS

Revised WHO classification of brain tumors in childhood
(Pediatric Brain Tumor Workshop (1985).)

Tumors	Characteristics
I Tumors of neuroepithelial tissue	
A Glial tumors	
1. Astrocytic tumors	
a Astrocytoma	Subtypes: fibrillary, protoplasmic, pilocytic, mixed-celled, xanthomatous
	Cystic/solid; infratentorial usually in cerebellum; supratentorial: diencephalon, optic nerve; prognosis of cerebellar tumors good
b Anaplastic astrocytoma	Cell content ↑, cells variable, pleomorphism, mitoses variable
c Subependymal giant cell tumors	Periventricular tubera in tuberous sclerosis
d Giant cell glioma	Bizarre, large astrocytes
2. Tumors of the oligodendroglia	
a Oligodendroglioma	Well differentated, macroscopically poorly circumscribed, calcification
b Anaplastic oligodendroglioma	Cell density ↑, necroses, vascular proliferation, mitoses
3. Ependymal tumors	
a Ependymoma	Grows in the area of the ependyma (inner ventricular system, central canal of the spinal cord), vascularization ↑, perivascular pseudorosette formation, dysplastic cartilagenous or bony tissue; glial fibrillary acidic protein (GFAP) + (see p. 386)
b Anaplastic ependymoma	Anaplasia: nucleus: plasma ratio ↑, atypical nuclei, number of nucleoles ↑, mitoses ↑
c Myxopapillary ependymoma	Always originates from conus medullaris or filum terminale

HEMATOLOGY/HEMOSTASIS/ONCOLOGY

4. Tumors of the choroid plexus

a	Plexus papilloma	Grows intraventricularly; despite mature tissue structure, colonizes the CNS
b	Anaplastic plexus papilloma	Spreading from plexus papilloma (4a) or *de novo* as a carcinoma in every ventricle, usually in one lateral ventricle

5. Mixed glioma

Two or three glial types, growing in the cerebrum

a	Oligoastrocytoma	Designation according to the dominating component. If a component is anaplastic, it is termed 'anaplastic'
b	Ependymoastrocytoma	Pseudorosettes, GAFP + (see p. 386), astrocytes
c	Oligoastroependymoma	All three glial types present
d	Oligoependymoma	
e	Subependymoma – subependymal astrocytoma	Mature cells, tumor nodes localized around the fourth ventricle, poor prognosis
f	Gliofibroma	Astrocytes + fibroblasts; a rare tumor

6. Glioblastoma

a	Multiform glioblastoma	Anaplastic tumor, perinecrotic pseudopalisades
b	Giant cell glioblastoma	Same as 6a, + usually multinuclear large cells
c	Glioblastoma with sarcomatous components	Glioblastoma + fibrosarcoma

7. Cerebral gliomatosis

Every type of glial cell, diffuse or arranged in nodes (glioblastoma)

B Neuronal tumors

1. Gangliocytoma

Grows in one hemisphere, cerebral seizures as first symptom, cyst formation, almost exclusively ganglion cells, some multinuclear

2. Anaplastic gangliocytoma

3. Ganglioglioma

Ganglion cells + astrocytoma cells, grows slowly, produces cysts

4. Anaplastic ganglioglioma

Anaplasia affects the glia (similar to multiform glioblastoma)

C 'Primitive' neuroectodermal tumors (PNET)

Origin of the cells unclear (?neural plate, ?early cerebellar anlage, ?late transformation), hence the descriptive classification. They metastasize in the CSF fluid space and, more rarely, extracranially as well as spinally.

1. 'Primitive' neuroectodermal tumor (PNET) (not further specified)	Small round nuclei, small plasma space, usually one chromatin-rich nucleolus, large cells with round or over nuclei Loacalization: cerebellar vermis, pineal gland or elsewhere
2. PNET with	Barely differentiated neuroepithelial cells + one of the points noted under a–f
a Astrocytes	Interspersed cell nests of astroglia, GFAP + (see p. 386)
b Oligodendroglia	Neoplastic oligodendrocytes: local cellular increase; GFAP –; rarely anaplasia
c Ependyma cells	Old term: ependymoblastoma; rosette formation
d Nerve cells	Variable proportions of mature and immature ganglion cells
e Other cells (mesenchymal, melanocytes)	Rare tumors, neoplastic signs recognizable only electron microscopically
f Mixed-cell forms	Cells under 2a–e
3. Medullary epithelioma	Pleomorphic 'embryonic' tumor, grows mainly in the cerebral hemispheres, subarachnoid metastasizing
a Medulloepithelioma, not further specified	Structures such as the neural tube, mitoses ↑
b Medulloepithelioma with 1. Astrocytes 2. Oligodendrocytes 3. Ependymal cells 4. Ganglion cells 5. Other cells (mesenchymal, melanocytes) 6. Cells 3b 1–5	

HEMATOLOGY/HEMOSTASIS/ONCOLOGY

D Pineal cell tumor — To be differentiated from other tumors (IA–C) that can grow in the pineal gland
two forms: teratoma-like germ cell tumors; parenchymal tumors from neuroepithelial anlage of the pineal gland (pineoblastoma, pineocytoma)

1. Pineoblastoma — Structure like PNET; differentiation towards a retinoblastoma possible; metastasizing possible

2. Pineocytoma

   a Pineocytoma, not further specified — Small and large cells, lobular structures as in the pineal gland

   b Pineocytoma with ganglion cells

   c Pineocytoma with astrocytes — Neoplastic astrocytes

II Tumors of the meninges and associated tissues

A Meningioma — On the dura and nerve sheaths

1. Meningioma, not further specified — rarely mitoses; subtypes: syncytial (meningoepitheliomatous), fibroblastic, angiomatous, cystic, psammomatous; calcification

2. Papillary meningioma — Histologically not malignant, yet often recurs and metastasizes

3. Anaplastic meningioma — Penetrates into the brain tissue

B Sarcomatous tumors of the meninges

1. Meningeal sarcoma, not further specified — Diffuse growth in the subarachnoid space

2. Rhabdomyosarcoma — (Or leiomyosarcoma), in posterior cranial cavity

3. Mesenchymal chondrosarcoma — Predominantly in the anterior cranial cavity, recurs, invades cerebrum

4. Fibrosarcoma — Anaplasia, spindle-shaped cells

5. Other sarcomas — Xanthosarcoma, fibroxanthosarcoma

MEMORIX PEDIATRICS

C Primary melanocytic tumors

1. Malignant melanoma — Focal or diffuse, intracranial or intraspinal
2. Melanomatosis — Hamartoma: nests of melanocytes
3. Melanocytic tumors — Pigmented meningioma or melanocytic schwannoma or melanocytic neurofibroma. Localized usually in the spinal cord

III Tumors of the nerve sheath

A Neurilemmoma — (Schwannoma, neurinoma) Tumor capsule: sometimes cystic; Schwann cells form pallisades; nerve fibres not in but on the tumor

B Anaplastic neurilemmoma — Mitoses ↑

C Neurofibroma — Schwann cells + fibroblasts; components of Recklinghausen's disease

D Anaplastic neurofibroma — Neurofibrosarcoma; sometimes complications of Recklinghausen's disease

IV Primary malignant lymphoma

V Tumors of vascular tissues

A Hemangioblastoma — Rarely anaplasia; can appear as part of Hippel–Lindau angiomatosis

B Hemangiopericytoma — Aggressive growth, mitoses ↑; reticular fibers

C Neoplastic angioendotheliosis (angiosarcoma) — Vascular formation < cell density; originates also in other organs

VI Germ cell tumors — Originates in the neuroaxial centre

A Germinoma — Large round cells with one to two eosinophilic nucleoli as in testicular seminomas or dysgerminomas of the ovary. Abundant lymphocytes in the stroma, single multinucleated giant cells

HEMATOLOGY/HEMOSTASIS/ONCOLOGY

    B Embryonic carcinoma

    C Choriocarcinoma   Very malignant, cells same as syncytiotrophoblasts

    D Endodermal sinus tumor α_1-fetoprotein +

    E Teratoma
        1. Immature teratoma   Malignant tumor
        2. Mature teratoma   Tissue derivatives from two or three germ layers
        3. Teratocarcinoma   Teratoma with anaplastic epithelial nests

    F Mixed germ cell tumors

VII Malformation tumors

    A Craniopharyngioma: Growth: → hypothalamus or third ventricle

    B Cysts of Rathke's pouch: Intrasellar

    C Epidermoid cyst

    D Dermoid cyst

    E Colloid cyst: Grows in third ventricle near the foramen of Munro

    F Enterogenic/bronchogenic cyst

    G Other cysts   Arachnoid cyst among others

    H Lipoma   Grows in the interhemisphere cleft, quadrigeminal bodies, hypothalamic, around the cauda equina (+ dysraphia)

    I Granular cell tumor: Posterior pituitary lobe

    J Hamartoma
        1. Neuronal hamartoma   Usually in the hypothalamic region
        2. Glial hamartoma   near the infundibulum and optic tract
        3. Neuronoglial hamartoma   Glia + ganglion cells of abnormal composition
        4. Meningoangioneurinomatosis   Neuroectodermal dysplasia with arachnoidal and Schwann cells

VIII Neuroendocrine tumors

A Pituitary tumors

        1. Pituitary adenoma   Further classified according to hormone production
        2. Piuitary adenocarcinoma   Anterior pituitary lobe

B	Paraganglioma	Growth direction intraspinal and intracranial, rarely a primary intracranial growth

IX Locally displacing or infiltrating tumours from near the central or peripheral nervous systems

X Metastasizing tumors: → CNS

XI Unclassified tumors

Note: Tumor classification usually possible only electron microscopically. GFAP = glial fibrillary acidic protein (demonstrated by antibody marking); NFP = neurofilament protein (in ganglion cells).

Stages of cerebral medulloblastoma
(After Harisiadis and Chang (1977).)

Stage

T1	Tumor <3 cm Ø, limited to the vermis region, the roof of the fourth ventricle, or to one cerebellar hemisphere
T2	Tumor >3 cm Ø, grows into a bordering structure or partly fills the fourth ventricle
T3 A	Tumor invades two adjacent structures, fills the fourth ventricle completely, breaks into the aqueduct, Magendie's foramen, or the foramen of Luschka; obstructive hydrocephalus
T3 B	Tumor grows out from the floor of the fourth ventricle or the brain stem and fills out the fourth ventricle
T4	Tumor penetrates through the aqueduct into the third ventricle or midbrain or grows towards the cervical cord
M0	Macroscopically not metastasizing in the subarachnoid space or hematogenous spread
M1	Microscopic tumor cells in the CSF
M2	Nodular seeding in the ventricular system or the subarachnoid space
M3	Nodular metastasis in the spinal subarachnoid space
M4	Extraspinal metastases

HEMATOLOGY/HEMOSTASIS/ONCOLOGY

MAPS classification of primitive neuroectodermal tumors (PNET, medulloblastomas) of the posterior cranial cavity
(After Laurent, Chang and Cohen (1985).)

Stage: M = metastasis; A = age; p = pathology; S = surgery.

M0	No metastasis
M1	Tumor cells in meninges or CSF
M2	Supratentorial metastatic nodes (CT)
M3	Spinal metastases (myelogram)
M4	Combined metastases in two compartments: supra- and/or infratentorial and/or spinal
M5	Extraspinal metastases
A1	<3 years
A2	>3 years
P1	Microscopy: tumor typical, benign. Well-differentiated tumor cells
P2	Microscopy: malignant, anaplastic tumor. Multiform cell lines
S0	No residual tumor
S1	Residual tumor <1.5 cm (greatest diameter)
S2	Residual tumor >1.5 cm Ø
S3	Residual tumor (any size) invading the medulla, pons, meso- or diencephalon
S4	Residual tumor (any size) growing in more than one compartment (supra-/infratentorial, spinal)

Evaluation:

Stage	Score
M0	0
M1–M5	1
A1	0
A2	1
P1	0
P2	1
S0	0
S1–S4	1

3 and 4: extremely unfavorable prognosis

MEMORIX PEDIATRICS

Tumors as a complication of diseases and syndromes
(Partly after Leiber (1981).)

Disease/syndrome	Characteristics	Tumor localization	Manifestation (C = children/juveniles, A = adults)	Remarks, further tumors
Carcinoma				
Familial disposition		Typical sex specific manifestations	A	
dermatomyositis			A	Sometimes also sarcoma
Werner's syndrome	Progeria		A	
EMG syndrome	Exomphalus, macroglossia, gigantism	Adrenals	C	+ Wilms' tumor (see p. 389)
Ulcerative colitis		Colon	A	
Cowden's disease	Multiple hamartomas, bird-face	Breast, thyroid	A	
Crohn's colitis		Small and large intestine	A	+ Abdominal lymphoma
Gardner's syndrome	Polyposis	Colon, adrenals, thyroid	A	+ Multiple osteomas and fibromas
MMN syndrome	Mucosal neurofibromas, endocrine adenomas	Thyroid, breast	A (?)	+ Pheochromocytoma
Oldfield's syndrome	Familial colonic polyposis, sebaceous cysts	Colon	A	Also chondrosarcoma
Pendred's syndrome	Hypothyroidism, inner ear deafness	Thyroid	A (?)	Very rare
Peutz–Jeghers syndrome	Mucosal pigmentation, ileal polyposis	Stomach, small intestine	A	
Colonic polyposis	Familial cumulative	Colon	A	
Sipple's syndrome		Thyroid	A	+ Pheochromocytoma
Turcot syndrome	Familial polyposis	Colon, rectum	A	+ Gliomas after puberty
Turner's syndrome	XO/OY mosaicism	Genitalia	A	+ Gonadoblastoma

HEMATOLOGY/HEMOSTASIS/ONCOLOGY

Disease/syndrome	Characteristics	Tumor localization	Manifestation (C = children/juveniles, A = adults)	Remarks, further tumors
Sarcoma				
Blue-rubber nevus syndrome	Multiple cutaneous and visceral hemangiomas	Fibrosarcoma	C	+ Medulloblastoma
Multiple exostoses	Phacomatoses	Chondrosarcoma Angioleiosarcoma (kidneys)	A C	Also retinoblastoma
Recklinghausen's disease type I	Neurofibromatosis	Fibrosarcoma	?C, A	+ Glioma
Ollier's disease	Enchondromatosis (unilateral)	Chondrosarcoma of long bones	A	
Leukemias/lymphomas				
Bloom's syndrome	Short stature, hypogonadism, immunodeficiency	Lymphatic malignoma	A	
Down's syndrome	Trisomy 21	Acute leukemia	C	
Fanconi's anemia	Short stature, aplastic anemia	Leukemias	C, A	Also hepatoblastoma
Klinefelter's syndrome	Hypogonadism	Acute lympatic leukemia	C, A	Also teratomas, dysgerminoma
Louis–Bar syndrome	Ataxia teleangiectasia	Leukemia, lymphosarcoma	C, A	Carcinoma of the breast
Poland's syndrome	Aplasia of the pectoral muscle, syndactyly	Acute lymphoblastic leukemia	?	
Wiskott–Aldrich	Immune defect, eczema, thrombocytopenia	Acute myeloid leukemia, Hodgkin's and non-Hodgkin's lymphoma	C, A	Also glioma, sarcoma
Wilms' tumor				
Beckwith–Wiedemann syndrome	EMG syndrome (see p. 388)	Nephroblastoma	C	+ Adrenocortical carcinoma, hepatoblastoma
Miller's syndrome	Aniridia	Nephroblastoma	C	
Sotos' syndrome	Cerebral gigantism	Nephroblastoma	C	Liver carcinoma

MEMORIX PEDIATRICS

Disease/syndrome	Characteristics	Tumor localization	Manifestation (C = children/ juveniles, A = adults)	Remarks, further tumors
Other tumors				
13q syndrome	Microcephaly, thumb aplasia	Retinoblastoma	C	
Deletion 14 syndrome	Amaurosis	Retinoblastoma	C	
Neurocutaneous melanosis		Skin: malignant melanoma	C	
Pigmented xeroderma	Short stature, oligophrenia xeroderma	Malignant melanoma	?C, A	Also basalioma, spinalioma

Stages of retinoblastoma
(After Reese (1976).)

Stage	Tumor growth
I	Single or multiple tumor(s) on or behind the equator of the eyeball. Size <4 pupillary diameter.
II	Single or multiple tumor(s) on or behind the equator of the eyeball. Size 4–10 pupillary diameter.
III	Tumor in front of equator (as seen by an observer) or single tumor >10 pupillary diameter
IV	Multiple tumors, partly >10 pupillary diameter, all behind the ora serrata
V	Tumors take up >50% of the retina

HEMATOLOGY/HEMOSTASIS/ONCOLOGY

Cytostatic agents/antimetabolites

Sites of action of cytostatic drugs

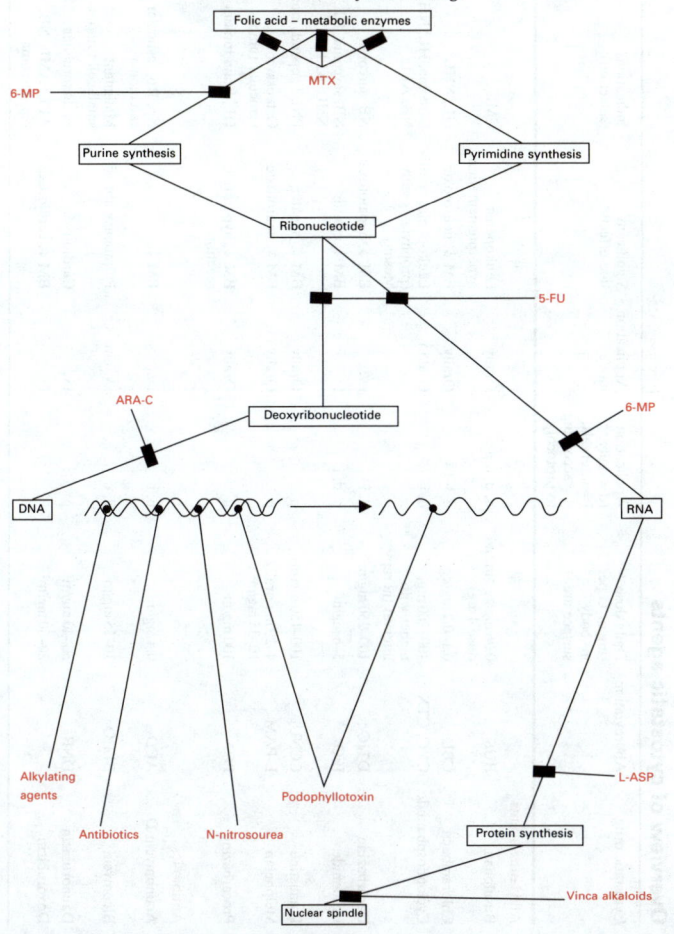

Overview of cytostatic agents

Cytostatic drug	Abbreviation	Daily dose (mg or U per m² body surface area)	Application (d = daily, i = intervals, p = according to protocol)	Application mode	Significant side-effects*	Indications (selection)†
Alkylating agents						
Busulphan	BUS	0.06 mg/kg (initial dose 4 mg)	n, d, i, p	Orally	Leukopenia, hyperpigmentation	CML
Chlorambucil	CBL	0.1–0.2 mg/kg	d 3–14	Orally	BM ↓, neurotoxic	HL, NHL
Cyclophosphamide	CYC, CTX	100–200 mg, higher with interval therapy	d, i	Oral/i.v.	Leukopenia, cystitis (prophylaxis with Mesna)	Sarcoma, HL, NHL NB, ALL
Dacarbazine	DTIC	100–250 mg/m²	d, i	i.v.	BM ↓, hepatotoxic	NB, sarcoma
Ifosfamide	IFO	5–6 mg/m²	p, d, i	i.v.	BM ↓, cystitis	NB, sarcoma, HL, NHL, ALL
Lomustine	CCNU	100–150 mg/m²	p	Orally	BM ↓, hepatic	PNET, ependymoma
Melphalan	L-PAM	4–20 mg orally 10–35 mg/m² i.v.	p	Orally/i.v.	BM ↓, neurotoxic	Osteosarcoma, testicular tumors
Procarbazine	PCA	100 mg/m²	d	Orally	BM ↓, hyperergic reaction	HL, brain tumors
Antibiotics						
Actinomycin D	ACD	0.4 mg/m²	p, i	i.v.	BM ↓	Np, Rb, testicular carcinoma
Bleomycin	BLEO	10–15 mg/m²	d, i	i.v, i.m., s.c.	Pulmonary fibrosis	Malignant small-cell tumors
Daunorubicin	DNR	30–40 mg/m²	p	i.v.	Cardiotoxic	as doxorubicin
Doxorubicin		20–60 mg/m²	i	i.v.	BM ↓, cardiotoxic	ALL, AML, NB, Np, sarcoma

HEMATOLOGY/HEMOSTASIS/ONCOLOGY

Antimetabolites					
Cytarabine	ARA-C	75–200 mg standard treament, 3000 mg high dose 30 mg intrathecal	p	BM ↓, hepatotoxic, neurotoxic	ALL, AML, NHL
Fluorouracil	5-FU	15 mg/kg weekly (max 1 g/d)	d	BM ↓	Carcinoma
Mercaptopurine	6-MP	50–75 mg/m²	orally	BM ↓, hepatotoxic	ALL, CLL, ANLL, NHL
Methotrexate	MIX	3.3 mg/m² i.v. or 30 mg/m² o/i.m.	d, p 2/week	BM ↓, pulmonary fibrosis, antidote: calcium folinate	ALL, ANLL, NHL, osteosarcoma, cerebral tumors
Alkaloids					
Etoposide	VP-16	60–150 mg/m²	d, i	BM ↓, neurotoxic	ALL, NHL, NB, cerebral tumors
Teniposide	VM-26	30–250 mg/m²	d, i	BM ↓, hyperergic reactions	HL, histiocytosis
Vinblastine	VLB	3–6 mg/m²	i, p	BM ↓, neurotoxic,	ALL, ANLL, NB, HL, sarcoma
Vincristine	VCR	1–2 mg/m²	i	As for vinblastine	ALL, NHL, HL, histiocytosis
Vindesine	VSD	2–4 mg/m²	i	As for vincristine	ALL, NHL
Others					
Asparaginase	L-ASP	5000 U	i	Hyperergic reaction	ALL, NHL
Cisplatin	CIS-Pt	50–100 mg/m²	i	BM ↓, nephrotoxic, neuro- and ototoxic	Sarcoma
Mitoxantrone	MXN	12–16 mg/m²	i	BM ↓, cardiotoxic	ALL, ANLL, NHL

*BM ↓ = (bone marrow) myelopoiesis depressed; Mesna = sodium-2-mercaptoethane sulfonate.
† CML = chronic myelogenous leukemia; HL = Hodgkin's disease; NHL = non-Hodgkin's lymphoma; ALL = acute lymphoblastic leukemia; PNET = primitive neuroectodermal tumor; AML = acute myeloblastic leukemia; Rb = rhabdomyosarcoma; CLL = chronic lymphocytic leukemia; ANLL = acute nonlymphocytic leukemia.

Definitions of dysmaturity

Description	Synonym	Definition
Gestational age	–	Age from first day of the last menstruation in weeks of pregnancy (PW)
Conception age	–	Gestation age minus two weeks (approximate value)
Mature neonate	Term infant	38–41$^{6/7}$ PW
Premature neonate	Immature neonate	Gestational age ≦37$^{6/7}$ PW
Postmature neonate	Postterm infant	42 PW
Eutrophic neonate (mature, immature)	Appropriate for gestational age (AGA)	Birth weight between 10th and 90th percentile
Large for date baby	Large for gestational age (LGA)	Neonate (mature, immature) with birth weight >90th percentile
Macrosomal neonate		birth weight ≧4500 g
Underweight neonate	Low birth weight infant (LBW)	Birthweight ≦2500 g
Very underweight neonate	Very low birth weight infant (VLBW)	Birthweight ≦1500 g
Extremely underweight (+ immature) neonate	Extremely low birth weight infant (ELBW)	Birth weight ≦1000 g (<28 PW)
Dystrophic neonate	Small for date baby Light for date baby Small for gestational age (SGA)	Neonate (mature, immature) with birth weight <10th percentile

Evaluation of newborn: Apgar score
(After Apgar (1953).)

Test criteria	Score		
	0	1	2
Skin color	White to dark blue	Limbs blue, trunk rosy	Rosy complexion
Heart rate per minute	0	<100	>100
Reflex response/ irritability to stimulus	None	Moderate: only facial distortion	Good: grimaces, sneezes or coughs
Muscle tone	Limp, no movements	Some limb flexion	Well flexed; active movements
Respiratory effort	Apnea	Slow, irregular, gasping, weak	Regular (screams)

Assessment of fetal maturity of neonates
(After Ballard, Novak and Driver (1979).)

External signs of maturity

Points	0	1	2	3	4	5
Skin	Red, transparent	Smooth pink, venous markings	Superficial scaling + reddening, few veins visible	Pale, cracked areas, few venous markings	Pigmented, deep cracks, no venous markings	Leather-like, wrinkled, cracked
Lanugo (shoulder)	None	Abundant	Sparse	Free areas	Almost none	
Sole creases (extended foot)	None	Thin red lines	Only anterior transverse crease	Creases in distal 2/3 of sole	Creases in the whole sole	
Nipple	Breast hardly recognizable	No nipple, only flat areola	Nipple diameter 1–2 mm, areolar point	Nipple 3–4 mm, areola raised	Nipple >5 mm, areola fully developed	
Ear	Earlobe flat, remains folded	Earlobe edge slightly rolled in, soft, reforms slowly	Well rolled-in lobe edge, soft, reforms quickly	Earlobe firm, reforms at once	Earlobe stiff, cartilage firm	
Female genitalia	Clitoris + labia minora prominent		Labia minora and labia majora similar	Labia majora broader than labia minora	Labia majora completely cover clitoris and labia minora	
Male genitalia	Scrotum not folded, empty		Testes descending, little folding	Testes down in scrotum, good folds	Testes movable in scrotum, deep folds	

NEONATOLOGY

Neuromuscular signs of maturity

Points	0	1	2	3	4	5
Spontaneous body posture						
Hypothenar–forearm angle	90°	60°	45°	30°	0°	
Arm recoil	180°		100°–180°	90°–100°	<90°	
Popliteal angle	180°	160°	130°	110°	90°	<90°
Scarf sign						
Heel to ear						

Assessment (*sum of scores on this page and p. 396*)

Points	5	10	15	20	25	30	35	40	45	50
Gestational age	26	28	30	32	34	36	38	40	42	44

Testing for neuromuscular signs of maturity
(After Dubowitz and Dubowitz (1977).)

Avoid the use of force.

Hypothenar–forearm angle (square window): Bend the arm of the child to 90° at the elbow; the upper arm lies on the bed. The examiner flexes his or her hand against the child's forearm until natural resistance is felt. The examiner's index finger (or thumb) is placed on the distal forearm and his/her thumb (or index finger) is placed on the back of the child's hand, over the metacarpal joints. The ulnar angle can now be estimated.

Arm recoil: Place the child in the supine position and flex his/her forearm for approximately 5 seconds. Then grasp the child's hands and fully extend them, suddenly releasing your grip. Estimate the angle to which the lower arm recoils.

Popliteal angle: The examiner places the child in the supine position and grasps the sides of the child's knee joint between his/her thumb and index finger, placing the index finger of his/her other hand on the child's Achilles' tendon. The child's leg is flexed at the hip joint and extended at the knee joint with gentle pressure.

Scarf sign: Place the child in the supine position. Grasp his/her hand and place the arm in front of the neck, pulling towards the opposite shoulder. Calculate how far the elbow joint can be pulled over the midline.

Heel to ear: Place the child in the supine position. Hold his/her trunk against passive rolling movements. Grasp the child's forefoot with your other hand and pull towards the ipsilateral ear until natural resistance is felt.

NEONATOLOGY

Finnström method of calculating fetal maturity from external characteristics
(After Finnström (1977).)

Characteristics	Assessment score			
	1	2	3	4
Skin transparency	Numerous veins, small veins and branchings visible, particularly over abdomen	Veins + branching	Few large veins in abdominal skin	Few large indistinct vessels on abdomen or none visible anymore
Breast diameter	<5 mm	5–10 mm	>10 mm	
Nipple growth	Nipple hardly identifiable, no areola	Nipple well defined, areola present but not prominent	Nipple well defined, border of areola prominent	
Head hair	Delicate, woolen, downy, individual strands hardly separable	Strong, silky, individual hairs identifiable		
Cartilage of ear (palpation)	Not palpable in antitragus	Palpable in antitragus	Present in antihelix	Palpable in dorsocranial part of antihelix
Fingernails	Fingertips not reached	Fingertips reached	Fingertips reached or overgrown, distal borders fully developed	
Plantar skin creases (permanent ones only)	None	Distal transverse creases only	Some creases in distal 2/3 of sole	Creases over whole sole

Calculation

Total points																
7	8	9	10	11	12	13	14	15	16	17	18	19	20	21	22	23
27 +2	28 +2	29 +1	30 +1	31	32	32 +6	33 +6	34 +5	35 +5	36 +4	37 +4	38 +3	39 +3	40 +2	41 +2	42 +2
Duration of pregnancy (weeks and days)																

MEMORIX PEDIATRICS

Intrauterine growth in body length and weight
(After Lubchenco et al. (1963).)

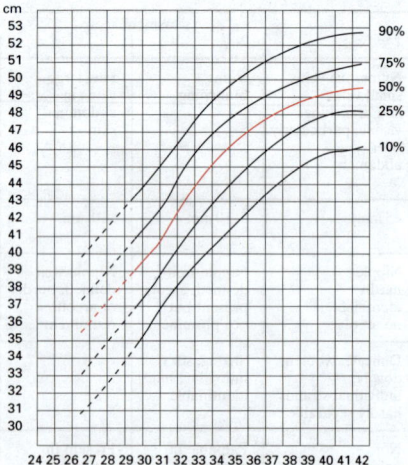

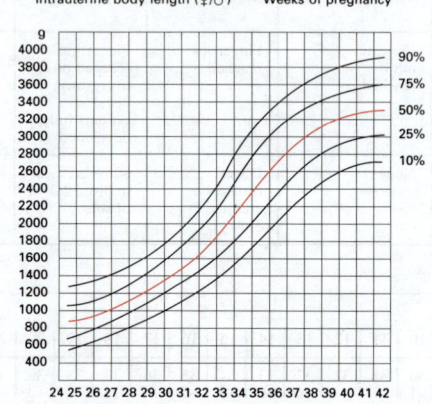

NEONATOLOGY

Intrauterine head circumference (♀/♂)

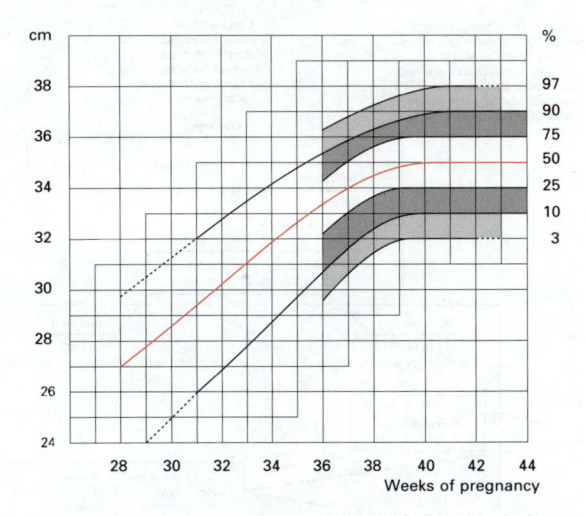

(Reproduced by kind permission of Milupa AG, Friedrichsdosf.)

Infant respiratory distress syndrome (IRDS)

Radiological differential diagnosis

Stage		Differential diagnosis
I	Lung transparency hazy, lung structure finely granular	Amniotic fluid residue (wet lung disease), pneumonia
II	Lung opacity a little more than in stage I; air bronchogram overlaps the heart shadow	Streptococcal-B pneumonia
III	Increasing opacity, heart shadow and diaphragm just about recognizable; air bronchgram positive	Congested lung: hypoplastic left heart, anomalous venous connection
IV	Homogeneous ('white') lung opacity, heart and diaphragm not recognizable; air bronchogram	Pulmonary vein atresia

MEMORIX PEDIATRICS

Differential diagnosis of neonatal jaundice

HC = hematocrit; Hb = hemoglobin; Ery. = erythrocytes; MCV = mean cell volume; CRP = C-reactive protein; γGT = γ-glutamyl transpeptidase; SGOT = serum glutamic oxaloacetic transaminase; SGPT = serum glutamic-pyruvic transaminase; CMV = cytomegalovirus; HSV = herpes simplex virus.

History:
Child weaned?
Fetofetal transfusion?
Maternal infection?
Maternal diabetes?
Maternal lupus erythematosus?
Medication?

Findings:
- Asphyxia
- Congestion
- Anemia
- Cephalohematoma
- Pale stools
- Hepato (spleno) megaly
- Shock

Measurement of total bilirubin / Bilirubin differentiation

| Unconjugated (= indirect) ≥85% → prehepatic causes | Conjugated (= direct) ≥15% → hepatic and/or posthepatic causes |

Further investigations

Blood picture:
- Cell count ↑, HC ↑
- Dehydratation
- Polycythemia

- Leukocytes ↕ ↑, Platelets ↓
- CRP ↑, IgM ↑, γGT, SGOT, SGPT ↑
- Sepsis Hepatitis

Blood culture / Viral isolation / Serology:
Gram-negative bacteria, *Staphylococcus aureus*, CMV, hepatitis B virus, other viruses, rubella, toxoplasmosis, *Listeria*, HSV

Blood group Mother/child:
Coombs' test ±
blood group incompatibility
(A-O/Rh etc.)

Blood film/automatic cell analysis:
Hb ↓ ery. ↓, MCV ↕
Abnormal erythrocyte forms and staining

Reticulocyte count:
Greatly raised
Hemolytic anemia
① ② ③

Sonography:
④ ⑤ Intrahepatic / Extrahepatic } structural abnormality

Histology:
Neonatal idiopathic hepatitis

Specific diagnosis:
⑥ Metabolic diseases

402

NEONATOLOGY

Hyperbilirubinemia

Specific diagnosis in persistent hyperbilirubinemia

1. Erythrocyte membrane protein defect
2. Erythrocyte enzyme defect
3. Hemoglobinopathies
4. Arteriohepatic dysplasia (Alagille's syndrome)
   Polycystic nephropathy (infantile type)
   Caroli's disease (cystic bile duct dilatation)
   Intrahepatic bile duct atresia
5. Extrahepatic hypoplasia/atresia of bile ducts
   Common bile duct stenosis/cyst
6. Metabolic:
   α_1 antitrypsin deficiency
   Hypothroidism
   Mucoviscidosis
   Galactosemia
   Fructose intolerance
   Glycogen storage disease types III/IV
   Tyrosinemia
   Glutaricaciduria type II
   Acid-lipase defect (Wolman's disease)
   Niemann–Pick disease type IA
   Enzyme defect of bile acid synthesis
   Copper/iron poisoning
   Zellweger syndrome

Bilirubin levels as indications for treatment

Indication for phototherapy — Total serum bilirubin mg/dl (µmol/l)	Risk group	Birth weight (g)	Indication for exchange transfusion — Total serum bilirubin mg/dl (µmol/l)
15 (257)	I	≥2500	20 (342)
112 (205)	II	1500–2500 Group I + R	18 (308)
10 (171)	III	<1500 Group II + R	16 (274)
10 (171)	IV	<1500 + R	12 (205)

R additional risk factors: hypoxia, acidosis, Hb <12 g/dl, hypoglycemia, hypoalbuminemia, sepsis

Further indications for exchange transfusion: Blood group incompatibility
Failure of high dosage gammaglobulin treatment in Rh incompatibility
Sepsis
Leukemia at birth
Neonatal myasthenia

MEMORIX PEDIATRICS

Umbilical vein catheter

Position of umbilical vessels

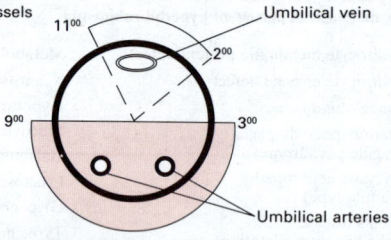

The length of umbilical catheter necessary to place its tip at the required level is dependent on the shoulder–umbilicus distance, measured from the upper lateral end of the clavicle perpendicular to the umbilicus.
(After Dunn (1966).)
The tip of the catheter should be placed between the diaphragm and the left atrium.

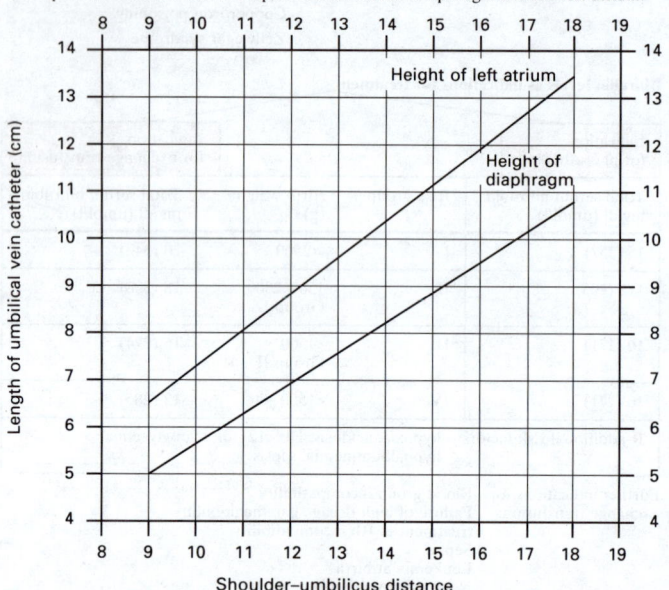

NEONATOLOGY

Umbilical artery catheter

The length of umbilical catheter necessary to place its tip at the required level is dependent on the shoulder–umbilicus distance, measured from the upper lateral end of the clavicle perpendicular to the umbilicus.
(After Dunn (1966).)
The tip of the catheter should lie above the diaphragm even though the complication rate from lower and higher positions is not significantly different.

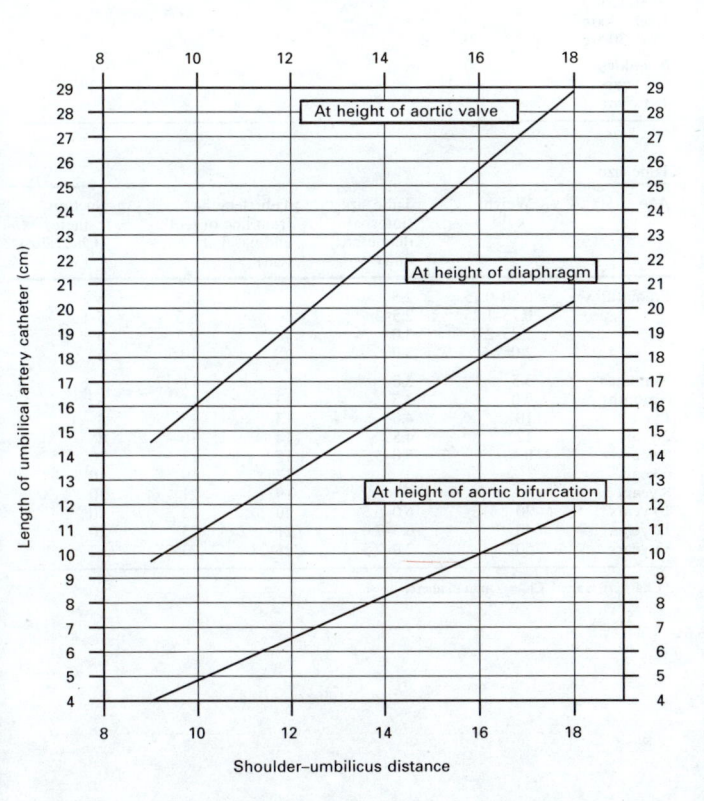

Neonatal respiration: masks, endotracheal tubes and laryngoscopes

Ventilation

Age	Mask size (after Rendell–Baker)	Laryngoscope
Prematures		
≤1000 g	0	0
1000–1250 g	0	0
1200–2500 g	0	0
2500–3000 g	0	0
Neonates	0	0–1
1–3 years	1–2	1–2
4–8 years	2–3	2

Tube size

Age	Weight (kg)	Tube size (internal diameter, mm)	Tube length from line of teeth and nasal ala (cm)	Suction catheter (Charrière)*
Prematures	0.50–0.75	2.5	7.5	5
	0.75–1.25	2.5–3	8.5	5–6
	1.25–2.0	3.0	9.5	6
	2.0–2.5	3.0	10.5	6
Neonates	3.5	3.0	11–12	6–8
6 months	7.0	3.5	13 15	8
1 yr	10	4.0	13 15	8
2 years	12	4.5	14 16	8
5 years	8	5.0–5.5	15 17	10
6 years			17 19	10
8 years			19 21	10
10 years	30	6.0–6.5	20 22	10
12 years	40	6.5–7.0	21 23	10
14 years	50	7.0–7.5	21–23 23–25	12

* Charrière scale: 1 Ch. = $1/3$ mm diameter.

NEONATOLOGY

Approx. feeding tube sizes

Tube size (>2 years): ID mm = $4 + \dfrac{\text{age (years)}}{4}$

French size: $18 + \text{age (years)}$

Tube thickness: approximately the diameter of the patient's little finger
Tube length

Oral (cm): $12 + \dfrac{\text{age (years)}}{2}$

Nasal (cm): $15 + \dfrac{\text{age (years)}}{2}$

Test to distinguish HbA from HbF

1. Wash out stool with water until the supernatant is a pale pink.

2. Centrifuge and take up the supernatant.

3. Add one part of 0.25 N NaOH to five parts of the supernatant.

4. After 1–2 min read off the color reaction:
    yellow–brown (maternal blood)
    pink (child's blood).

Neonatal seizures

Idiopathic

① Benign neonatal seizures

② Benign familial neonatal seizures

Symptomatic

③ Early infancy epileptic encephalopathy

③ Early infancy myoclonic encephalopathy

Causes

①	②	③	④
?	Genetic	CNS malformations Tuberous sclerosis Sturge–Weber syndrome Meningitis, encephalitis (pre/postnatal) Intracerebral/subdural hemorrhage Asphyxia Metabolic imbalance (electrolytes, hypoglycemia) Drug withdrawal Pyridoxine requirement	Genetic metabolic defects: Respiratory chain Pyruvate metabolism Hyperglycinemia Aciduria Peroxisomal defects

Treatment:
1. Causal
2. Anticonvulsant drugs

	Initial	Maintenance
– Phenobarbitone	20–40 mg/kg	3–5 mg/kg/d
– Pyridoxine	50 mg	
– Phenytoin	10–20 mg/kg (1 mg/kg/min)	4–8 mg/kg/d

Note: If attacks are unresponsive to treatment they may be controlled with lignocaine 2 mg/kg/min during EEG monitoring.

Once the convulsions have ceased, return to treatment with phenytoin or phenobarbitone.

NEONATOLOGY

Nutrition of the premature infant

Initial levels for individualized nutrition

Oral nutritional buildup

Energy requirement = 130–150 kcal/kg/d   Energy density = 65–85 kcal/ml

$$\text{Energy density of nutrition} = \frac{\text{energy}_{\text{required}}\,(\text{kcal/kg})}{\text{fluid}\,(\text{ml/kg})} = \frac{\text{kcal}}{\text{ml}}$$

Nutrition: breast milk, feed for prematures

Supplements: calcium gluconate + calcium glycerophosphate as necessary up to the calculated date of birth. Check: alkaline phosphatase, calcium and phosphorus excretion in urine

vitamin D_3 1000 U/d

vitamin K_1 2 × 0.1–0.2 mg s.c.

Procedure: feeding trial 2–4 h postpartum with 1–2 ml of 5% glucose

stomach residue before next meal <2 ml

nutrition in prematurity (see p. 297): 1–2 ml every 2 h

transition to breast milk from the start

increase quantity daily: 1 ml/meal (children <1500 g)
2 ml/meal (children >1500 g)

Adjuvant parenteral nutrition. If from day 3 ≤60 kcal/kg can be taken orally. Example of oral buildup + infusion:

Day	Infusion quantity of which: ml/kg	Amino acids g of amino acids/kg	Glucose (10% solution) ml/kg	Fat (10% solution) g/kg
1	50	0.5	40	0.5
2	65	1	45	1
3	75	1.5	45	1.5
4	85	1.5	50	2
5	Continue as day 4 or implement adjusted reduction depending on the increase in fluid taken by mouth			

MEMORIX PEDIATRICS

Exclusively parenteral nutrition

Fluid requirement (ml/kg/d)

Number of days postpartum	Prematures <1000 g	Prematures 1000–1500 g	Prematures >1500 g	Mature neonates
1	70	70	60	60
2	90	90	80	80
3	110	100	100	90
4	120	110	110	110
5–7	130	130	120	130
>7	150–180	140–170	130–160	130–160

Prospective correction of fluid balance

Fluid volume raised in:

- fever (+20% to 30%)
- phototherapy (+20%)
- tachypnea (+20%)
- weight loss >15%
- suspected hypovolemia (urine amount <0.5 ml/kg per h)
- increased diuresis (glycosuria, caffeine citrate)

Fluid reduction:

- on ventilator (−20% to 30%)
- double-walled incubator + air humidity 80 to 100% (−20%)
- to 50–60 ml/kg/d after asphyxia in cardiac failure, in persistent ductus arteriosus, if no weight loss in the first few days
- to 30 ml/kg/d + urine amount if inadequate antidiuretic hormone secretion (edema, diuresis ↓, hematocrit ↓, Na ↓, K ↓) and in renal failure

NEONATOLOGY

Calculation of parenteral nutrition

Aim: Total energy 80–90 kcal/kg/d
  Proportions: 40–45% carbohydrate
    40% fat
    10–15% amino acids

Composition of infusion (amount per kg and day)

	Initial amount (g)	Starting on day	With increases/d (g)	To a total daily amount (g)
Carbohydrate*	5	1	1	15
Fat[†]	0.5 1	2 (1) 1*	0.5 0.5[‡]	2 3.5[‡]
Aminoped 10%	0.5	1	0.5 (<1500 g) 1.0 (>1500 g)	2.5–3
Sodium (NaCl)	2 mmol	2	After testing	
Potassium (KCl)	1 mmol	2	After testing	
Calcium gluconate	1–2 mmol	1	–	
Glucose-1-phosphate-Na	1–2 mmol	3	–	
Vitamins A, D, K[§] Vitamin E	1 ml 5 drops orally	2 From the beginning of oral nutrition	–	Maximally 4 ml
Water soluble vitamins	1 ml	2	–	
Trace elements	0.5 ml			

* Blood sugar >50/≤150 mg/dl; [†] in separate infusion, give half if 20% solution used;
[‡] for mature neonates; [§] add to lipid fluid.

Laboratory tests

Several times/d	**Once/d**	**Twice/d**	**Once/week**
Blood gases	Electrolytes →		Creatinine
Blood sugar	Triglycerides →		Urea
Specific gravity (urine) →		Total protein →	
	Bilirubin →		Transaminases
	Blood picture →		Alkaline phosphatase
			Serum magnesium
			Serum phosphate

MEMORIX PEDIATRICS

Drug dosages for immature and mature neonates

Drug	Single dose per kg body weight	Number of single doses per day	Administration	Remarks
Acyclovir	10 mg	3	i.v.	For 8 days
Adrenaline	0.01 ml of 1:1000		Endotracheally	Can be repeated
	0.1 ml of 1:10 000	SD	i.v.	
Albumin 5%	500 mg	SD	Short infusion	Volume load
20%	250 mg	4	Short infusion	Electrolyte check
Aminophylline	Initially 8 mg, then 1.5 mg	2	Orally	Serum level 7–13 µg/ml
Atropine sulphate	0.01–0.02 mg	1	i.v.	
Carbimazole	0.25–0.5 mg	2	Orally	
Caffeine	Initially 10 mg then 2.5 mg	1	Orally, i.v.	Serum level: 10–15 µg/ml
Clonidine	3–5 µg	3	Orally, i.v.	
Dexamethasone	0.1–0.5 mg	2	i.v.	
Dobutamine	1–10 µg/kg/min		Infusion	
Dopamine	0.1–0.2 mg/h		Infusion	
Fentanyl	10 µg	SD	i.v.	
Furosemide	1 mg	3–6	i.v.	⎫ Maximally
	2 mg	2–3	Oral	⎭ 10 mg/kg/d
Heparin	100 U/kg	1	Infusion	
Indomethacin	0.2 mg	2	Orally	
Lignocaine	1–2 mg/h	SD	Infusion	
Magnesium sulphate	50 mg	2	i.v.	
	0.65 mg	2–4	Orally	
Naloxone HCL	0.01 mg	(SD)	i.v.	Can be repeated
Pancuronium bromide	40 µg 0–7 d		i.v.	
	60 µg 7–21 d			
	90 µg > 21 d			
Phenobarbitone	Initially 20 mg, then 3–5 mg	1	i.v., orally	Serum level: 15–40 µg/ml
Phenytoin	2.5–5 mg	1	Orally, i.v.	Drug of last choice
Prednisolone	0.5 mg	1–4	i.v.	
Propafenone	0.5–1.0 mg		i.v.	Not with NaCl
Propranolol	0.01–0.015 mg	4	i.v.	
	0.25 mg	2–4	Orally	
Prostaglandin E$_1$	0.01–0.1 µg/kg/min		Infusion	
Protamine HCl	1 mg/100 U heparin		i.v.	
Thyroxine	25 µg	1	Orally	
Vecuronium bromide	0.1 mg	SD	i.v.	
Verapamil	0.1–0.3 mg	SD	i.v.	

SD = only as a single dose.

NEONATOLOGY

Antibiotics in the neonatal period

	Neonates <7 days		Neonates >7 days	
	Daily dose mg/kg	Number of doses/d	Daily dose mg/kg	Number of doses/d
Aminoglycosides[*,†]				
Amikacin	15	2	20	3
Gentamicin	5	2	7.5	3
Netilmicin	5	2	6	3
Tobramycin	4	2	6	3
Other				
Chloramphenicol[†]	25	1	25–50	2–3
Imipenem	50	2	50–75	2–3
Isoniazid	5–10	1	5–10	1
Metronidazole	15	2	15	2
Vancomycin	20–30	2	30–45	3
Cephalosporins				
Cefotaxime	100	2	150	3
Cefuroxime	50–100	2	100–150	3
Ceftazidime	25–50	2	25–60	2
Penicillins				
Ampicillin	50–100	2	100–200	3–4
Flucloxacillin	40–80	2	40–100	3–4
Penicillin G	50 000–100 000 IU	2	100 000 IU	3
Piperacillin	150–200	2	200–300	3

[*] Prematures: ≤1500 g half the daily dose, 1500–2000 g three-quarters the daily dose, as starting doses.
[†] Measure serum level after 2–3 days.

Approximate timetable for motor development

(After Flehmig (1971) and Schulte (1989).)

Reflex/reaction	Conception age; length of pregnancy (weeks) 28–40	Age of infant (months) 1–14
Flight reflex		
Automatic reaction		
Pupillary reaction to light		
Doll's eye phenomenon		
Grasp reflex: palmar		
Grasp reflex: plantar		
Seek reflex		
Walking movement		
Crossed extensor		
Placing reaction		
Glabellar		
Head lifting in prone position		
Galant's reflex		
Moro startle		
Symmetrical tonic neck reflex (STNR)		
Asymmetrical tonic neck reflex (ASTNR)		
Neck positioning		
Labyrinth positioning		
Body positioning		
Landau reaction		

--- Motor reaction still immature and/or not constant: reactions in the first two to three days postpartum unreliable.

NEUROPEDIATRICS

Neurological investigation in neonates and infants

Investigative conditions: ambient temperature for neonates 27–30 °C, for infants ≥20 °C. No investigation in a neonate if obviously asleep, crying, or showing spontaneous excitement.

Investigation procedure

1. Observation — Behavior, position at rest taking account of the birth position, spontaneous movement (intensity, symmetry, athetoid movements, clonus (= shivering, paresis, mimicry, 'startles').
2. Palpation — Muscular development. Muscle tonus: measurement of passive resistance during slow extension of the limbs and flexion of the trunk.
3. Investigation of the autonomic nervous system — Skin color, breathing and heart rate, pupil width.
4. Investigation of movement — Always look for symmetrical head and body posture. To stabilize the trunk symmetrically, the child's hands should be held across his/her chest.

Reflexes and reactions

B = behavioral state; P = initial position of child; I = investigative procedure; R = reflex/reaction; D = diagnosis

Automatic reaction

B: any.
P: prone.
I: child lies with his/her face on the mattress.
R: head turned to side (to free air passages), extending the body at the same time.
D: absent in cases of CNS damage.

Tonic labyrinth reflex (TLR)

B: any.
P: first prone, then supine.
I: place child in each position in turn.
R: in prone position, generalized hypertonic flexion, which competes with the automatic reaction and often prevents it; opisthotonus when in supine position.
D: always a pathological reflex in cases of CNS damage.

Lip reflex

B: quiet, eyes open or closed.
P: supine.
I: briefly tap on the red part of the upper or lower lip with the index finger.
R: contraction of orbicularis oris muscle = lips pouting.
D: normally present; delayed or absent in CNS damage.

415

MEMORIX PEDIATRICS

Oral sucking reflex

- B: quiet, not satiated.
- P: supine.
- I: touch the perioral skin with a finger.
- R: distortion of mouth and turning of head to the stimulated side.
- D: reaction weak to absent in acute CNS damage; absent in satiated child.

Sucking reflex

- B: quiet, awake.
- P: supine.
- I: place teat or finger 1.5–2 cm into the mouth.
- R: sucking movements.
- D: Weaker in the first 2–3 days than later; weakened if CNS damage.

Glabella (orbicularis oculi) reflex

- B: quiet.
- P: supine.
- I: Quick tap on the glabella (between the two eyebrows) with the index finger.
- R: rapid closure of the eyelids.
- D: increased if hyperexcitable; delayed or absent if CNS damage.

Abdominal skin reflex

- B: quiet, relaxed abdominal muscles.
- P: supine.
- I: lightly stroke the skin of the four quadrants of the abdominal wall from lateral to medial with a pointed object.
- R: ipsilateral abdominal muscle contraction.
- D: significant if always asymmetrical.

Cremasteric reflex

- B: any.
- P: supine.
- I: stroke the inguinal region or the inner side of the thigh with a blunt probe.
- R: muscular contraction and testis drawn upward.
- D: absent in spinal cord injuries at L1 and L2.

Anal reflex

- B: any.
- P: supine.
- I: lower legs held up and moved towards the abdomen, the perineal skin stroked with a probe.
- R: contraction of the external anal sphincter.
- D: absent in lesions of S4 and S5.

Galant's (infantile) reflex

- B: quiet.
- P: held in prone.
- I: supporting the child with one hand under his/her abdomen, the skin around the renal region is stimulated.
- R: vertical column flexion and pelvic rotation.
- D: normal up to nine months.

NEUROPEDIATRICS

Chvostek's sign
B: quiet, eyes open.
P: supine.
I: Short tap on the parotid with the index finger.
R: phasic contraction of the ipsilateral facial muscles.
D: normal, absent, increased in hyperexcitability.

Blink reflex
B: quiet.
P: supine.
I: 1. optical: light flashes (not too strong), alternating between eyes.
   2. acoustic: clap at 30 cm from the side of the head (avoid draughts).
R: lids close.
D: absent in lesions of the optic tract.

Corneal reflex
B: quiet, eyes open.
P: supine.
I: touch with cotton wool ball.
R: lids close.
D: significant only if absent.

Doll's eye test
B: quiet, eyes open.
P: supine.
I: slow rotation of head to right and left.
R: eyes move opposite to direction of rotation.
D: absent in abducens paralysis.

Rotation test
B: quiet, eyes open.
P: vertical.
I: variant 1:   child held with hands under the his/her arms, fixing the child's hands across his/her chest with one's thumbs;
   variant 2:   child held with the inner surface of the examiner's hands on the child's trunk; thumbs grasp under the child's arms from behind, while the index and middle fingers support the child's head;
   variant 1 + 2: slow rotation of the examiner on the same axis to right and left, variant 1 before variant 2.
R: variation 1:   child turns its head in the direction of the rotation;
   variation 2:   with the head fixed the eyes turn in the direction of the rotation.
D: asymmetry in abducens paralysis; absent in vestibular disorders.

Recoil of arms
B: quiet.
P: supine.
I: grasp the child by the hands, stretch out the arms, then suddenly let go.
R: recoiling of the arms into flexion.
D: asymmetry significant.

MEMORIX PEDIATRICS

Grasping reflex
- B: quiet.
- P: supine.
- I: hands: examiner's hand placed into the palm of the infant's hand from the ulnar side;
  foot: thumb pressure against the sole of the foot.
- R: grasping movement of fingers/toes.
- D: weak reaction in all limbs in acute CNS damage; unilaterally weak reaction of hand or foot = peripheral paresis (no facilitated reflex response when simultaneously sucking).

Foot clonus
- B: quiet.
- P: supine.
- I: quickly press the front of the foot from its plantar surface back against the thigh.
- R: clonus.
- D: physiological; prolonged in hyperexcitability.

Babinski's sign
- B: quiet.
- P: supine.
- I: stroke the lateral margin of the sole of the foot from toes to heel.
- R: tonic hyperextension of the big toe; spreading and plantar flexion of the second to fifth toes.
- D: physiological; normally disappears after six months; unilaterally absent in spinal cord lesion.

Magnet reflex
- B: quiet.
- P: supine.
- I: with the legs flexed, exert soft pressure with the thumb on the sole of the feet.
- R: child extends legs if the thumb remains in contact with the soles.
- D: absent in spinal cord lesion.

Bauer reaction
- B: quiet.
- P: prone.
- I: pressure on the soles of the feet.
- R: child extends legs, then makes crawling movement.
- D: weak to absent in paresis; absent in acute CNS injuries.

Checking head control
- B: quiet, possibly spontaneous movement, eyes open.
- P: first supine, then prone.
- I: first: child held by his/her wrists and raised symmetrically to a sitting position;
  second: body stabilized with one hand.
- R: first: head is briefly held up; arm muscles tonic;
  second: observe head tilting.
- D: absent in hypotonia.

418

NEUROPEDIATRICS

Placing reaction

B: quiet, eyes open.
P: vertical.
I: child held up from behind; head held up supported by index finger and thumb; child held at the edge of the examination table so that the back of the foot just touches it.
R: foot is raised and placed on the examination table ('ready to stand').
D: Note any asymmetry; absent in hypotonia, paresis.

Step reaction

B: quiet, eyes open.
P: vertical.
I: this examination follows the placing reaction. The neonate must touch the mattress with one sole, possibly slightly inclining the body forward.
R: the leg is extended, the other leg is flexed and then extended, but no continuous stepping movements.
D: persistence after three months is noteworthy.

Neck reflexes

Moro reflex

B: quiet, awake.
P: supine.
I: body lies on the volar side of a forearm, the head supported with the other hand; look out for straight alignment and symmetrical holding of the head; head holding hand is quickly dropped by ca. 4 cm.
R: first phase: abduction and stretching of arms, spreading of the fingers, opening of the mouth;
second phase: subsequent mouth closure, flexion of arms and their movement towards trunk.
D: may be absent in CNS damage, but always asymmetrical or persisting.

Symmetrical tonic neck reflex (STNR)

B: awake.
P: supine.
I: 1st, flexion: head bent on chest;
2nd, extension: trunk a little raised and head extended.
R: 1st, flexion: symmetrical tonic arm bending and stretching of both legs to the toes, slight adduction and internal rotation of legs;
2nd, extension: complete extension of the arms and leg flexion.
D: pathological: persistence beyond six months (interferes with four-footed stance).

Asymmetrical tonic neck reflex (ATNR)

B: quiet.
P: supine.
I: head slowly turned to one side and held there for several seconds.
R: after some seconds, extension of the limbs on the side the face is turned to and flexion of the other (fencing posture).
D: as for STNR.

Neck position reflex

B: quiet.
P: supine.
I: head of child turned slowly sideways.
R: trunk of child follows the rotation, in the first few weeks in a rolling movement, then in a screw-like motion.
D: pathological if there is no body rotation and, later, if there is persistence of the rolling motion.

Body position reflex to the head

B: quiet.
P: supine.
I: child held by the legs, then turned into the prone position by crossing the legs.
R: at first child turns as a whole; turning becomes increasingly screw-like from second month onward.
D: retraction of the upper shoulder during the turning is pathological.

Positional reflexes (center of gravity control, spatial orientation)

Labyrinth position reflex (LPR)

B: quiet, awake.
P: prone.
I: child lies on the examination table or is placed in different positions by holding the trunk.
R: infant tries to bring his/her head into the right position for spatial orientation.
D: weak or absent in CNS damage.

Head-hanging reaction (Peiper–Isbert reflex)

B: quiet, awake.
P: supine.
I: child held by thighs and lifted up into the head-hanging position.
R: up to three months: stretching and abduction of the arms, then symmetrical straightening of the arms on the mattress, and labyrinth position reflex of the head, i.e. extension or flexion in an attempt by the child to right him- or herself.
D: pathological if asymmetrical, no arm movement and head reaction absent.

Axillary suspension reaction

B: quiet, awake.
P: vertical.
I: child held up high by the trunk, then slight forward and backward pendular movement of the legs.
R: slight flexion of the legs; from three months onward, active leg flexion; from six months onward, nimble leg stretching; symmetrical swinging.
D: stretch synergy and crossing of legs and asymmetrical swinging (difference in muscle tone in the two legs) is abnormal.

Traction reaction

B: quiet, awake.
P: supine.
I: examiner's index finger is placed on the ulnar side of the child's palm, and at the same time the distal forearm is grasped with the third and fourth fingers; the child is pulled up to ca. 45°.
R: general flexion from six weeks; less marked leg flexion and active pulling up by the infant into sitting position from six months.
D: persistence of pure flexion and asymmetry are abnormal.

NEUROPEDIATRICS

Landau reaction

B: awake, quiet.
P: vertical after horizontal.
I: child held with both hands by the trunk and brought into the horizontal position.
R: after the sixth week the head is held in the plane of the body; from four months it is held above it (spatial orientation); from six months symmetrical body stretching and, with appropriate leg stretching, active center of gravity control.
D: pathological: absent or weak head erection; asymmetrical position of legs; overextension of one or several limbs.

Oblique position reaction

B: awake, quiet.
P: vertical.
I: child loosely held by lower trunk and slowly tilted sideways to 45°.
R: head placed vertically in the oblique position; center of gravity correction = stretching of the upper arms and legs + adduction of the lower hanging limbs.
D: insufficient control of center of gravity and head positioning is pathological.

Side tilting reaction

B: quiet, awake.
P: vertical.
I: child held as in oblique position test, then rapidly turned sideways to 90°.
R: up to four months, nimble flexion of the upper arm and leg, and stretching of the forearm and leg; up to seven months, slight symmetrical leg flexion, then as in the oblique position test.
D: delay in the age-related reactions is significant, as are abnormal limb positions and differences between sides.

Collis reaction (horizontal)

B: quiet, awake.
P: lying horizontally on the side.
I: child held distal from the shoulder and hip joints of one side, and then lifted from the supine position and suspended horizontally.
R: until the fourth month, nimble flexing of the lower (hanging) limbs; from six months support reaction with the lower arm; and from nine months support reaction with the lower arm and leg; from six months simultaneous raising of the head above the horizontal.
D: absent head control, abnormal limb posture and differences between sides are pathological.

Collis reaction (vertical)

B: quiet, awake.
P: supine.
I: child grasped by the thighs and held head down.
R: First six months, flexion of the free legs at the hip and knee joints, then nimble stretching at the knee joint.
D: persistence of flexion of the free limbs and constant differences between sides are significant.

MEMORIX PEDIATRICS

Ready to jump

B: quiet, awake.
P: prone, sitting.
I: child held at the trunk from behind, lifted into the suspended horizontal position and moved towards the mattress.
R: straightening of the limbs for support on the mattress with extension of the hands and feet; head extension (6–12 months).
D: pathological: absence of the reaction and asymmetrical position of the limbs.

Idiomuscular reflexes

Biceps tendon reflex (BTR)

B: quiet.
P: supine.
I: place index finger on the biceps tendon, stretch the forearm a little with the fourth finger of the same hand; trigger the reflex by striking the index finger with a reflex hammer or a finger of the opposite hand.
R: muscle contraction.
D: differences between sides are significant.

Patella tendon reflex (PTR)

B: quiet.
P: supine.
I: place a leg over one hand, lift it somewhat and with a finger of the other hand or a reflex hammer tap the tendon below the patella.
R: as for BTR.
D: as for BTR.

Achilles tendon reflex (ATR)

B: quiet.
P: prone.
I: hold forefoot, leg slightly flexed and with it the tendon stretched; tap tendon with finger or reflex hammer.
R: as for BTR.
D: as for BTR.

NEUROPEDIATRICS

Milestones in motor development
(Compiled after Michaelis, Krägeloh-Mann and Haas (1989).)

Age	Milestones
1 month	Holds head for several seconds in the plane of the trunk while in suspended prone position.
3 months	Lying prone, stable head lifting and supporting on the forearm
6 months	Flexing of the arms and fixing the head in the plane of the trunk when being lifted up into sitting position.
9 months	Stable unsupported sitting with a straight back.
12 months	Stands holding on to furniture.
18 months	Free stable walking, controlling balance.
2 years	Firm running, can run around obstacles.
3 years	Hopping, with legs apart, from low step.
4 years	Well coordinated turning of pedals and steering of tricycle.
5 years	Walking up and down stairs without holding on.
6 years	Fluent one-legged hopping with good balance control.

MEMORIX PEDIATRICS

Motor development: erect gait
(After Brandt (1983).)

Median (month)	Milestone
1.0	Can repeatedly hold up head for at least 3s
3.0	Supports itself on forearms, lifts head 50–90°
3.7	With support, pulls itself up from supine position, bending head forwards
6.0	Pushes itself up from prone position on outstretched arms, lifts head at least 90°
6.1	Turns from supine to prone position
6.1	If put into a sitting position, can sit unsupported by leaning forward and steadying itself
8.0	Sitting up, can support itself with arms and hands to one side
8.2	Lifts body from prone to four-limbed position
9.2	Pulls itself up against a firm object and stands unsupported by holding on
9.7	Coordinated crawling on hands and knees
10.0	Sits up by itself from the four-limbed position without holding on
10.0	Stands up securely by itself and makes sideways steps

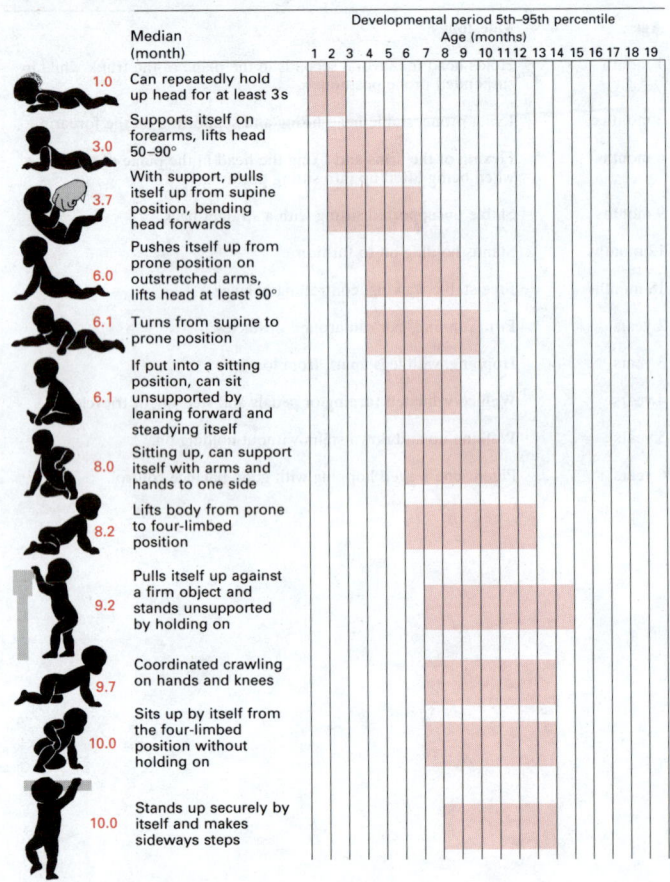

Developmental period 5th–95th percentile, Age (months) 1–19

NEUROPEDIATRICS

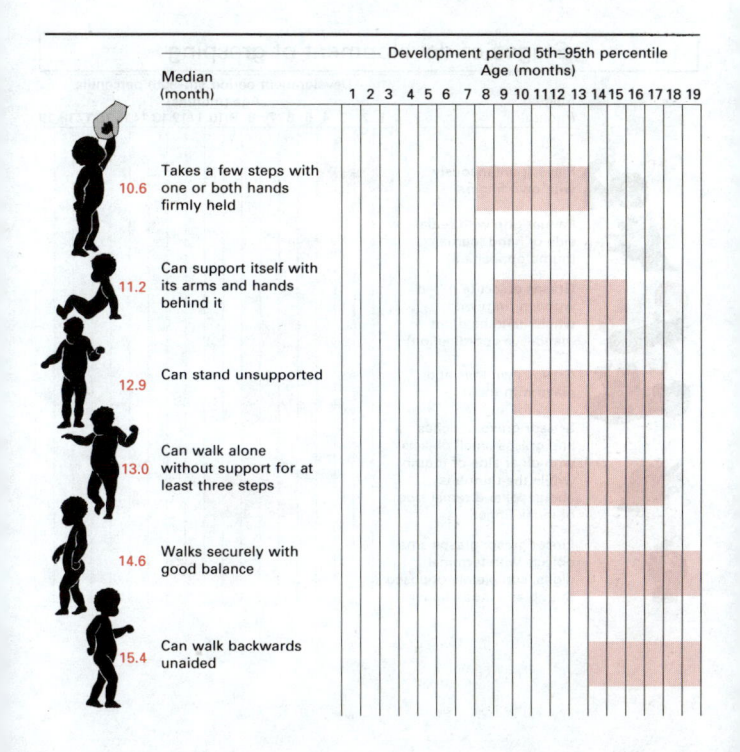

Median (month)	Milestone	Development period 5th–95th percentile Age (months)
10.6	Takes a few steps with one or both hands firmly held	8–13
11.2	Can support itself with its arms and hands behind it	9–14
12.9	Can stand unsupported	10–15
13.0	Can walk alone without support for at least three steps	11–15
14.6	Walks securely with good balance	12–17
15.4	Can walk backwards unaided	13–18

MEMORIX PEDIATRICS

Motor development: grasp

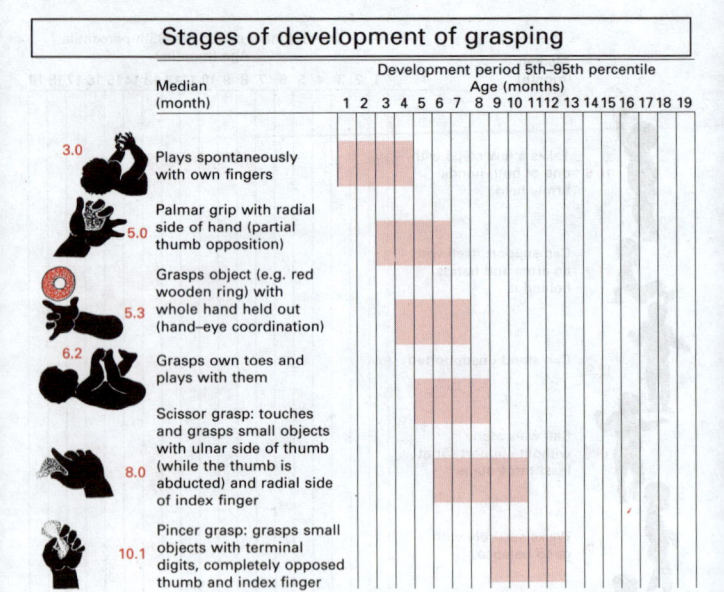

Stages of development of grasping

Median Age (month)	Description	Development period 5th–95th percentile (months)
3.0	Plays spontaneously with own fingers	1–4
5.0	Palmar grip with radial side of hand (partial thumb opposition)	3–7
5.3	Grasps object (e.g. red wooden ring) with whole hand held out (hand–eye coordination)	4–7
6.2	Grasps own toes and plays with them	5–9
8.0	Scissor grasp: touches and grasps small objects with ulnar side of thumb (while the thumb is abducted) and radial side of index finger	6–11
10.1	Pincer grasp: grasps small objects with terminal digits, completely opposed thumb and index finger	9–13

Grading of the gross strength of the voluntary musculature (inverse: grades of paresis)

Grade
0: No activity possible
1: Few muscular movements visible/ contractions palpable
2: Active movements after compensating for gravity
3: Gravity can be offset or surmounted
4: Active movement against resistance
5: Normal muscular strength

NEUROPEDIATRICS

Diagnostic EEG

Electrode positions

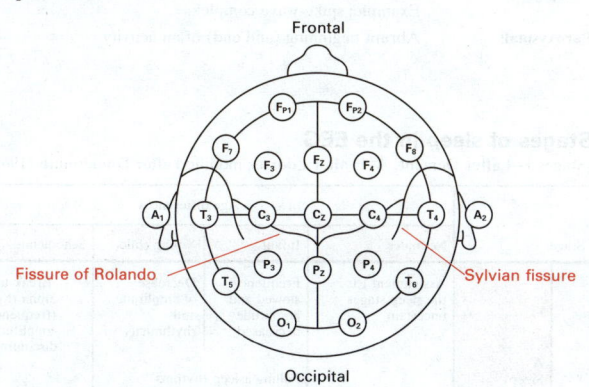

Symmetrical electrode positions according to the 10–20 system. In prematures and neonates there is a variable reduction in the number of electrode positions (mostly two each occipital, frontal and temporal, plus two to three central electrodes).

Description of EEG

Definitions

Waves: potential difference between different electrode positions.
Characteristics: polarity (positive downwards, negative upwards), amplitude, duration, form

Wave types	Frequency	Duration (ms)
Subdelta	1/s	1000
Delta	1–3/s	250–1000
Theta	4–7/s	125–250
Alpha	8–13/s	75–125
Beta	14–30/s	35–75

Potential (transient): particularly pronounced waves.

Activity: sequence of waves.

Basic activity: Optically registered continuous activity (background activity), to be distinguished from separately recognizable normal or abnormal waves.

MEMORIX PEDIATRICS

Rhythm: Regular sequence of similar waves.
Example: alpha rhythm, beta rhythm, theta rhythm.

Complex: Combination of different waves.
Example: spike-wave complex.

Paroxysmal: Abrupt beginning (and end) of an activity

Stages of sleep in the EEG

(Stages 1–4 after Dement, A–E after Loorris; modified after Dumermuth (1965).)

Stage		Age differences				
		Neonates	Infant	Young child	Schoolchild	Adult
1	A Sleepy	Assignment to the sleep stages uncertain	Frequency slowed and amplitude decreased	Decrease of amplitude and rhythmicity	Break-up of alpha rhythm (frequency ↓, amplitude ↓, discontinuity)	
			Falling asleep rhythms			
			– particularly precentral, parietal –			
		Slowing of frequency and increase in amplitude	Continuous 2–4/s	Paroxysmal 4–6/s	Frontal theta group	
	B Falling asleep		Activity (optional) ↑		Low voltage	
			Diffuse theta–delta activity	Diffuse theta–delta activity	Or low theta activity	
			Steep to sharp vertex potential			
2	C Light sleep	Polymorphic delta activity, with discrete 13–15/s spindles	Central 14/s spindles, 'sleep spindles'			
			Intermittent delta bursts		Frontal 12/s spindles (optional)	
3	D Medium–deep sleep	High polymorphic delta activity	**Spindles reduced**			
			Polymorphic diffuse delta activity			
			Theta superposition		Theta–alpha superposition	
4	E Deep sleep		High bilateral synchronous delta activity			

Pathological EEG variations

Criterion	Variation	Causes
Generalized		
Basic activity	Slowing (= general changes)	Hypoxia Ischemia Cerebral edema Hyper-/hypoglycemia Contusion Encephalitis Meningitis Acute infectious diseases Electrolyte imbalance Anticonvulsives Neuroleptics
	Diffuse beta wave activation	Neuroleptics Barbiturates Benzodiazepines
	Suppression in premature and mature neonates (extremely flat EEG, burst suppression pattern)	Metabolic disorders Infections Asphyxia
Focal		
Delta wave focus	1. Structural lesion 2. functional disorder	All CNS injuries
	EEG focus and CNS structure not necessarily identical	
Local depression	(+ frequency ↓, amplitude ↓)	Epidural/subdural hematoma Porencephaly
Basic rhythm activation	(Amplitude ↑, frequency ↓)	Interval stage in the healing of focal processes
Intermittent beta rhythm		Brain stem: trauma encephalitis hemorrhage 'absence' epilepsy
Paroxysmal slow wave		Between seizures

MEMORIX PEDIATRICS

Pathological EEG patterns

With spikes and/or sharp waves
(continuous, paroxysmal, generalized or focal occurrence)

Type	Features	Occurrence
Hypsarrhythymia	High polymorphic theta–delta waves Spikes and sharp waves with changing interspersed localization	West's syndrome
Spike wave variant pattern	Complex of steep and slow waves, 1.5–5 complex(es) Polymorphism of complexes	Myoclonic–astatic seizures
3/s spike wave paroxysms	Spikes + slow wave complex Frequency 2.5/s–3.5/s, usually 3/s, generalized rhythm duration	'Absence' epilepsy
Polyspike wave paroxysms	Spikes + slow wave complex Variability of frequency: spikes to 15/s, waves to 4/s	Impulsive petit mal
Irregular spike wave paroxysm	SW complexes, frequency (2.5/s–3.5/s), amplitude and form variable within a paroxysm	Symptomatic/idiopathic epilepsy
Sharp and slow waves	Sharp and slow wave complex Frequency in the rhythms 1.5/s–2/s	Twilight state, atypical 'absences'
Periodic complexes, steeper and slower waves (Radermecker)	Sharp wave, followed by 1/s–2/s slow waves; complex duration 1s; repetition at almost regular intervals	Subacute sclerosing panencephalitis
Periodic spike wave complexes	Spikes or sharp waves, optionally coupled with polymorphic 2–3/s waves; variable complex; temporal appearance	Herpes simplex encephalitis

Points potential

- Spike
- Polyspike complex
- Sharp wave
- Spike wave pattern
- Double spike wave complex
- Polyspike wave complex
- Sharp slow wave complex

NEUROPEDIATRICS

Evoked potentials

The form of the evoked potential is dependent on:

- Stimulation modality
- Neuronal excitation (Anatomical structures)
- Site of the electrode placement
- Lead technique
- Sex of patient
- Maturity of the nervous system and sensory organs
- Vigilance and cooperation of the child or juvenile
- Medication

Visual evoked potential (VEP)

Nomenclature: polarity as in EEG; positive (P) amplitude directed to the vertex = deflection downwards; negative (N) amplitude directed upwards.
Latency = stimulus → peak time in milliseconds.
Stimulus lead time = latency difference between two peaks (peak–peak interval).
Amplitude count: (1) consecutive numbering $P_0, N_1, P_1, N_2, P_2, N_3, P_3$, or (2) description with the corresponding average latency, e.g. N 80, P 100, N 120, P 300.

Development phenomena: latency decrease, depending on stimulus, up to the seventh year.
Differentiation of the potential components P_1, N_2, N_3 up to adolescence.

Diagnostic criteria:
Latency increase
Amplitude reduction
Variation in potential duration and form
Interocular comparison.

Indications for investigations:

A If diagnosis suspected

Ocular diseases:
- refraction disorders
- amblyopia

Diseases of the optic nerve:
- neuritis
- glioma
- hereditary atrophy:
  spinocerebellar ataxias
  Friedreich's ataxia
  optic atrophy
  (Leber's disease)

Intracranial processes:
- trauma
- tumors with visual disorders
- space-occupying lesions
- all demyelinizing diseases, neurometabolic storage diseases; toxic neuropathies
- encephalitis (borreliosis, *Treponema*, viruses)
- AIDS
- hereditary ataxia
- vascular diseases (hypoxia, migraine, brain death)

Psychogenic visual disorder

B For follow-up checks

Visual evoked potential

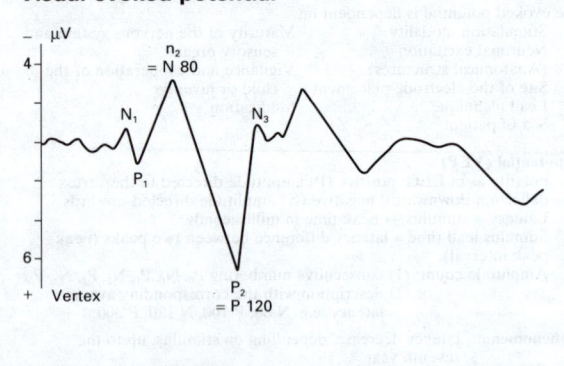

Acoustic evoked potential (AEP)

Component of AEP	Abbreviation	Latency range (ms)	Site of origin
Electrocochleogram (= very early AEP)	E CochG (VEAEP)	<1	Cochlea
Early AEP:	EAEP	1–10	
Wave I		1–2	Cochlea, acoustic nerve
Wave II		2–3	Acoustic nerve, medulla
Wave III		3–4	Neurons of the cochlear nuclei (pons)
Wave IV		4–5	Cochlear and olivary nuclei, lateral lemniscus (pons)
Wave V		5–6	Lateral lemniscus, inferior quadrigeminal body
Wave VI		6–8	? Midbrain
Wave VII		6–10	? Auditory radiations
Mean AEP Waves N_o, P_o, N_a, P_a, N_b	MAEP	10–50	Midbrain-cortex, nuchal muscle
Late AEP	LAEP	50–300	Cortical acoustic projection fields
Very late AEP	VLAEP	>300	Cortical event-correlated potential

Peripheral lead time (pLT) = peak–peak interval of waves I and II.
Central lead time (cLT) = peak–peak interval of waves II and VII.

NEUROPEDIATRICS

Developmental phenomena: The latencies of EAEP are reduced in the first three years to adult levels while simultaneously the amplitudes are increased
Early maturation of the inner ear (nearly the same pLT in the neonate as in the adult)

Diagnostic criteria: Latency, amplitude, potential pattern, comparison of the two sides

Indications for investigation (preponderantly EAEP as brain stem potential):

A if diagnosis suspected

Differentiation of hearing disorders
Localization of brain stem lesions: tumors, meningoencephalitis, demyelinizing diseases

B as follow-up and check after purulent meningitis

Acoustic evoked potential

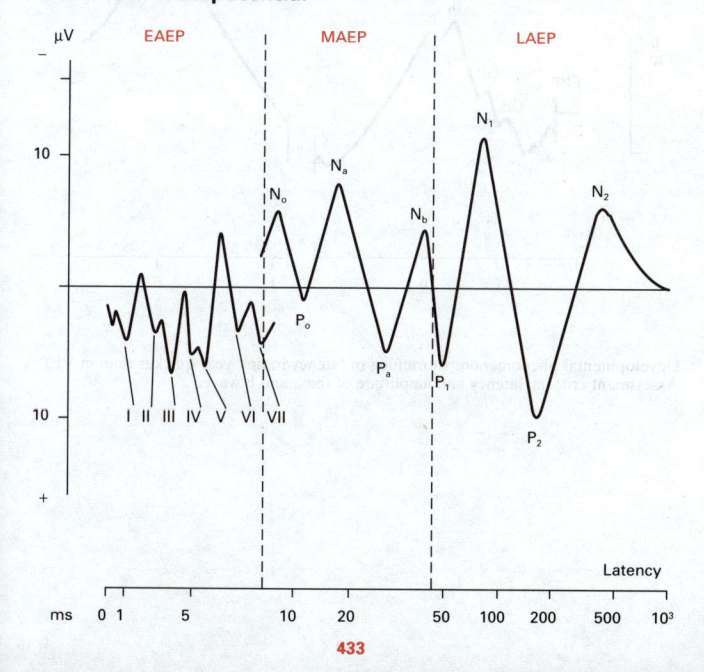

Electroretinogram (ERG)

Nomenclature: polarity with positive direction to the anterior eye pole = deflection upwards

Potential components
early receptor potential (ERP)
a_1 wave
a_2 wave
oscillatory potentials (OP)
b_1 wave
b_2 wave
c wave

Site of origin
outer receptor segment
cones ⎫ inner receptor segment
rods ⎭
inner nuclear layer
cone-activated ⎫ bipolar cells
rod-activated ⎭
pigmented epithelium

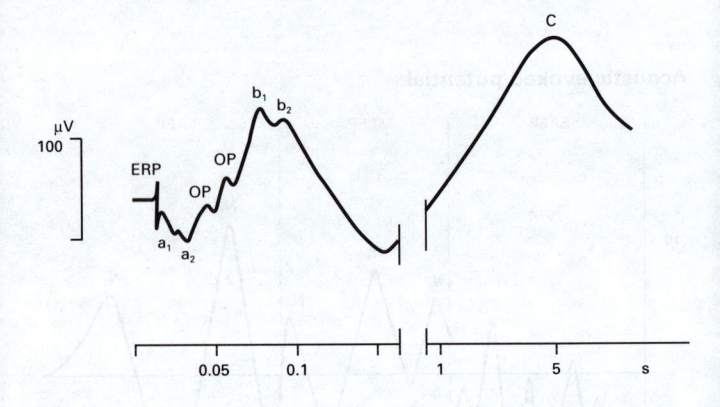

Developmental phenomenon: shortening of latency in first year quicker than in VEP
Assessment criteria: latency and amplitude of the a and b waves

NEUROPEDIATRICS

Retinopathies

Indications for investigation:

A If diagnosis suspected

Hereditary tapetoretinal dystrophies:
Vitreoretinal dystrophies
Chorioretinal dystrophies
Retinal dystrophies:
 diffuse, central, peripheral
Syndromes:
 Alström's
 Bardet–Biedl
 Cockayne's
 Forsius–Eriksson
 Graefe–Sjögren's
 Ito's
 Jeune's
 Joubert's
 Klippel–Feil
 Laurence–Moon–Biedl
 Mauriac's
 Saldino-Mainzer
 Sjögren–Larsson
 Thevenard's
 Usher's

*With cherry-red spots

Pseudoretinitis pigmentosa:
Prenatal infections:
 rubella, cytomegaly, toxoplasmosis, syphilis
Postnatal uveitis
Spinopontocerebellar ataxias
Myotonic dystrophy
Hereditary metabolic defects:
 Sphingolipidoses:
  Sphingomyelin lipidosis (Niemann–Pick disease)*
  Glucosylceramide lipidosis (Gaucher's disease)*
  G_{M1} gangliosidosis (Landing's disease)*
  G_{M2} gangliosidosis (Tay–Sachs disease)*
  G_{M2} gangliosidosis (Sandhoff's disease)*
  Metachromatic leukodystrophy[(*)]
  Lipogranulomatosis (Farber's disease)*
  Multiple sulfatase deficiency*
  Mucolipidosis type IV
 Mucopolysaccharidoses (types I-H, I-S, II, III)
 Ceroidlipofuscinosis
 Cystinosis
 Hyperornithinemia
 Peroxisomal disorders:
  Zellweger syndrome
  Adrenoleukodystrophy (neonatal)
  Refsum's disease (infantile form)
 Abetalipoprotinemia
 Wolman's disease
 Enteropathic acrodermatitis

B follow-up checks

Somatosensory evoked potential (SSEP)

Nomenclature: positivity with the exploring electrodes compared with the indifferent one = deflection downwards; naming the components in the manner of numbering VEP with average corresponding latency

Indications for investigation: plexus damage, all lesions near the spinal cord and spine
objectifying sensory functions from neonates to preschool age

Diagnostic criteria: absolute latencies, interpeak latencies, amplitudes

MEMORIX PEDIATRICS

Electromyography (EMG)

Motor unit = motor anterior horn cell + axon of anterior horn cell + synaptically connected group of muscle fibres

Electromyographic patterns

EMG recording conditions: at rest with light–strong–maximal voluntary innervations

Spontaneous activity	Pattern	Method of generation	Characteristics	Significance
Normal	Action potential	On inserting needle electrode	Begins with negative amplitude (direction upwards)	
	Potential of motor end-plate			
Pathological	Fibrillation potential	Spontaneous	Two-/three-phasic, potential duration <5 ms, begins with positive amplitude, irregular/rhythmic occurrence	Neurogenic + + + Myogenic + Especially myositis
	Positive sharp waves	Spontaneous	Begins with positive amplitude, slow negative late deflections	Neurogenic + + + Myogenic +
	Fasiculation potential	Spontaneous in interference area of motor units	Amplitudes higher Rhythmic appearance at times	Spinal muscle atrophy
Abnormal voluntary activity	Myotonic discharge	Voluntary, after percussion of the muscles, after needle insertion	Potential series with decreasing amplitude, changing frequency of the series	Myotonias
	Polyphasic discharge	After innervation	Base line exceeded by potential 4 times	Myopathies

NEUROPEDIATRICS

Clinical forms of myasthenia gravis

Effects and course of characteristics	Low grade	Medium grade	High grade	Fulminant	Ocular	Transitory neonatal
Paresis:						
Eye muscles	+++	+++	++	+	+++	++
head/neck muscles	++	+++	+++	+++	−	++
Other skeletal muscles	+	++	+++	+++	−	++
Thymoma	−	−	+	+	−	−
Progression	+	+	+++	+++	−	−

Diagnosis of myasthenia

1. Edrophonium test: 0.1 mg edrophonium chloride as cholinesterase inhibitor.
   Result: improvement of the paresis for a few minutes.
2. EMG with repeated stimulation of a peripheral nerve.
   Result: amplitude reduction of the action potential during the first five stimuli.
3. Demonstration of antibodies against acetylcholine receptors.

Electrophysiological differences between neuropathies and myopathies

Criterion	Neuropathy Axonal	Neuropathy Myelinated	Myopathy
EMG:			
Action potential duration	↑	↑	↓
With maximum muscle tension:			
Amplitude			↓
Interference pattern	Thinned out	Thinned out	Full
Polyphasia	(+)	(+)	+++
Fibrillation potential / Positive sharp waves	+++	(+)	(+)
Fasciculations	+	(+)	−
Nerve conduction velocity (NCV)	n	↓ → ↓↓↓	n

Hereditary sensorimotor neuropathies (HSMN)

Type Characteristics	HSMN I (Charcot–Marie–Tooth disease)	HSMN II –	HSMN III (Déjérine–Sottas disease)
Mode of inheritance	Autosomal dominant	Autosomal dominant	Autosomal recessive
Disease onset	First year	Later childhood	Infancy
Motor function	Muscular atrophy Stork legs Stepping gait	Muscular atrophy Legs > arms	Muscular atrophy Muscle hypotonia Coordination disorder
Muscle reflexes	↓	(↓)	Ø
Sensory function: Touch/pressure Vibration Pain/temperature	n/(↓) ↓ n	n/(↓) (↓) n	} ↓↓↓
Deformities	Pes cavus Coxa valga Kyphoscoliosis	(+)	Pes equinovarus (club foot)
Diagnosis: EMG injury pattern NCV motor/sensitivity	Neurogenic ↓	Neurogenic n/(↓)	Neurogenic ↓↓↓
Morphology (sural nerve)	Axonal dystrophy Onion-skin myelin hypertrophy + Demyelinization (peripheral nerves, spinal cord)	Axonal dystrophy No myelin hypertrophy	Abnormal Myelin formation Onion skin CSF protein ↑

Note: heredopathic atactic polyneuritis (Refsum's disease = phytanic acid storage disease) is sometimes also described in the literature as HSMN type IV.
EMG = electromyography; NCV = nerve conduction velocity.

NEUROPEDIATRICS

Summary of the hereditary sensory neuropathies (HSN)

(Modified after Moser (1992).)

	HSN I	HSN II	HSN III	HSN IV
Synonyms	Familial ulceromutilating acropathy	Congenital sensory neuropathy	Riley–Day familial dysautonomia	Congenital sensory neuropathy with anhydrosis
Mode of inheritance	Usually autosomal dominant	Autosomal recessive, sporadic	Autosomal recessive	Autosomal recessive
Disease onset	2nd or 3rd decade	From birth	At birth	At birth
Disorder of sensory modality				
touch	+	+++	–	–
pressure	+	++	–	–
vibration	++	+++	–	–
pain	+++	++	Analgesia	+++
temperature	+++	++	–	+++
Localization of sensory disorder	Lower leg, forearm	Chiefly limbs	Generalized	Generalized
Sense of taste	Normal	Normal	Impaired or absent	Occasionally absent
Deafness	Frequent	Sporadic	None	None
Muscle reflexes	↓	n/(↓)	↓	↓
Disorder of autonomic function	None	None	Fever bouts, absent tears, drop in blood pressure, pathological pupillary reaction	Sensation of pain absent, fever, ptosis
Perspiration	Absent in affected areas	Absent in affected areas	Increased	Absent
Intelligence	n	n	n	↓
Nerve conduction velocity (NCV)				
motor	↓	n/(↓)	n/(↓)	n
sensory	↓	↓	n/(↓)	n
Nerve biopsy	Changes in the nonmedullated and small caliber myelinated fibers	Reduction in nonmedullated fibers, axonal changes	Reduction in nonmedullated fibers, 'onion skin'	Normal
CNS pathology	None	None	Atrophy of posterior tracts, loss of cells in certain nuclei	Atrophy of certain zones and of spinal cord pathways

439

MEMORIX PEDIATRICS

Percentile growth curves for head circumference: boys 0–6 years
(From Brandt (1986), with acknowledgements to Milupa AG, Friedrichsdorf.)

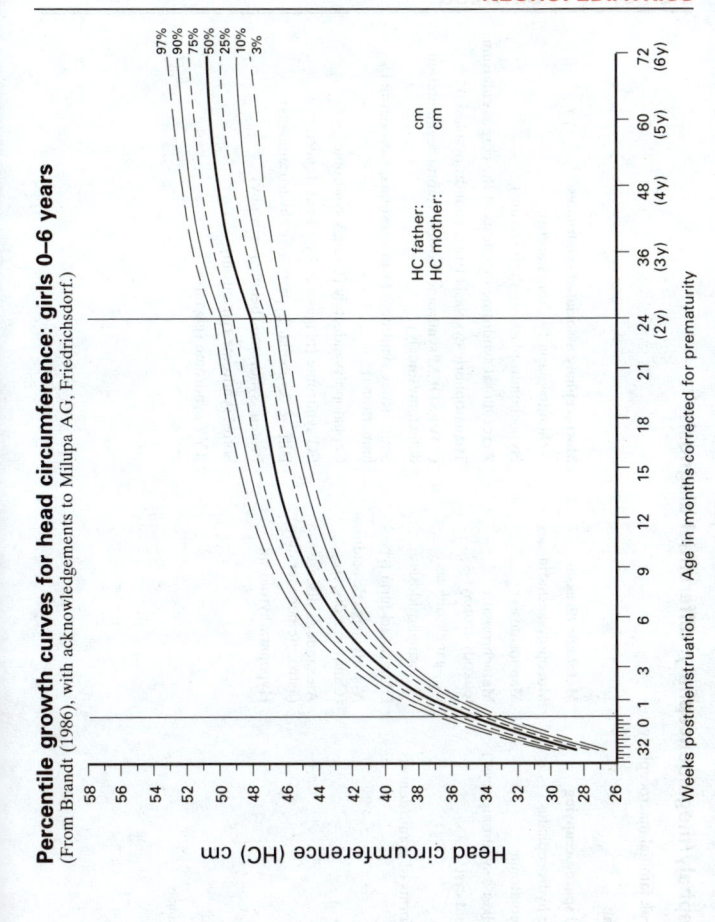

Percentile growth curves for head circumference: girls 0–6 years

(From Brandt (1986), with acknowledgements to Milupa AG, Friedrichsdorf.)

HC father: cm
HC mother: cm

Macrocephaly/megaloencephaly: differential diagnosis

Physiological: familial macrocephaly

Pathological:

Intracranial space-occupying	Metabolic diseases*	Macrocephaly associated syndromes
Obstructive hydrocephalus	Mucopolysaccharidoses	Achondroplasia (+ short stature)
Subdural hematoma	Mannosidosis	Hypochondroplasia (+ short stature)
Dandy–Walker's syndrome (cyst)	Metachromatic leukodystrophy	Acrocallosal syndrome (agenesis of the corpus callosum)
Subarachnoid cyst	G_{M1}-gangliosidosis	Thanatophoric dysplasia (osteochondrodysplasia)*
Tumors	G_{M2}-gangliosidosis	COVESDEM syndrome (costovertebral segmentation defect, mesomely)
Particular forms of craniostenosis	Glutaric aciduria type 1	Smith-Riley syndrome (+ macrosomia, mesodermal hamartoma)*
	N-acetylaspartic aciduria (Canavan's disease)	Cephalopolysyndactyly (Greig's syndrome)
	Alexander's disease (astrocyte degeneration)	FG syndrome (plagiocephaly + anal stenosis)*
	Hypoparathyroidism	Diffuse cerebellar hypertrophy (hydrocephalus)
		Proteus syndrome (hemihypertrophy)
		Sotos' syndrome (gigantism)
		XYY syndrome (gigantism)

* Megaloencephaly.

NEUROPEDIATRICS

Classification of the clinical types and diagnostic criteria of the neurofibromatoses

Type 1	NF1	Classic form = von Recklinghausen's disease	≥ five *café-au-lait* spots, diameter ≥5 mm, after pubery ≥15 mm
			Freckle-like hyperpigmentation in the axillary and inguinal regions
			Optic glioma
			Two or more neurofibromas or one plexiform neurofibroma
			Two or more iris nodules (Lisch nodules)
			Osseous dysplasias (sphenoid, cortex of marrow bones)
			A parent and/or sibling with proven NF1

For diagnosis, at least two criteria must be definitely present

Type II	NF2	Central form = familial acoustic schwannoma	Bilateral acoustic schwannoma (proven by MRI, CT or histology)
			A parent or sibling with NF2 or an acoustic tumor
			A parent or sibling with NF2 and two of the following criteria: neurofibroma, meningioma, glioma, juvenile posterior subcapsular lens opacity

Type III	NF3	mixed form = NF1 + 2	Multiple CNS tumors

Encephalofacial angiomatosis (Sturge–Weber syndrome)

Type 1
a One or bilateral port-wine stain (flame nevus) prominent at least in the first branch of the trigeminal area

b Glaucoma

c Angiomatosis of the veins, usually of one hemisphere (radiological evidence of perivenous cirsoid (varicoid) calcification)

d focal cerebral seizures, or seizure focus in EEG

Diagnosis allowed if criteria a–d, a + b, a + c or a + d are met.

Type 2   Port-wine stain (flame nevus) as in type 1 ± glaucoma, without signs of intracranial angiomatosis

Type 3   Isolated leptomeningeal and cortical angioma

MEMORIX PEDIATRICS

CSF–blood barrier

Synopsis of the interpretation of raised protein concentration in the CSF
(After Reiber (1980).)

Albumin ratio → indicator for disorder of the blood–CSF barrier

IgG ratio → indicator of inflammation in the CNS

Measurements in the range of	Interpretation	Clinical examples
⓪	Does not occur	–
①	Normal range	–
②	Increased permeability of blood–CSF barrier, filter function still present	High fever After a seizure Systemic diseases
③	a) Raised permability with decreased filter function for plasma protein b) Disorder of barrier function with local IgG production	Absorptive inflammation After subarachnoid bleeding After artificial bleeding Acute meningitis
④	Barrier disrupted + local, often oligoclonal IgG production	Chronic meningitis, meningoencephalitis, encephalitis (e.g. subacute sclerosing panencephalitis, multiple sclerosis)
⑤	Local IgG synthesis in the CNS, barrier normal	Slow-virus encephalitides

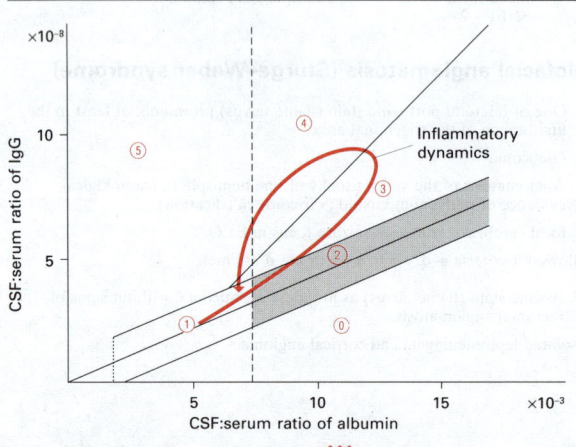

NEUROPEDIATRICS

International classification of epileptic seizures
(International League Against Epilepsy (1981).)

I **Focal (local, partial) seizures**
EEG: focal contralateral discharges beginning over the representative cortical areas.

   A **Single focal seizures (without impairment of consciousness)**

   1. With motor symptoms (motor (Jacksonian) seizures with/without 'march', partial continuous epilepsy, displaced seizures, vocalization seizures).

   2. With sensory symptoms (visual, acoustic, olfactory and gustatory hallucinations, vertigo, falling sensation).

   3. With autonomic symptoms (nausea, pallor, sweating, coldness, flushing, etc.).

   4. With psychological symptoms (anxiety, *déjà vu* events, dreamy states).

   B **Complex focal (partial) seizures with impaired consciousness (psychomotor seizures)**
   EEG: usually asynchronous local discharges, temporal, frontotemporal, unilateral or bilateral.

   1. Begins as a single focal seizure (see A1–4) with subsequent impairment of consciousness or automatism.

   2. Begins with impaired consciousness or automatism.

   C **Focal seizures with subsequent generalization**
   EEG: primary focal discharges that rapidly become generalized

   Generalized tonic–clonic, tonic or clonic seizures that arise from a single focus (IA), complex foci (IB) or from IA via IB.

II **Generalized seizures (convulsive or nonconvulsive)**

   A 1. **Absences** (briefly impaired consciousness + a motor autonomic or automatic component of mild degree).
   EEG: generalized spike and slow wave (SW) complexes, usually 3 Hz, less frequently 2–4 Hz during seizures. Predominantly normal between seizures.

   2. **Atypical absences** (additional components more clearly marked than in IIA1, begin and end less abruptly).
   EEG: heterogeneous during seizure, usually with paroxysmal activity between seizures.

   B **Myoclonic seizures (single or multiple convulsions)**
   EEG: ictal, interictal, polyspike wave, spike-wave or sharp and slow wave complexes.

   C **Clonic seizures**
   EEG: rapid seizure activity ($\geq 10/s$) and slow waves, sometimes SW pattern. SW or polyspike wave discharges between seizures.

   D **Tonic seizures**
   EEG: low amplitude seizure activity, rapid discharges or rhythms.

E Tonic–clonic seizures (grand mal)
EEG: in the tonic phase, discharges (≥10/s) with increasing frequency and rising amplitude; in the clonic phase, interspersed slower waves. SW or polyspike wave complexes between seizures.

F Atonic seizures (astatic or myoclonic astatic seizures)
EEG: polyspikes and waves (during or between seizures), low amplitude rapid discharges (during seizures).

III Unclassified attacks

International classification of epilepsies and epileptic syndromes
(International League against Epilepsy (1985).)

Definitions
Idiopathic epilepsies: genetic disposition, onset age-related, characteristic clinical and EEG findings.

Cryptogenic epilepsies: cause unknown + age-related.

Symptomatic epilepsies: cause known or obviously based on a disease.

1 Localization-related (focal, local, partial epilepsies and syndromes)

1.1 **Idiopathic**
Benign epilepsy of childhood with centrotemporal spikes (3–13 years).
Childhood epilepsy with occipital seizures (2–17 years).

1.2 **Symptomatic**
Variable according to the location of the cause of the seizure (see p. 445 for seizure types).

2 Generalized epilepsies and syndromes

2.1 **Idiopathic with age-related onset**
Benign familial fits of the newborn (2–3 days).
Benign fits of the newborn (1–7 days).
Benign myoclonic epilepsy of early childhood (0.5–3 years).
Absence epilepsy of childhood (pyknolepsy) (5–8 years).
Juvenile absence epilepsy (10–17 years).
Juvenile myoclonic epilepsy (impulse petit mal epilepsy) (12–18 years).
Early grand mal epilepsy (10–25 years).
Other generalized idiopathic epilepsies.

2.2 **Cryptogenic or symptomatic**
West's syndrome (jack-knife salaam seizures, infantile spasm) (3–8 months).
Lennox–Gastaut syndrome (petit mal variant) (1–7 years).
Epilepsy with myoclonic astatic seizures (1–9 years).
Epilepsy with myoclonic absences (6–7 years).

2.3 **Symptomatic**

2.3.1 **Nonspecific etiology**
Early infancy myoclonic encephalopathy.
Early infancy epileptic encephalopathy with burst suppression pattern.

2.3.2 **Specific syndromes**
Seizures as the dominant sign of various diseases (CNS malformations, congenital metabolic diseases with variable age manifestation).

3 **Epilepsies and syndromes without definite attachment to focal or generalized seizures**

3.1 **With generalized as well as focal seizures**
Neonatal fits.
Severe myoclonic epilepsy of early childhood (0.5–3 years).
Epilepsy with persisting SW discharges in synchronized sleep (bioelectric status epilepticus in non-REM sleep (2–10 years).
Epilepsy–aphasia syndrome (2–8 years).

3.2 **No definite classification among epilepsies**
e.g. sleep grand mal.

4 **Special syndromes**

4.1 Occasional attacks.
Febrile convulsions.
Seizures that only occur under specific pathophysiological conditions.

4.2 Oligoepilepsy.

4.3 Reflex epilepsy.

4.4 Continuous progressive partial epileptic seizures of childhood.
( ) = Age of manifestation in age-associated seizures.

Febrile convulsions

Definitions: Average epilepsy risk 3–4%
Simple febrile convulsion: no rise in epilepsy risk
Complicated (= risk-associated) febrile convulsions: increased risk of epilepsy

Risk factors
Familial history of epilepsy
First febrile convulsion before the first and after the fourth birthday
Several convulsions during the same infection
A total of ≥4 febrile convulsions
Duration of convulsion ≥15 min
Signs of previous cerebral damage
Focal neurological signs during and/or after seizures
Focal changes in the EEG after seizures
Persistence of EEG changes after seizures (focal signs, hypersynchronous discharges, abnormal rhythms)

Acute treatment: clonazepam/diazepam (i.v./rectal)

Long-term treatment: phenobarbitone/primidone/(sodium valproate)

Indications for long-term treatment
Febrile convulsions always last for 15 minutes or more
Serial seizures
Focal or unilateral signs during and/or after seizures

Treatment of epilepsy

Type of epilepsy	Antiepileptics First choice	Second choice
Generalized epilepsy		
Early childhood absence Pyknolepsy Juvenile absence	Sodium valproate	Ethosuximide/phenobarbitone*/ primidone
Myoclonic astatic seizures in early childhood	Sodium valproate	Ethosuximide[†]/ACTH
Impulsive petit mal	Sodium valproate	Phenobarbitone/primidone/ ethosuximide[†]
Waking-up grand mal	Sodium valproate	Phenobarbitone[†]/primidone/ ethosuximide
Other grand mal types	Sodium valproate	Phenobarbitone/primidone/ potassium bromide/ carbamazepine/phenytoin
West's syndrome (jack-knife salaam seizures)	ACTH (dexamethasone)	Sodium valproate/clonazepam/ pyridoxine
Lennox–Gastaut syndrome	Sodium valproate	ACTH/clonazepam/ethosuximide[†]/ phenobarbitone[‡]/primidone[‡]
Partial (focal) epilepsy		
Idiopathic benign partial epilepsy	Carbamazepine	Phenytoin/phenobarbitone
Simple/complex focal seizures (± secondary generalization)	Carbamazepine	Phenytoin/primidone/ phenobarbitone/vigabatrin
Landau–Kleffner syndrome		ACTH/sodium valproate/ primidone
Bioelectric status epilepticus		ACTH/sodium valproate/ primidone

* = As protection against grand mal.
[†] = In combination with medication of first choice.
[‡] = In tonic cases.
SVP = Sodium valproate; ACTH = adrenocorticotropic hormone (corticotropin).

MEMORIX PEDIATRICS

Antiepileptics

Drug	Infants	Monotherapy – daily dose Young children	Schoolchildren	Dose frequency	Effective plasma concentration (µg/ml)	Steady state after days	Effect on serum concentration of other drugs
First choice							
Carbamazepine (CBZ)	–	20–25 mg/kg	15–20 mg/kg	3–4	3–12	4–6	phenobarbitone ↓, phenytoin ↓, sodium valproate ↓
Clonazepam (CZP)	<1 y 1–3 mg	1–5 y 3–6 mg	6–12 y 4–8 mg	3	25–75	5–7	
Ethosuximide (ESM)	–	30 mg/kg	20 mg/kg	3	40–120	4–10	phenytoin ↑, sodium valproate ↑
Phenobarbitone (PB)	4–5 mg/kg	4 mg/kg	3–4 mg/kg	2	15–40	14–21	carbamazepine ↓, phenytoin ↕, sodium valproate ↓
Phenytoin (PHT)	–	7 mg/kg	5 mg/kg	2	5–20	5–14	carbamazepine ↓, phenobarbitone ↕, sodium valproate ↓
Primidone (PRM)	20 mg/kg	20 mg/kg	15 mg/kg	3	4–12	2–4	carbamazepine ↓, phenytoin ↕, sodium valproate ↓

| Drug | Monotherapy – daily dose | | | Dose frequency | Effective plasma concentration (µg/ml) | Steady state after days | Effect on serum concentration of other drugs |
	Infants	Young children	Schoolchildren				
Sodium valproate (SVP)	30–80 mg/kg	30–100 mg/kg	20–50 mg/kg	2–3	30–120	2–6	carbamazepine ↑, phenobarbitone ↑, phenytoin ↕
Vigabatrin (VB)	50–100 mg/kg	50–80 mg/kg	50 mg/kg	2			
Second choice							
Acetazolamide	–	10–15 mg/kg	10–15 mg/kg	2–3	8–14	2	

List of aids to resuscitation

Mask no.	Endotracheal tube* (Internal diameter (mm))	Age	Weight (kg)	Adrenaline 1 ml = 1 mg 1:10 diluted (ml)	Sodium bicarbonate (8.4%) 1 ml = 1 mmol to be diluted if at all possible (ml)	Atropine 1 ml = 0.5 mg (ml)	Lignocaine (2%) 1 ml = 20 mg (ml)	Defibrillation initially (J)
0	3.0	Neonates	3.0	0.4	4	0.4	0.2	10
0	3.5	6 months	7.0	0.7	7	0.7	0.35	20
1	4.0	1 year	9	0.9	9	0.9	0.45	20
1–2	4.5	2 years	12	1.2	12	1.2	0.6	20
2–3	5.0–5.5	5 years	19	1.9	19	1.9	0.95	40
3	6.0	9 years	30	3.0	30	3.0	1.5	60
3–4	6.5–7.0	12 years	40	4.0	40	4.0	2.0	80
4	7.0–7.5	14 years	50	5.0	50	5.0	2.5	100
		Dosage		0.1 ml/kg	1 ml/kg	0.1 ml/kg	0.05 ml/kg	Maximally 4 J/kg

For intermediate body weights the exact dosages can be calculated from the dosage guidelines.
* Either curved or straight-bladed laryngoscopes are used for the intubation of infants and children.

EMERGENCIES

Ventilation
Classification of forms of ventilation in relation to the work of breathing:

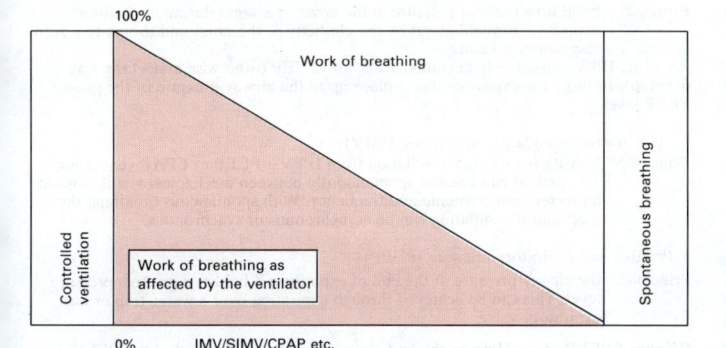

Controlled ventilation:
Ventilation with positive pressure in which the ventilator provides a given volume at a pre-set stroke frequency independent of the work of breathing by the patient. All the work of breathing is done by the ventilator.

True spontaneous respiration:
All respiratory effort is made by the patient.

Between these two lie various mixed types (assisted ventilation), in which the particular division of the work of breathing depends on the type and extent of the mechanical support.

Most frequently used abbreviations:
CMV	controlled mechanical ventilation
CPAP	continuous positive airway pressure
CPP	continuous positive pressure ventilation
HFPPV	high frequency positive pressure ventilation
HFJV	high frequency jet ventilation
HFOV	high frequency oscillatory ventilation
IMV	intermittent mandatory (mechanical) ventilation
IPP	intermittent positive pressure ventilation
PEEP	positive end-expiratory pressure
SIMV	synchronized intermittent mandatory (mechanical) ventilation
SIPPV	synchronized intermittent positive pressure ventilation.

MEMORIX PEDIATRICS

Frequently used types of ventilation

1 Intermittent positive pressure ventilation (IPPV)

Principle: build up a positive pressure in the airway passages during inspiration; expiration brought about by the elasticity of the lungs and thorax to a zero respiratory pressure.

As a rule IPPV is used only in combination with PEEP (otherwise atalectasis may develop). In this case, expiration takes place up to the airway pressure of the pre-set PEEP level.

2 Intermittent mandatory ventilation (IMV)

Principle: transitional form of ventilation from IPPV + PEEP to CPAP ventilation. The patient can breathe spontaneously between mechanical ventilations at a pre-set stroke volume and frequency. With spontaneous breathing the mechanical ventilation can be asynchronous or synchronous.

3 Positive end-expiratory pressure (PEEP)

Principle: the airway pressure at the end of expiration is held at a positive pressure level. This can be achieved through expiration over a water-trap or an expiratory valve.

Effects of PEEP (depending on the underlying disease and the level of the PEEP:
 – enlargement of the functional residual capacity of the lungs
 – prevention of alveolar collapse
 – reduction of any intrapulmonary right–left shunt.

4 Continuous positive airway pressure (CPAP)

Principle: setting a positive pressure level (above atmospheric) in the airway of a spontaneously breathing child.

Effects and side-effects correspond to those of PEEP.

Parameters that have to be set or controlled during mechanical ventilation:

1. Oxygen supply (Fi_{O_2})
2. CPAP/PEEP level (cmH_2O)
3. Peak inspiratory pressure (Pip/Pin; cmH_2O)
4. Ventilation rate (l/min)
5. Ratio of inspiratory to expiratory time (I:E), or in- and/or expiratory time (in s; as a percentage of the respiratory cycle)
6. Respiratory minute volume or inspiratory stroke volume (l/min; ml)
7. Mean airway pressure.

Ventilators are classified according to which physical parameter ends the supply of the respiratory volume to the patient or causes the ventilator to switch from inspiration to expiration:
 – time controlled
 – pressure controlled
 – volume controlled.

Pressure controlled ventilation is especially used in neonates, while volume controlled ventilation is usual in older children.

EMERGENCIES

Effects of mechanical ventilation

Comparison between pressure controlled and volume controlled ventilation
(After Rogers (1987).)

	Pressure controlled	Volume controlled
Advantages	Avoidance of very high inspiratory pressure Less risk of barotrauma	Constant stroke volume High ventilatory pressure indicates changes in lung mechanics
Disadvantages	Variable stroke volume Changes in compliance or resistance are not recognized	Possibility of producing a very high inspiratory pressure Increased risk of barotrauma

Side-effects of CPAP/PEEP
(After Rogers (1987).)

Reduced cardiac output
    Reduced systemic venous return
    Raised pulmonary vascular resistance
    Shift of the interventricular septum
    Neural and/or humoral depression of the left ventricle
    Reduced myocardial blood flow

Reduced cerebral perfusion pressure
    Raised intracranial pressure
    Systemic hypotension

Changes in renal blood flow
    Reduction in and redistribution of renal blood flow
    Reduced clearance of free water and creatinine
    Reduced sodium excretion

Reduced blood flow in the splanchnic region
    Reduced intestinal and hepatic blood flow

Alveolar overdistension
    Air-leak syndrome (pneumothorax, -mediastinum, -pericardium, cutaneous emphysema)
    Increased physiological deadspace

MEMORIX PEDIATRICS

Indications for mechanical ventilation

1. Acute respiratory arrest.
2. Acute respiratory failure = all conditions involving inadequate alveolar ventilation or arterial oxygenation, or both together.
3. The ratio of deadspace to tidal volume (V_D/V_T) >0.6.
4. Any condition where there is a threat of respiratory failure.
5. Any condition requiring secure control of the respiratory pattern and breathing function (e.g. in raised intracranial pressure; in cardiac failure).
6. All conditions where a reduction in the work of breathing is desirable (e.g. severe cardiac failure, chronic respiratory failure).

Guidelines for the initial setting of the ventilator when ventilating children
(After Rogers (1987).)

Adequate ventilation:
Ventilation rate: as near to physiological for age as possible
Ventilator stroke volume: 12–15 ml/kg
I:E ratio: aim at an I:E ratio of ≥1:2; in obstructive diseases, the duration of expiration should be increased

Immediate check for adequate ventilation:
thoracic excursion; auscultation for breath sounds; Pa_{CO_2} = 35–45 mmHg.

Adequate oxygenation:
Fi_{O_2}* = 1.0
PEEP = 3–5 cmH$_2$O, higher if necessary and hemodynamically tolerated.

Immediate check for adequate oxygenation:
skin color; Pa_{O_2} > 70 mmHg.
Check for hemodynamic side-effects: blood pressure; peripheral perfusion.

*Fraction of inspired oxygen.

In premature and mature neonates, in whom, as a rule, ventilation is not volume controlled but pressure and time controlled, the following initial settings may be used:

Ventilator rate: 40/min
Inspiratory peak pressure: 20–25 cmH$_2$O
PEEP: 4–5 cmH$_2$O
Flow ≈ 8 l/min

Target systemic arterial blood gas levels: Pa_{O_2} = 65–95 mmHg
Pa_{CO_2} = 35–45 mmHg

EMERGENCIES

Neonatal ventilation

Advantages and disadvantages of using inspiratory peak pressure and ventilator rate when ventilating neonates
(After Fox (1988).)

Peak pressure	Advantages	Disadvantages
Low	Fewer side-effects, especially in bronchopulmonary dysplasia and pulmsnary air leak	Inadequate ventilation Low Pa_{O_2} if setting too low Possibly development of generalized atelectasis
High	Possibly re-opening of atelectases High Pa_{O_2} Low Pa_{CO_2}	Increased risk of side-effects Impaired venous return

Ventilator rate	Advantages	Disadvantages
Low <40/min	Possibly better oxygenation, higher $P_{A_{O_2}}$ levels Useful in weaning off ventilator and for ventilation with reversed I : E ratio	High peak pressure may be necessary to obtain adequate ventilation Relaxation may be necessary
High >60/min	Lower peak pressure may be necessary; lower mean airway pressure; if hyperventilation is desired, e.g. if persistent fetal circulation is present	Because of the duration of expiration for lung emptying → 'air trapping' and respiratory alkalosis is possible

Advantages and disadvantages of using PEEP when ventilating neonates
(After Fox (1988).)

PEEP level	Advantages	Disadvantages
Low 0–3 cm H_2O	Maintenance of lung volume in prematures with low functional residual capacity	Possibly too low to support adequate lung volume CO_2 retention
Medium 4–7 cm H_2O	Stabilizing of areas with atelectasis Raised lung volume in surfactant deficiency	Possible hyperinflation
High 8–10 cm H_2O	Prevention of alveolar collapse in surfactant deficiency Improved ventilation distribution	Increased risk of pneumothorax Reduced compliance Impaired venous return Increased pulmonary vascular resistance CO_2 retention

Criteria of acute respiratory failure

(After Toro-Figueroa, Morriss and Levin (1990) and Rogers (1987).)

1. Clinical criteria
   Tachypnea; apnea; expiratory groan; stridor; flared nostrils; inspiratory rib retraction; tachycardia; bradycardia; cyanosis; restlessness; clouded consciousness.

2. Laboratory data:
   $Pa_{O_2} < 50\,mmHg$ if $Fi_{O_2} > 0.5$
   $Pa_{CO_2} > 55\,mmHg$ in acidosis or
   $Pa_{CO_2} > 40\,mmHg$ in severe respiratory impairment
   Vital capacity $< 15\,ml/kg$.

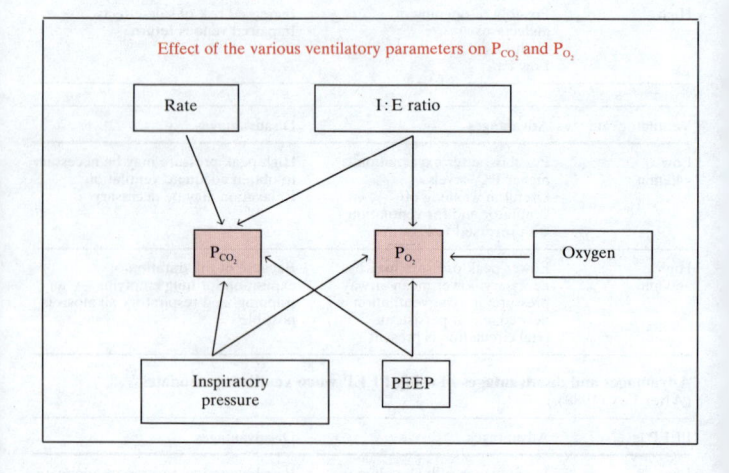

Effect of the various ventilatory parameters on P_{CO_2} and P_{O_2}

EMERGENCIES

Complications of assisted ventilation

Pulmonary complications – Air leak syndrome
(After Perelman (1986).)

Acute interstitial emphysema
Chronic persistent interstitial emphysema generalized/localized
Pneumothorax
Pneumomediastinum
Pneumopericardium
Pneumoperitoneum
Subacute emphysema
Retroperitoneal air accumulation
Air embolism

Complications of endotracheal intubation
(After Macpherson et al. (1988).)

Acute	Chronic

Traumatic
  Perforation of nasopharynx,
  oropharynx or hypopharynx
  Hemorrhage
  Laryngeal edema, etc.
 	
Mechanical
  Malposition (esophagus, main bronchus)
  Obstruction
  Accidental extubation
  Tube kinking
 	
Other
  Apnea
  Hypoxia
  Aspiration
	Abnormal primary dentition
	Acquired cleft palate
	Choanal stenosis
	Gingival furrow
	Subglottal stenosis
	
	Granuloma
	Tracheal necrosis
	Necrotizing tracheobronchitis
	Tracheomegaly

Complications of endotracheal aspiration
(After MacDonald et al. (1986).)

Hemorrhage
Unintended extubation
Perforation of lung or main bronchus
Bronchopulmonary fistula
Hypoxia
Bradycardia
Increase in cerebral blood flow and intracranial pressure
Rise in blood pressure

MEMORIX PEDIATRICS

Resuscitation

Confirm apnea: – absence of chest and/or abdominal excursion
    – absent air stream

Confirm cardiac arrest: – absent heart action
    – absence of pulse (in the brachial artery in infants, in the common carotid artery in young children)

Confirm loss of consciousness: – no response on being spoken to

↓

Call for additional help

↓

Positioning: supine on a hard flat surface

↓

Commence resuscitation

↓

Assisted ventilation
- Clear the air passages
- Lift the chin and slightly extend the head; suction
- Ventilation without mechanical aid:
    Neonates/infants: mouth to mouth and nose
    Young children/older children: mouth to mouth
- Ventilation with mechanical aid:
    Mouth to nasopharyngeal or oropharyngeal tube
    Ventilator bag and mask
    Ventilator bag to nasopharyngeal or oropharyngeal tube
    Ventilator bag to endotracheal tube
- Ventilation rate:
    Neonates   40–60/min
    Infants   20/min
    Children   15–20/min

External cardiac massage
Neonates/infants:

Compress the middle third of the sternum with two or three fingers, or with both thumbs after encircling chest
Rate: 120/min in neonates
           100/min in infants

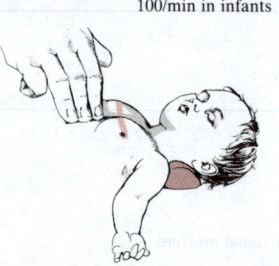

EMERGENCIES

Young children up to school age:
> Compress vertically the lower third of the sternum with the ball of one hand
> Rate: 80–100/min

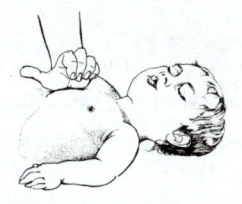

Schoolchildren:
> Place the ball of one hand on the lower third of the sternum. Lay the other hand on it and press
> Rate: 80/min

Ratio of number of external compressions to ventilations:
> Neonates   3:1
> Infants/children   5:1

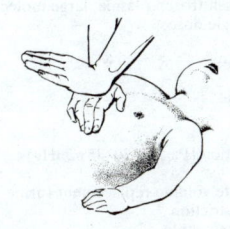

MEMORIX PEDIATRICS

Medication: application

Access:
- Peripheral vein
- Endotracheal
- Intraosseous (tibial head)
- Intracardiac

Medication:
- Oxygen (100% if possible)
- Adrenaline 0.01–0.05 mg/kg i.v. (= 0.1–0.5 ml/kg of a 1:10000 solution) repeat after 5 min
- Sodium bicarbonate 1 mEq/kg = 1 ml/kg 8.4% solution i.v. diluted 1:1 with distilled water in neonates
- Atropine 0.01–0.03 mg/kg i.v. (always >0.1 mg/single dose)

Extended resuscitation medication

- Calcium 5–10 mg/kg i.v. (calcium gluconate 10% solution = >0.5 ml/kg; 1 ml = 10 mg) in hypocalcemia, hyperkalemia, hypermagnesemia; overdose of calcium antagonist
- Lignocaine 1 mg/kg i.v. in ventricular tachycardia, flutter or fibrillation; repeat dosage 0.5 mg/kg i.v.; recurrence prevention: 20–50 µg/kg/min
- Volume replacement in hypovolemia: (blood; crystalloid solutions (NaCl 0.9%, Ringer-Lactate); colloidal solutions (human albumin 5%, fresh frozen plasma, large molecular colloids)) 5–10 ml/kg/single dose

Treatment principles in the postresuscitation phase

- Adequate oxygenation (Pa_{O_2} = 100 mmHg)
- Normal ventilation to moderate hyperventilation (Pa_{CO_2} = 30–35 mmHg)
- Adequate organ perfusion
- If reduced intravascular volume, give adequate volume replacement (urine production >1 ml/kg/hour); otherwise fluid restriction

  Catecholamines:
  - dobutamine   5–20 µg/kg/min
  - dopamine   2–20 µg/kg/min
  - adrenaline   0.1–1.0 µg/kg/min
  - noradrenaline   0.1–5.0 µg/kg/min

  Correction of disorders of the electrolyte and acid–base balance
- Treatment of seizures:
  - diazepam   0.3–0.5 mg/kg i.v.
  - clonazepam   0.05–0.1 mg/kg i.v.
  - phenobarbitone   5–10 mg/kg i.v.
  - phenytoin   10–15 mg/kg i.v.
- Positioning: upper part of body raised 30°, head in midposition

EMERGENCIES

Disorders of consciousness: diagnostic procedures

Note: before any other measures are taken, it is most important to safeguard the vital functions → emergency ABC (airway, breathing, circulation)

History pointers:
Acute onset?
Trauma, maltreatment?
Fever?
Vomiting?
Diarrhea?

Medication?
– anticonvulsives?
– antihypertensives?
– insulin?
Previous illness?

Investigation of disorders of consciousness

Pulse:	radial artery, carotid artery
Pupils:	size, symmetry, movement
Heart:	rate, rhythm, sounds, blood pressure
Respiration:	rate, amplitude, pattern, ratio of inspiration to expiration, stridor, sounds, impairment
Fetor:	alcohol, acetone, uremia
Skeleton:	fractures (swelling, hematoma, crepitation)
Skin:	pallor (the unconscious child is pale except in diabetic coma and encephalitis), cyanosis, jaundice (sclera), hematoma, injection sites (arms, thighs, abdomen), electric shock burns
Fontanelles:	tense, protruding
Temperature:	rectal
Movements:	spontaneous movements, muscle tone (note any laterality)
Eyes:	eye position, deviation (conjugated, disconjugated), eye-rolling movements; pupillary reaction to light (direct, consensual) corneal reflex
Coma scale:	repeat from time to time
Meningismus:	Brudzinski' sign (test only if trauma eliminated), Kernig's sign

Relationship between site of damage and pupillary reaction

Site of the disorder	Pupil size and reaction
Cerebral hemispheres, subcortical white matter, posterior thalamic nuclei	Normal
Diencephalon	Constricts to light
Midbrain	Midposition; slightly dilated or unequal, or markedly dilated; nonreactive
Pons	Constricted, nonreactive

Additional diagnostic measures

	Blood gas analysis	Serum electrolytes osmolality	Creatinine, urea-N	Bilirubin, γ-glutamyl transpeptidase, ammonia, bleeding time, Quick's test, prothrombin time, thrombin time
Blood pressure, blood picture, hematocrit, C-reactive protein, glucose, urine, skin perfusion				
→	→	→	→	→
Shock (hemorrhage, sepsis) CNS infections Febrile fits Hypertensive crisis Hemolytic–uremic shock Hypo-/hyperglycemia	Hypoxia Hypercapnia Hypocapnia Heart/kidney/liver failure Intoxication Metabolic acidosis in enzyme defects of intermediary metabolism	Hypo-/hypertonic Dehydration Adrenal cortical insufficiency	Uremic coma	Hepatic coma, clotting disorder

CSF – bacteriology – cytology	EEG, sonography, Doppler sonography, X-rays (skull), CT (skull), MRI (CNS)			ECG, sonography, X-rays (chest)
→	→			→
Meningitis Meningoencephalitis Subarachnoid hemorrhage	Cerebral seizures Intracranial space-occupying lesions: cerebral edema, hemorrhage, tumor, metastases, encephalitis, abscess, embolism, thrombosis, angioma			Arrhythmias Cardiac failure Chest trauma Aspiration

EMERGENCIES

The Glasgow Coma Scale and age-related modifications
(After Teasdale, Jennet and Jakobi, cited in Yager, Johnston and Seshia (1990).)

		Score
Eye opening (E) (all age groups)	spontaneous	4
	to speech	3
	to pain	2
	no eye opening	1

Motor responses (M)

Older child	obeys movement commands promptly (e.g. deliberate grasping)	6
Child <2 years	normal spontaneous movements	
Older child	purposive reaction to pain stimulus (can localize the pain site)	5
Child <2 years	purposive movement after pain stimulus	
Older child/ child <2 years	nonpurposive movement after pain stimulus (withdraws)	4
Older child/ child <2 years	nonpurposive flexor movements (arms) after pain stimulus + tendency to stretch legs (decortication position)	3
Older child/ child <2 years	stretching of all limbs after pain stimulus (decerebration position)	2
Older child/ child <2 years	no movements after pain stimulus	1

Verbal response (V)

Older child	knows its surroundings (is orientated), understands speech	5
Child <2 years	recognizes familiar person, fixates, follows objects, smiles	
Older child	is confused, disorientated, confused conversation	4
Child <2 years	uncertain recognition, just cries, inconsistent fixation and following of objects	
Older child	replies inadequate, speaks incoherently using inappropriate words	3
Child <2 years	only arousable for a time, does not eat or drink, cries miserably	
Older child	makes only incomprehensible sounds	2
Child <2 years	cannot be aroused, restless movements at times, no verbal sounds	
Older child	no verbal sounds	1
Child <2 years	does not react to any stimulus	

Coma score = E + M + V

    Minimum score = 3, maximum score = 15
    Scores of 6 or less: condition life-threatening
    Score of 15: no disorder of consciousness

Intracranial pressure

Cerebral perfusion pressure = mean arterial pressure minus intracranial pressure
Autoregulation: cerebral blood flow is constant at a perfusion pressure of between 50 and 150 mmHg
At a perfusion pressure <50 mmHg there is a rapid fall in cerebral perfusion
Loss of autoregulation (e.g. after trauma): reduction in cerebral blood flow even with a perfusion pressure >50 mmHg

Normal intracranial pressure
(lying quietly in a horizontal position):
- Neonates → ca. 2 mmHg
- Infants ca. 5 mmHg
- Young/preschool children ca. 6–13 mmHg
- Schoolchildren ca. 15 mmHg

Measures to be taken in cerebral edema/swelling

I   Checking of the vital functions
    Establishment of the Glasgow Coma Scale score

II Fundoscopy, EEG and CT
    Decision on intracranial pressure measurement
    Exclude obstructive hydrocephalus, intracranial hemorrhage

III **Special measures against pressure build-up**

Prevention	Advantages	Disadvantages
Positioning: head and upper body +30°	Increased pressure gradient to right atrium	Only possible with a stable circulation
Relaxation: pancuronium bromide 0.04–0.1 mg/kg	Controlled ventilation possible	Doing without establishing/following complete neurological status
Hyperventilation: Pa_{CO_2} to be held at 30–25 mmHg Pa_{O_2} > 100 mmHg Respiratory pressure to be held low	Reduction of intracranial blood compartment, respiratory compensation of any potential metabolic acidosis pressure gradient to heart	Hypocapnia reduces cerebral blood flow —
Dexamethasone, 1 mg/kg/d i.v. in 6 doses over 3–7 days (depending on tendency to edema), reducing over a further 3 days	Stabilized blood–brain barrier	Great danger of infection/delayed wound healing with higher dosages
Rectal temperature to be lowered to 36.5–35°C	Reduced cerebral metabolic activity	—
Fluid supply ca. 2/3 of normal maintenance requirement (using as measures: mean weight, hematocrit 30–40%, urinary excretion >2 ml/kg/h)		

EMERGENCIES

Procedures for pressure reduction

Osmotic therapy:		
– Furosemide, 2–5 mg/kg	Aids mannitol infusion, appropriate in recurrent tendency to edema	
– Mannitol (brief infusion), 0.25–1 g/kg over 10 min – Serum osmolality not above 310 mosmol/l	Reduces intracranial pressure within a few minutes	Effect lasts only 2–4 h
Phenobarbitone, initially 10–15 mg/kg for first hour, then maintenance with 2–3 mg/kg Serum level 25–40 mg/l	Reduces cerebral blood flow, reduces energy-consuming electrical activity	With higher dosage (barbiturate coma) danger of fatal summation of causal brain damage and circulatory depression

Burns

At place of accident: children up to 14 years: burnt surface area (%)
= X × surface area of child's hand (1%)
juveniles: Wallace's rule of nines

```
      9
   9 / \ 9
  18     18
      1
  18 / \ 18
```

In hospital:

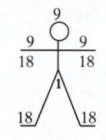

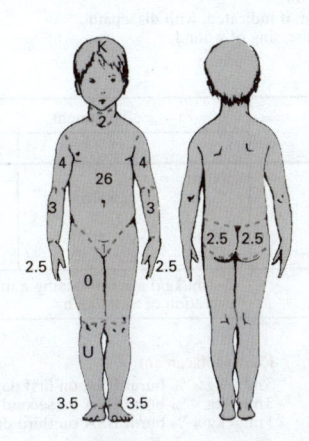

Front: K, 2, 4, 4, 26, 3, 3, 2.5, 0, 2.5, 2.5, 2.5, U, 3.5, 3.5

467

MEMORIX PEDIATRICS

Percentage division of body surface area in the assessment of burns
(After Lund and Browder (1944).)
The growth-dependent regions are:

Age in years	<1	1	3	5	7	10	12	15	>15
Body region (%)									
H head	19	17	15	13	12	11	10	9	7
T (1) thigh	5.5	6.5	7	8	8.5	8.5	9	9	9.5
L (1) leg	5	5	5.5	5.5	5.5	6	6	6.5	7

Estimation of fluid loss in first 24 h:

ml/kg body weight/% burned body surface	
wound exudate	~0.7
edema	~2.0
evaporation	~1.5

Grade of severity:
- low grade burns = <5% (except face, hands, external genitalia, feet)
- medium–severe burns = ≤15% (grade II)
- severe burns = >15% (of which 5% grade III)

Treatment at site of accident: Secure vital functions
- in case of smoke inhalation: corticosteroids by aerosol or i.v.; early assisted ventilation
- shock and pain:
    pethidine 1–2 mg/kg i.v.
    infusion: NaCl (0.9%) + glucose (5%) as 1:1 solution (60 ml/h ~20 drops/min or more)

Gastric tube
Sedation, if indicated, with diazepam
Sterile dressing of wound

Infusion treatment in hospital
(After Butenandt and Coerdt (1979).)

Infusion solution Composition	Treatment 1	Treatment 2	Treatment 3
NaCl (0.9%) + glucose (5%) = 1:1	500 ml		
NaCl (0.9%) + glucose (5%) = 1:2		500 ml	
NaCl (0.9%) + glucose (5%) = 1:4			500 ml
Human albumin (20%)	50 ml	50 ml	50 ml
Na bicarbonate (8.4%) (ml = mmol)	15 ml		
KCl (7.45%) (ml = mmol)	2–4 ml/kg/d after obtaining a urinary excretion of >1 ml/kg/h		

Amount of infusion per day:

Maintenance requirement   +   Fluid replacement

Up to 10 kg BW: 100–150 ml/kg
Up to 20 kg BW: 80–100 ml/kg
Up to 40 kg BW: 60–80 ml/kg

5 ml × kg × % burnt BSA on first day
3 ml × kg × % burnt BSA on second day
1 ml × kg × % burnt BSA on third day

From the fourth day reduce the total quantity to maintenance requirements.

BW = body weight; BSA = body surface area.

EMERGENCIES

Status epilepticus
Definition: Serial cerebral attacks: the end of individual attacks is marked by regained consciousness
Status of cerebral seizures: consciousness does not return between attacks

Types	Main symptoms
Grand mal	Clouded consciousness/unconsciousness/clonus
Petit mal	Clouded consciousness/motor automatism/clonus
Status of simple partial attacks	Clonus (continuous partial epilepsy)/twilight state
Status of complex partial attacks (rare)	Twilight state
Bioelectrical status in non-REM sleep	Developmental arrest and regression/speech disorders (ESES: electrical status epilepticus during slow sleep)

Diagnostic aids: EEG or long-term EEG (→ ESES)

Treatment of grand mal:
Diazepam, rectal 5 mg (infants)
  10 mg (older children)
 when possible intravenously: diazepam 2 mg (infants)
  20 mg (juveniles)
  or clonazepam 0.25 mg (neonates)
  0.5 mg (child)
  1–4 mg (older child)

Slow injection until seizures cease

First choice for newborn: phenobarbitone 15–20 mg/kg.
In the tonic attack states, avoid benzodiazapines and start with phenobarbitone or phenytoin straight away.

– Wait 5 min for the effect, lay the patient down, insert an intravenous line, give oxygen; blood-gas analysis

If no anticonvulsant effect:
  Have intubation instruments ready
– phenobarbitone 20 mg/kg i.v. (slowly)

If no effect:
– phenytoin, initially 15 mg/kg i.v.; effect sets in after 10–15 min

If no effect or inadequate breathing (Sa_{O_2} < 90%):
– mechanical ventilation
– anticonvulsive treatment with thiopental sodium, 2–4 mg/kg, then 2–8 mg/kg/h

▶ Additional measures: antipyretics (physical, paracetamol)
  dexamethasone 1 mg/kg
  furosemide 1–3 mg/kg

Treatment of petit mal: clonazepam, as for grand mal
  continue long-term treatment at higher dosage

Continue diagnostic measures → causes of status epilepticus:
Neonates: see p. 408 (lactate and ammonia to be measured first on the day after the end of the attacks)
Older children: infection (particularly meningitis, encephalitis)
  intoxication
  tuberous sclerosis
  hypoglycemia
  intracranial hemorrhage

Types of shock

General object of treatment: optimization of tissue perfusion.

Generally valid treatment principles:
- treatment of the basic disease
- prevention of hypoxia (Sa_{O_2} 95–99%, hematocrit 35–40%)
- correction of disorders of acid–base balance
- removal of respiratory 'derailment'
- improvement in cardiovascular function: heart rate, stroke volume, preload and after-load
- further supportive treatment:
  steroids
  treatment of abnormal renal function
  prophylaxis and treatment of a consumptive coagulopathy.

Hypovolemic shock

Definition: reduced intravascular volume with consecutive diminution of venous return to the heart and resulting diminished preload.

Signs: reduced peripheral perfusion (gradient between rectal and skin temperatures >10°C).
Tachycardia, diuresis ↓, high urinary specific gravity, narrow pulse pressure, but normal systolic blood pressure.
Central venous pressure ↓, pulmonary capillary wedge pressure ↓, systemic vascular resistance ↓, cardiac output ↓.

Shock signs in acute blood loss:

Loss <15%	→	raised heart rate (10–20%), blood pressure normal, capillary filling time normal
Loss 15–25%	→	tachycardia >20%, tachypnea, pulse pressure amplitude ↓, capillary filling time prolonged, oliguria
Loss 25–35%	→	+oliguria/anuria, change of consciousness
Loss 38–50%	→	'corpse-like' appearance, pulse impalpable, coma, possibly bradycardia.

Treatment
- Adequate volume replacement:
  Substitution fluid according to type of loss:
  if blood loss → blood (hematocrit → >30%)
  with Hb ≧ 10 g% and hematocrit → >30%:

→ plasma, human albumin (5%)	2–5 ml/kg over 15 min
Ringer's solution	10–20 ml/kg over 15 min
plasma substitute	1–2 ml/kg of Rheomacrodex (10%)

EMERGENCIES

Cardiogenic shock

Definition: reduced cardiac performance with subsequent congestion of the left and right heart resulting in increased preload and systemic hypotension.

Signs:
Compensated: reduced peripheral perfusion (cold limbs, gradient T >10°C); tachycardia, reduced diuresis with high specific gravity; pulse amplitude small, systolic blood pressure normal, central venous pressure ↑, pulmonary capillary wedge pressure ↑, systemic vascular resistance ↑, cardiac output ↓.

Decompensated: pulmonary edema, generally reduced perfusion, hypotension, multiorgan dysfunction.

Treatment:
– increasing contractility, improved perfusion with catecholamines (dobutamine, dopamine)
– decreased preload: nitroglycerine, furosemide
– if clouded consciousness → assisted ventilation
– if pulmonary edema → hemofiltration
– no cardiodepressive medication.
Watch out for inadequate additional volume replacement.

Anaphylactic shock

Signs:
breathlessness from laryngeal edema, bronchospasm, pulmonary edema and/or vascular collapse;
cutaneous reactions: pruritis and urticaria with/without angioedema; nausea, vomiting, diarrhea, abdominal cramps.

Treatment:
– immediate stop to administration of the antigen
– resuscitation if cardiac or respiratory arrest:
  adrenaline 0.001–0.01 mg/kg as a single dose, then infusion with 0.01–0.1 µg/kg/min
  (β receptor stimulation → bronchodilatation)
– oxygen administration, assisted ventilation
– volume replacement
– steroids: prednisolone 1–2 mg/kg every 4–6 hours
– antihistamines: clemastine 0.025–0.05 mg/kg as single dose i.v.
– anticonvulsive treatment with diazepam 0.2–0.5 mg/kg as single dose i.v.

Septic shock

Definition: circulatory failure in sepsis due to Gram-negative or Gram-positive bacteria, viruses or fungi.

Clinically:
in the compensatory phase of septic shock, the cardiac output and the heart rate are raised; because of the reduced vascular resistance, the blood pressure is normal and there is a metabolic acidosis ('hyperdynamic shock'). With increasing failure, circulatory centralization and respiratory failure develop. In the end-stage there is the complete picture of circulatory shock with lowered cardiac output and blood pressure, centralization, clouded consciousness and/or coma ('hypodynamic stage'). However, this applies only to older children – there is no hypodynamic stage in neonates or young infants.

Treatment:
- treatment of the respiratory failure
- antibiotic treatment according to the causative organism, usually in combination with an aminoglycoside
- catecholamines (dobutamine, dopamine)
- volume replacement with fresh frozen plasma
- compensate for the acidosis
- steroids: 20–30 mg/kg triamcinolone or methylprednisolone as a brief infusion (three times at intervals of six hours)
- immunoglobulins.

EMERGENCIES

Pulmonary edema

Etiology:

Left heart failure	e.g. myocarditis, cardiomyopathy
Congenital heart defects	
– with raised pulmonary venous pressure:	hypoplastic left heart, cor triatriatum, mitral stenosis
– with left heart failure:	critical aortic stenosis, aortic coarctation, large arteriovenous fistulae
– with increased pulmonary flow:	ventricular septal defect, patent ductus arteriosus; iatrogenic (aorto–pulmonary) shunts (Waterston shunt)
Severe undernutrition	
Extensive burns	
Nephrosis, protein losing enteropathy	
Airway obstruction	epiglottitis, asthma, bronchiolitis
Pneumonia and other infections	
Goodpasture's syndrome, allergic pneumonia,	lupus erythematosus
Hypervolemia	
Poisoning	barbiturates, narcotics, alcohol, paraquat, adrenaline, hydrocarbons, gases, prussic acid, smoke
Endotoxins	
Neurogenic pulmonary edema with raised intracranial pressure	
Staying at high altitude.	

Pathophysiological components:
  Equilibrium between intravascular and interstitial hydrostatic and colloid-osmotic pressures, vascular permeability and lymphatic drainage.

Signs and symptoms:
  Tachypnea, cough (brownish sputum), dyspnea, chest pain, groaning; pallor or cyanosis;
  fine rales (first auscultatory and radiological signs when amount of extravascular and interstitial fluid has doubled or trebled);
  radiologically: perhaps Kerley A and B lines, low diaphragm (obstruction) (other pathological lung processes can overlay or conceal signs of pulmonary edema).

Principles of treatment

Aim	Measures
Elimination of the hypoxia	Oxygen administration, perhaps mechanical ventilation
Improvement of cardiac performance	Diuretics: furosemide, 1 mg/kg i.v.
Reducing plasma volume	Digitalis, catecholamines
Lowering the after-load	Venous dilatation
Elimination of the hypoalbuminemia	Colloidal solutions
Reducing O_2-consumption	Sedation, analgesia

Status asthmaticus

Status asthmaticus = a very severe asthma attack.
Definition: severe bronchial obstruction, not improved by inhalation of β-adrenergic agents.
Dyspnea, prolonged expiration, tachypnea >50/min, cyanosis, tachycardia >150/min, paradoxical pulse.

Management

A Monitor: heart rate, pulse oxymeter, blood gas analysis, peak flow.

B Treatment
1. Inhalation trial with inhaler (nebulizer):
   Children >18 months: salbutamol, 2.5 mg up to four times per day; may be increased to 5 mg if necessary, but consider medical assessment as alternative therapy may be indicated; clinical efficacy uncertain in children <18 months.
   + ipratropium bromide, 100–500 µg up to three times per day (children 3–14 years)
   +2 ml NaCl (0.9%)
   at intervals of 30 min to 2 h until relieved.

2. → Oxygen administration (with humidifier) initially 30–50%. Indication: O_2 saturation ≤95%.

3. → Parenteral fluid administration:
   in first hour 10–15 ml/kg of half-isotonic solution.
   Maintenance requirement: 50–70 ml/kg/d (ca. 2000–2500 ml/m^2) one-third isotonic
   solution containing: 5% glucose plus 2 mmol/l potassium and 3 mmol/l sodium in 100 ml of the solution.

4. Glucocorticoids:
   methylprednisolone i.v., initially 3 mg/kg, then four times 2 mg/kg/d.

5. Theophylline (in bypass):
   initially 5–6 mg/kg. If previously treated, 3 mg/kg slowly i.v. or by short infusion.
   Maintenance dose: 1 mg/kg/h (children <10 years)
   0.8 mg/kg/h (juveniles) } in bypass with glucose (5%)
   0.7 mg/kg/h (juveniles >15 years)

6. β-adrenergic drugs i.v. if the previous measures produce no improvement.
   Salbutamol initially   1 µg/kg/min
               maintenance: after 10 min   0.2 µg/kg/min
   If ineffective: increase every 20 min by   0.1 µg/kg/min
                   maximum: 50 µg/min
   Alternatively:
   Fenoterol   initially and for maintenance: 2 µg/kg/h

7. Sodium bicarbonate (8.45%) (if pH ≤ 7.3): base excess × kg × 0.3 (diluted 1:1 with distilled water)

C Further diagnostic aids: blood picture, C-reactive protein, electrolytes, chest X-ray.

9. Antibiotics if C-reactive protein >0.5 mg/dl and/or lung infiltrate present.

10. Indication for mechanical ventilation: exhaustion of child, Pa_{O_2} < 60 mmHg Pa_{CO_2} > 65 mmHg

D Further checks: heart rate maximum 200/min
                    O_2 saturation >95%
                    electrolytes (perhaps osmolality) every 8 h
                    fluid balance
                    theophylline serum level (after 2, 4, 8 h).

EMERGENCIES

Diabetic coma
Initial assessment

Criterion	Diabetic coma	Hypo-glycemia	Convul-sions	Intox-ication	Trauma	Shock from other causes	Uremic coma
Onset of clouded consciousness	Slow	Quicker	Sudden	Slow	Rapid	Rapid	Slow
Fetor	Acetone	–	–	?/Alcohol	–	–	Urine
Skin	Dry Red Warm	Moist Pale/red Warm/cold	Moist Pale Cold	~/Moist ~ ~	~ Pale Cold	Moist Pale Warm/cold	Dry Pale Warm
Respiration	Deep	n	Irregular/Slow	~	Irregular Slow	Frequent	Deep
Pulse rate	↑	n	~	~	~	↑	n

~ = variable findings; n = normal.

First measures: check vital functions.
In case of doubt, give glucose, **not insulin**.

Laboratory tests: blood count, erythrocyte sedimentation rate, C-reactive protein, blood sugar, blood gas check, electrolytes, osmolarity, urine.

Diabetic ketoacidosis: blood sugar ↑, pH < 7.25, plasma bicarbonate <20 mmol/l, osmolarity >300 mosm/l.

Treatment:
Fluid substitution: NaCl (0.9%) – no hypotonic solutions.
Quantity: maintenance requirement (see p. 295) + backlog requirement (90–130 ml/kg/d).
Backlog requirement according to degree of dehydration, estimated by weight loss (see p. 295) ~3000 ml/m^2.
Infusion rate: 1. One-third in 4–5 h
2. One-third in 8 h
3. One-third in 10 h.

Normal insulin by infusion pump in bypass.
0.1 IU/kg per hour diluted in 0.9% NaCl plus human albumin (0.5%) (blood sugar falls around 80 mg/dl/h).
NaHCO$_3$ (8.4%) only if pH < 7.15. Dosage: base excess × 0.15 × kg, diluted with four parts distilled water.
Potassium substitution: ca. 30–40 mmol/l infusion quantity as equal parts of KCl and KH$_2$PO$_4$.

Checks: at first, hourly blood sugar, blood gas, serum osmolarity, electrolytes, urine excretion.

Consequences: blood sugar to ca. 250 mg/dl → reduce insulin to 0.05 U/kg/h. With further rapid fall in blood sugar, give isotonic glucose with one-quarter 0.9% NaCl, then give further normal insulin subcutaneously. With a pH of ≥7.30, no further buffering required, but electrolyte check and substitution as needed.
After return of consciousness and normal serum osmolarity, change from parenteral fluid replacement to oral feeding.

MEMORIX PEDIATRICS

Poisoning: common symptoms
Nausea, retching, vomiting, tachypnea, foul-smelling breath, cardiovascular collapse, shock, excitability, confusion, hallucinations, tremor, ataxic choreaform movements, stupor, coma, convulsions.

Directions for treatment of poisoning
- Immediate treatment without loss of time
- Accurate information concerning the substance taken and its toxicity
- Symptomatic treatment in life-threatening conditions before eradicating the poison
- Elimination of the poison
- Specific measures ('antidote therapy')
- Avoid overtreatment.

Possible forms of poison elimination
1. Primary elimination
   - Induction of vomiting
     - mechanical stimulation of the posterior pharyngeal wall
     - ipecacuanha (pediatric emetic mixture)
     - apomorphine
     - avoid hypertonic cooking salt
   - Gastric lavage.

2. Secondary elimination
   - Acceleration of bowel evacuation ('artificial diarrhea')
   - hyperventilation
   - forced diuresis
   - extracorporeal procedures:
     - hemo- or peritoneal dialysis, hemofiltration
     - hemoperfusion
     - plasma separation
     - exchange transfusion.

3. Antidote treatment.

Practical measures for poison elimination

1. Medically-induced vomiting
   Pediatric ipecacuanha emetic mixture (ipecacuanha liquid extract 0.7 ml, hydrochloric acid 0.025 ml, glycerol 1 ml, syrup to 10 ml)

   Dose: 6–18 months   10 ml
           older children   15 ml (30 ml adults)

   Procedure:
   1. The dose is followed by a tumblerful of water, and repeated after 20 min if necessary.
   2. If still no vomiting after a further 30 min → wash out stomach to eliminate the emetic and the toxin.
   3. If necessary, send the vomitus for toxicological investigation.

EMERGENCIES

Contraindications to induction of vomiting:
- infants under nine months
- clouded consciousness
- convulsions
- ingestion of: foam-producing substances
  corrosive substances
  organic solvents.

Side-effects of ipecacuanha syrup:
- persistent vomiting
- diarrhea
- fever
- excitability
- cardiotoxic effect in high doses: arrhythmias.

Technique of gastric lavage

1. Insert an intravenous line.
2. Intubate and ventilate if necessary.
3. Place patient on the left side with the head lowered by 15°, or in prone position with the head low and turned to the side (watch out for malposition of the endotracheal tube).
4. Give atropine 0.01–0.025 mg/kg i.v. (at least 0.01 mg).
5. Push rubber wedge between the teeth.
6. Lubricate and insert stomach tube (size = age-related) perorally.
   Length of tube: distance from nostrils to the xiphoid + 10 cm.
7. Check position of tube by air insufflation. pH measurement of aspirate.
8. Empty the stomach as completely as possible by aspiration and retain contents.
9. Wash out stomach with lukewarm water or NaCl solution (0.9%) until the emergent solution is clear.
   Washout quantity: 5–10 ml/kg
10. Before removing the stomach tube instill a specific antidote or
    0.5–1.0 g/kg charcoal preparation
    0.5 g/kg Glauber's salt (sodium sulfate Na_2SO_4) as laxative
    3 ml/kg of paraffin oil if ingestion of organic solvents
11. Clamp or pinch off stomach tube, before removing it, to prevent aspiration.

Contraindications to gastric lavage

Lavage after a previous intubation only if:
- disorder of consciousness
- respiratory failure.

Ingestion of mineral products.
Ingestion of organic solvents.
Parenterally administered substances.

Complications of gastric lavage

- aspiration, aspiration pneumonia
- esophageal injury
- laryngospasm.

Antidotes to poisoning and overdosage

Poison	Antidote
Atropine, antihistamines, anticholinergics	Physostigmine, 0.02–0.06 mg/kg **slowly** i.v.
Ethylene glycol	Ethanol, 0.7 g/kg as loading dose, then 125 mg/kg/h as maintenance dose (infusion rate adapted to the desired serum level of 100 mg/100 ml)
Benzodiazepines	Flumazenil 0.005–0.02 mg/kg i.v.
Lead	EDTA,* up to 40 mg/kg twice daily
β-blockers	Glucagon, 0.05 mg/kg as a bolus, then 0.005–0.01 mg/kg/h by infusion Dopamine or adrenaline by infusion given according to effect
Digoxin	Digitalis Fab fragment antibodies
Iron	Desferrioxamine orally; i.v. 20 mg/kg then 15 mg/kg/h, maximum 80 mg/kg per day
Isoniazid	Pyridoxine (vitamin B_6); dose: 20 mg/100 mg isonicotinic acid hydrozide
Carbon monoxide	Oxygen
Amanita mushroom	No specific antidote
Coumarin	Vitamin K_1, 0.3 mg/kg i.v., i.m, or orally
Methanol	Ethanol (for dosage see ethylene glycol)
Methemoglobinemia (nitrite)	Methylene blue, 0.2 ml/kg in a 1% solution Thionine: infants, 3 mg; young children, 7 mg
Opiates, opioids	Naloxone, 0.01 mg/kg i.v. or i.m.
Organic phosphate	Atropine, 1–2 mg (<2 years 0.05–0.1 mg/kg) i.m. or i.v., repeated every 10–15 min until the atropine effect is recognizable
Paracetamol	Acetylcysteine, initially 150 mg/kg diluted in 2–3 ml/kg glucose (5%) as short infusion over 15 min; then 50 mg/kg in glucose (5%) over 4 h; then 100 mg/kg in glucose (5%) over a further 16 h

* EDTA = ethylenediaminetetraacetic acid.

EMERGENCIES

Poison	Antidote
Cyanide	Sodium nitrite and sodium thiosulphate; dosage dependent on the hemoglobin level; overdosage can cause fatal methemoglobinemia

Hemoglobin (g)	Initial dose of 3% Na nitrite (ml/kg i.v.)	Initial dose of Na thiosulfate (25%) (ml/kg i.v.)
8	0.22	1.10
10	0.27	1.35
12	0.33	1.65
14	0.39	1.95

Poisons information services in the UK and the Republic of Ireland

Belfast	01232-240503
Birmingham	0121-507 5588/9
Cardiff	01222-709901
Dublin	Dublin 837 9964/9966
Edinburgh	0131-229 2477
Leeds	0113-243 0715 or 0113-292 3547
London	0171-635 9191 or 0171-955 5095
Newcastle	0191-232 5131

These centers provide information on poisoning, and some also advise on laboratory analytical services, which may be of help in the diagnosis and management of some cases.

MEMORIX PEDIATRICS

Reye's syndrome

The cause of Reye's syndrome is unknown.

Clinical features	Additional findings (according to CDC case definition 1980)	Differential diagnosis (exclude an etiologic explanation for hepato- and/or encephalopathy (Reye-simulating diseases))
Preceding virus infection ('trigger')	Serum levels three times > normal for enzymes SGPT/SGOT or ammonia	Acute liver failure caused by hepatitis, medication. (salicylates, valproate, Tuberculostatics, monoamine oxidase inhibitors)
Aspirin intake (additional risk)	Increased liver fat (biopsy)	Endotoxic shock Toxins (aflatoxin, etc.)
Acute onset with profuse vomiting, clouded consciousness → coma	Exclude other causes of hepato- and/or encephalopathies	Congenital enzyme defects: of the urea cycle, of fatty acid oxidation, hyperammonemia Hyperlysinemia, Organic acidemias (proprionic-, methylmalonic acid), of gluconeogenesis, of the respiratory chain

Treatment:

1. General aims
   - Exact restoration of fluid and electrolyte balance
   - O_2 saturation ≥95%
   - Mechanical ventilation if consciousness clouded
   - Stable peripheral perfusion
   - Temperature homeostasis
   - Prevent infection

2. Specific measures
   - Correct any hypoglycemia
   - Reduce plasma ammonia concentration
     - Stop protein intake
     - Prevent catabolism
       Glucose infusion (6–8 mg/kg/min) with blood sugar check, give insulin if required
       → Plasma lactate measurement; if raised, no glucose but:
     - Reduce ammonia with hemo- or peritoneal dialysis
     - Metabolic alkalosis with L-arginine-HCl (first 2 h ca. 2 mmol/kg, then 2 mmol/kg/d)
     - Intestinal sterilization
   - Anticonvulsives: phenobarbitone (maximum 50 mg/kg); if required, additional phenytoin (4–8 mg/kg)
   - Hemostasis: fresh frozen plasma 5–10 ml/kg, 5 mg Vit K_1 replacement

SGPT = serum glutamic-pyruvic transaminase; SGOT = serum glutamic oxaloacetic transaminase.

EMERGENCIES

Acute renal failure (ARF)

Definition
Acute reduction in renal function with a rise in urea and creatinine concentration in serum. Oliguria or anuria are usually, but not necessarily, present; polyuria can also be present.

Definition of oliguria: urine excretion ≤ 300 ml/m^2 daily, or 0.5–1 ml/kg/h

Etiology
1. Prerenal (inadequate renal perfusion)
   (a) Absolute and relative volume deficiency:
       dehydration, hemorrhage, fluid loss into 'third compartment', shock
   (b) Reduced cardiac output, cardiac failure, pericardial tamponade
   (c) Occlusion of the renal arteries: embolism, aortic thrombosis

2. Postrenal (obstructive uropathy)
   (a) Urethral obstruction
   (b) Disorder of bladder function: neurogenic bladder; tumor
   (c) Ureteric obstruction

3. Renal
   (a) Primary parenchymal (vascular and interstitial)
       Glomerulonephritis
       Interstitial nephritis, pyelonephritis
       Hemolytic–uremic syndrome (HUS)
       Renal vein thrombosis
       Systemic disease with renal involvement (e.g. lupus erythematosus)
       Congenital renal disease (polycystic renal degeneration, renal hypoplasia/dysplasia, juvenile nephronophthisis (medullary cystic disease)
       Tumors

   (b) Acute tubular necrosis
       Shock
       Perinatal asphyxia
       Nephrotoxins (drugs, heavy metals)
       Myoglobinuria, hemoglobinuria

Symptoms
Vertigo, nausea, vomiting, diarrhea, fetor, pruritus, apathy, lassitude, seizures, clouded consciousness
Hypervolemia with cardiac failure, pulmonary edema, generalized edema
Hypertension
Oliguria or anuria, but possibly also polyuria

Laboratory findings
Azotemia (urea, serum creatinine ↑; serum creatinine rises by 0.5–1.5 mg/dl/d, depending on muscle mass)
Hyperkalemia
Hyponatremia
Metabolic acidosis
Anemia
Hyperphosphatemia, hypocalcemia

MEMORIX PEDIATRICS

Diagnosis

Aim:
- Confirmation of the diagnosis of ARF
- Differentiation between pre-, post- and renal forms
- Differentiation between newly occurring disease and exacerbation of one previously present (progressive disorder? polyuria/polydipsia in the past? rachitic changes?)
- Recognition of acute life-threatening complications requiring immediate treatment

1. History and investigatory findings

2. Laboratory investigations:
   blood count, blood sugar, electrolytes, urea, creatinine, uric acid, phosphates, osmolarity, coagulation, acid–base state, transaminases

   Special investigations:
   blood culture, antistreptolysin titer, C_3/C_4-complement, antinuclear antibodies
   urine: sediment, blood culture, electrolytes, urea, creatinine, osmolarity, protein

3. Imaging procedures:
   kidney and bladder sonography i.v. pyelogram and micturition cystourethrogram as required chest X-ray (? pulmonary edema)

Indices for distinguishing prerenal from renal kidney failure

	Prerenal	Renal
Neonates/infants		
U_{Na} (mEq/l)	<30	>50
U_{osm} (mosm/kg H_2O)	>350	<300
$U/P_{osmolality}$	>1.0	<1.0
Renal failure index (RFI)	<2.5	>2.5
FE_{Na} (%)	<2.5	>2.5
Older children		
U_{Na}	<20	>50
U_{osm}	>500	<300
$U/P_{urea/N}$	>8	<3
$U/P_{creatinine}$	>40	<20
$U/P_{osmolality}$	>1.5	<1.5
FE_{Na} (%)	<1	>1
C_{H_2O}	−25 to −180 ml/h/1.73 m^2	−15 to +15 ml/h/1.73 m^2

Formulas:

$$RFI = \frac{U_{Na}}{(U/P)_{creatinine}}$$

$$FE_{Na} = \text{fractionated Na excretion} = \frac{(U/P)_{Na} \times 100}{(U/P)_{creatinine}}$$

EMERGENCIES

C_{H_2O} = free water clearance

$$\text{urine excretion (ml/h)} - \frac{\text{Urine excretion} \times U_{Osm}}{S_{Osm}}$$

General treatment guidelines

1. Restore exact fluid balance, with fluid restriction if necessary
   - daily weight check (in the normovolemic patient, body weight ideally remains constant or falls by 1%/day)
   - equalization of fluid balance
     insensible perspiration 10–20 ml/kg
     fever >38°C increases daily water loss by 10 ml/kg per 1°C above 38°C or 100 ml/m² per 1°C

2. Enhancement of diuresis
   - dopamine, 2–3 µg/kg per min
   - diuretics: furosemide 1–2 mg/kg (to a maximum 4 mg per single dose) i.v.

3. Adequate calorie intake
   Desirable calorie amount: 100–120 mcal/kg/d or 1200–1500 kcal/m²/d
   carbohydrate: 3–10 g/kg/d
   amino acids: 0.5–1 g/kg/d
   fat: 0.5–1 g/kg/d
   Because of the fluid restriction, high percentage glucose solution will usually have to be given.

4. Dosage is adjusted according to the drug treatment

5. Treatment of complications

6. Kidney substitution by peritoneal or hemodialysis, hemofiltration
   Indications for dialysis:
   - hyperhydration with persistent hypertension and cardiac failure
   - urea/nitrogen >100 mg/dl
   - hyperkalemia with K^+ > 7 mEq/l
   - uncorrectable metabolic acidosis
   - uremic encephalopathy or pericarditis
   - severe hypo- or hypernatremia

Treatment guidelines for fluid administration

1. In prerenal renal failure (renal hypoperfusion) with oliguria
   - correct hypovolemia caused by dehydration and other volume loss (e.g. hemorrhage) or shock by adequate fluid volume administration:
     depending on the type of loss, colloidal or crystalloid solutions (e.g. 20 ml/kg/h of half-isotonic NaCl solution) until adequate urine production is achieved and shock status is corrected (watch out for cardiogenic shock)
   - insert an indwelling bladder catheter
   - if urine production remains inadequate give furosemide 2(–4) mg/kg/dose
   - compensate for hyponatremia with isotonic NaCl solution or, if there is metabolic acidosis, with sodium bicarbonate

If these procedures are unsuccessful, three possibilities should be considered:
   (a) the volume loss has been underestimated
   (b) there is an obstructive uropathy
   (c) the prerenal renal failure has already led to renal failure

MEMORIX PEDIATRICS

Note: in anuria or oliguria volume replacement treatment should only be carried out with the utmost care and under constant monitoring of vital functions because it carries the possibility of producing a life-threatening hyperhydration which may require immediate correction (possible dialysis).

2. In normovolemic patients
   - try effect of furosemide
   - exact fluid balance is necessary
     total fluid supply = fluid loss + insensible perspiration

3. In hypervolemic patients
   - hypertension and cardiac failure are usually the dominant features
   - immediate fluid removal by dialysis is usually required
   - in clinically stable patients with mild hypervolemia, an attempt at a more rigorous fluid restriction may be made (not longer than 24 h; watch out for hypercatabolism)

Treatment of complications of ARF

1. Hyperkalemia
   (a) calcium gluconate (10%), 0.5 ml/kg i.v. (watch out for bradycardia)
   (b) compensate for acidosis: 1 meq/kg i.v.
   (c) glucose/insulin supply: 1 IU insulin/3–4 g glucose
   (d) cation exchange: 0.5–1.0 g/kg/d orally or by suppository
       (e.g. polystyrene sulphonate resins; watch out for hypernatremia) 1 g/kg binds about 1 meq of potassium
   (e) dialysis

2. Hyponatremia
   If $Na^+ < 120$ meq/l → cerebral symptoms (encephalopathy, convulsions)
   Correction of Na^+ loss:
     substitution amount (meq) = $(Na_{required} - Na_{actual}) \times 0.3 \times$ body weight
   Correction if excess fluid administration: fluid restriction

3. Metabolic acidosis
   Substitution if $HCO_3^- < 15$ meq/l
     substitution amount (meq) = $(HCO_{3\ required}^- - HCO_{3\ actual}^-) \times 0.3 \times$ body weight, of which half is given in one hour and the rest over around three hours

4. Hyperphosphatemia/hypocalcemia
   Acute correction of the hypocalcemia necessary only with tetany
   Phosphate binders (e.g. aluminium hydroxide, calcium carbonate)
   Reduce phosphate intake

5. Cardiovascular complications
   In pulmonary edema, uncontrollable hypertension, cardiac failure, arrhythmias, pericarditis and pericardial effusion, hemodialysis/hemofiltration is required

6. Cerebral complications
   Anticonvulsive treatment

7. In polyuria, extreme water and electrolyte loss is possible; this requires serum electrolyte checks several times a day

EMERGENCIES

Drug dosages in impaired renal function
(After Trompeter (1987).)

Drug	Elimination/metabolism	Half-life (h) normal/RF	Procedure	GFR (ml/min) >50	GFR (ml/min) 10–50	GFR (ml/min) <10
Antibiotics/antimycotics						
Amikacin	R	2–3/30	D I	60–90 All 12–18 h	30–70 All 12 h	20–30 All 24 h
Gentamicin	R	2/24–48	D I	60–90 All 8–12 h	30–70 All 12 h	20–30 All 24 h
Tobramycin	R	2.5/56	D I	60–90 All 8–12 h	30–70 All 12 h	20–30 All 24 h
Amphotericin B	NR	24/24	I	24 h	24 h	24–36 h
Flucytosine	R	3–6/75–200	I	6 h	12–24 h	24–48 h
Ketoconazole	H	1.5–3.3/1.8	D	None	None	None
Cefazolin	R	1.4–2.2/18–36	I	8 h	12 h	24–48 h
Cefotaxime	R (H)	1/2.6	I	6–8 h	8–12 h	12–24 h
Cefuroxime	R	1.6–2.2/17	I	8–12 h	24–48 h	48–72 h
Ceftazidime	R	1.8/3–5	D I	None 12 h	None 12 h	50 24 h
Chloramphenicol	H (R)	2–4/3–7	D	None	None	None
Erythromycin	H	1.2–2.6/4–6	D	None	None	None
Metronidazole	H (R)	6–14/8–15	I	8 h	8–12 h	12–24 h
Amoxycillin	R (H)	9–2.3/5–20	I	6 h	6–12 h	12–16 h
Ampicillin	R (H)	8–1.5/7–20	I	6 h	6–12 h	12–16 h
Penicillin G	R (H)	0.5/6–20	I	6–8 h	8–12 h	12–16 h
Piperacillin	R (H)	0.8–1.5/3.3–5.1	I	4–6 H	6–8 h	8 h
Vancomycin	R	6–8/200–250	I	24–72 h	72–240 h	240 h
Analgesics/antipyretics						
Paracetamol	H	2/2	I	4 h	6 h	8 h
Acetylsalicylic acid	H (R)	2–19/2–19	I	4 h	4–6 h	Avoid
Morphine	H	2.3/?	D	None	None	None
Sedatives						
Clonazepam	H	18–50/?	D	None	None	None
Diazepam (Valium)	H	20–90/?	D	None	None	None
Midazolam	H	1.5–3/?	D	None	None	None

RF = renal failure; R = renal; D = adaptation by dosage reduction (given as percentage of the normal dose); I = adaptation by varying the dose intervals; NR = not renal; H = hepatic; GFR = glomerular filtration rate.

Drug dosages in imparied renal function (continued)

Drug	Elimination/metabolism	Half-life (h) normal/RF	Procedure	GFR (ml/min) >50	10–50	<10
Cardiovascular drugs/antihypertensives						
Propranolol	H	3.5/2.3	D	None	None	None
Diazoxide	R (H)	17–31/>30	D	None	None	None
Hydralazine	H (NR)	2–4.5/7–16	I	8 h	8 h	8–16 h 12–24 h
Digoxin	R	36–44/80–120	D	100 24 h	25–75 36 h	10–25 48 h
Nifedipine	H	4–5.5/?	D	None	None	None
Verapamil	H	3–7/?	D	None	None	None
Diuretics						
Ethacrynic acid	H (R)	2–4/?	I	6 h	6 h	Avoid
Furosemide	R (H)	5–1.1/2–4	D	None	None	None
Spironolactone	R	10–35/10–35	I	6–12 h	12–24 h	Avoid
Anticoagulants						
Heparin	NR	0.3–2/0.5–3	D	None	None	None
Antiepileptics						
Carbamazepine	H (R)	35/?	D	None	None	75
Ethosuximide	H (R)	55/60	D	None	None	75
Phenytoin	H	24/8	D	None	None	None
Sodium valproate	H	12/10	D	None	None	None
Various						
Tubocurarine	R (H)	Triphasic 0.2; 1.2; 5/ Unchanged	D	None	None	None
Cimetidine	R	1.5–2/3.5	D	100	75	50
			I	6	8	12
Theophylline	H	3–12/?	D	None	None	None
Terbutaline	H (R)	1–1.5/?	D	None	50	Avoid

RF = renal failure; R = renal; D = adaptation by dosage reduction (given as percentage of the normal dose); I = adaptation by varying the dose intervals; NR = not renal; H = hepatic; GFR = glomerular filtration rate.

PEDIATRIC SURGERY/ORTHOPEDICS

Degrees of pain

'Smiley' scale for personal assessment of pain

Degree of pain

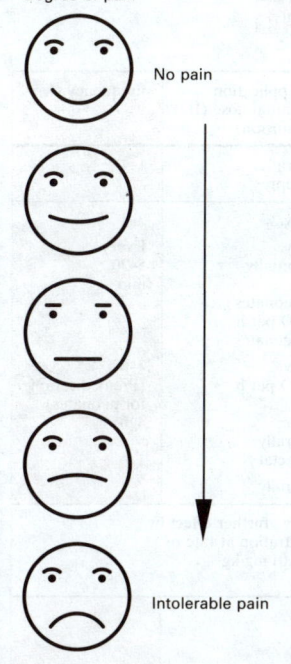

No pain

Intolerable pain

MEMORIX PEDIATRICS

Treatment of pain: WHO step schema for analgesic therapy

		Step 3	Strong opiates + step 1
	Step 2		Weak opiates + step 1
Step 1		Nonopiate analgesic (+ adjuvants)	

Pediatric examples

Step	Drug	Single dose (SD) mg/kg	Application (initial dose (ID) infusion)	Frequency
1	Paracetamol	20 mg/kg then 15 mg/kg/dose	orally, supp.	1–4
2	Buprenorphine	0.005–0.01	i.v.	3–4
	Fentanyl	0.003–0.015	i.v. initially	Every 5–20 min
		0.005–0.0125 0.001–0.003 0.0005–0.002	neonates ID per h neonates	
	Morphine	0.05–0.2 0.006–0.015	i.v. ID per h	4–6 (Premedication for neonates)
		0.15–0.3 0.2–0.6 0.15	s.c. orally rectal	4–6 1
	Pethidine	0.1–1.2	orally	
Antagonist for step 2	Naloxone	0.01 initially	i.v., further effect by titration at rate of 0.01 mg/kg	

Pain + inflammation			
	Acetylsalicylic acid (aspirin)	15–20	orally	4–6
	Diclofenac	0.1–1.5	orally	3
	Ibuprofen	2–10	orally	4
	Indomethacin	0.1–1–2	orally, supp.	3
	Naproxen	5–7.5–10	orally, supp.	2

Supp. = suppository.

PEDIATRIC SURGERY/ORTHOPEDICS

Diagnosis of appendicitis

1. **Spontaneous pain perception:** initially in umbilical region, later → McBurney's point

2. **Provoked pain (principle: passive movement of appendix)**

    Pain on pressure over right flank
    Recoil pain: slow contralateral abdominal wall pressure with sudden release
    Rovsing's sign: compression of descending colon in the left flank → propagation of pain into appendix
    Psoas sign: flex patient's right leg, then suddenly stretch it
    Hopping on right leg
    Chapman's sign: sudden sitting up
    Baldwin's sign: bending forward
    Obturator sign: pain on internal rotation (right leg)
    Ligate test: skin pinching → hyperesthesia in Sherren's triangle (umbilicus–right anterior superior iliac spine–symphysis pubis)

3. **Auscultation in Sherren's triangle:** reduced bowel sounds = positive sign

4. **Sonography:** inflammatory tumor; exclude urinary tract disease

5. **Blood picture:** leukocytosis + shift to left, C-reactive protein elevated

6. **Urine:** exclude urinary tract infection; hematuria if urinary calculus

MEMORIX PEDIATRICS

Differentiation of types of ileus

Criterion	Mechanical ileus		Functional (paralytic) ileus
	Obstructive ileus	Strangulation (volvulus, intussusception, incarceration)	
Onset of symptoms	Gradual	Sudden	Slowly, insidiously
Vomiting	Bilious/fecal, afterwards feeling better	Initially gastric juice, no improvement after vomiting	± Dependent on primary disease
Pain	+	+++	+
Feces	Increasing constipation	± Blood +Mucus	Ø
Abdomen	Distended	Normal (upper ileus) to distended (lower ileus)	Distended
Peristalsis	+++	+++	Ø ('deathly quiet')
Accompanying illness	±	± (Previous operation, hernia, acute enteritis, Henoch–Schönlein purpura)	Infections, hypokalemia, poisoning, drugs (Vinca alkaloids), temporary postoperative ileus, CNS trauma

Diagnosis in suspected ileus

History: Previous operation, chronic constipation, recurrent symptoms

Investigations: Inspection: shape of abdomen, intestinal contraction
Palpation: resistance, rectal tender point
Percussion: tympany, dullness
Auscultation: intensity, character of sounds

Laboratory results: blood picture, C-reactive protein, erythrocyte sedimentation rate, serum electrolytes, amylase, lipase, urine, blood sugar, serum creatinine, coagulation test

Sonography: free fluid, tumor, cysts, signs of intussusception, urinary tract

Radiography: plain X-rays (fluid levels, distribution of gas, 'free air'), excretion urography

PEDIATRIC SURGERY/ORTHOPEDICS

Types of esophageal atresia
Types I–IIIc after Vogt (1929).
Types A–D after Gross (1953).

Frequency: IIIb, 88%; II, 10%; the others ca. 1%. In types I, II, IIIa, abdomen in air-free plain X-rays.

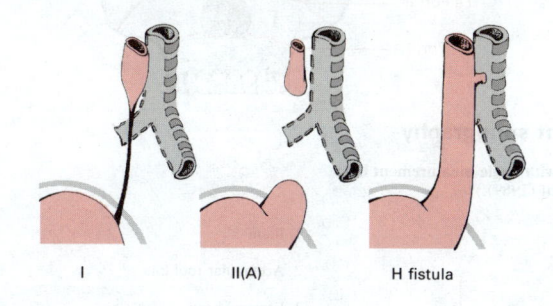

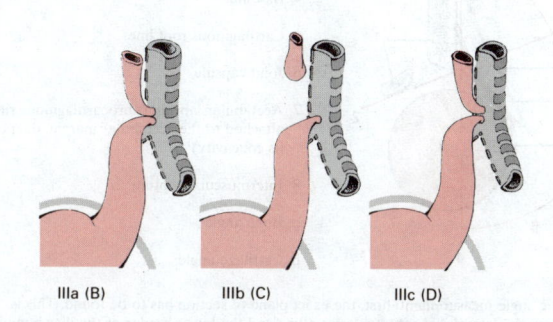

I

II(A)

H fistula

IIIa (B)

IIIb (C)

IIIc (D)

MEMORIX PEDIATRICS

Midfacial fractures (Le Fort's classification)

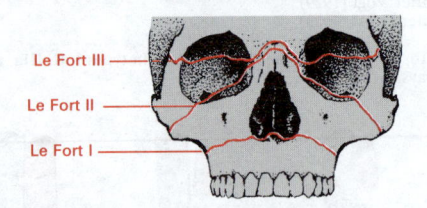

- Le Fort III
- Le Fort II
- Le Fort I

Hip joint sonography

Diagram with angle measurement lines
(After Graf (1989).)

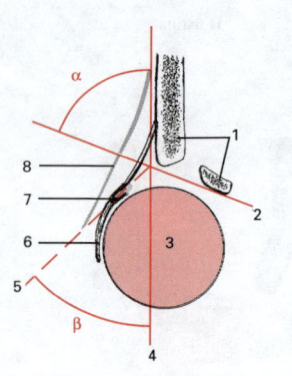

1 Ilium

2 Acetabular roof line

3 Femoral head

4 Base line

5 Cartilaginous roof line

6 Joint capsule

7 Acetabular labrum (fibrocartilaginous rim attached to the acetabular margin, deepening its concavity)

8 Intermuscular septum

α Bone angle

β Cartilage angle

Sonographic angle measurement: first, the exact plane of section has to be found. This is reached when the lateral ilial contour forms a line and the lower border of the iliac bone is clearly seen in the same plane. Measuring procedure: place a ruler on the lower margin of the acetabular fossa and turn it medially until it tangentially touches the echoes from the bony bay = acetabular roof line. The base line is drawn through the base of the cartilaginous acetabular roof to the ilium. If this contact line in the sonogram cannot be clearly defined, a line can be drawn to the medial border of the ilial echo. The base line is obtained by parallel lateral shifting to the proximal contact point of the acetabular roof cartilage with the periosteum of the ilium. The cartilaginous roof line and the acetabular roof line do not aways intersect on the bony bay. The cartilaginous roof line is drawn from the bony bay through the main echo of the acetabular labrum.

PEDIATRIC SURGERY/ORTHOPEDICS

Sonographic determination of maturation of the hip joint

(After Graf (1989).)

Classification	Descriptive findings			Angle		Consequence
Type	Bony structure	Bony bay	Cartilaginous bay	α	β	
Ia	Good	Angular	Wide overlap (pointed)	>60°	<55°	None, mature joint at any age
Ib	Good	Mostly curved	Short overlap	>60°	>55°	None
IIa (+) Physiological retardation of ossification	Adequate	Round	Overlap	50°–59°	>55°	Check only
IIa (–) As IIa (+) can last up to 3 months	Defective	Round	Overlap	50°–59°	>55°	Treatment by straddling or spreading apart, regular check
IIb Retardation of ossification	Defective	Round	Overlap	50°–59°	>55°	Straddling treatment, check
II 'e' or 'c' endangered or critical joint	Defective	Round flat	Still more overlapping	43°–49° (endangered region)	70°–77°	Found at all ages, treat with straddling trousers
D Decentralized joint	High grade defective	Round–flat	Displaced	43°–49°	>77° (Decentralizing region)	Immediate treatment for all ages
IIIa Dislocated joint	Poor	Flat	Displaced cranially; no structural disorder yet	<43°	>77°	Immediate teatment, repositioning
IIIb Dislocated joint	Poor	Flat	Displaced cranially with structural disorder	<43°	>77°	Immediate treatment, reposition with deep head placement
IV	Poor	Flat	Displaced cranially	<43°	>77°	Immediate treatment, repositioning

MEMORIX PEDIATRICS

X-ray diagnosis of the hip joint

Metric lines of the hip joint in the X-ray film

α   Acetabular roof angle.
cCD   Femoral neck shaft angle.
CE   Wiberg's 'CE' angle (center → end of the roof); measure for the lateral roofing of the femoral head. Measurement (after Wiberg): angle between perpendicular on to the femoral head center and the tangent from this center to the lateral margin of the acetabulum. Scoles' measurement: in children up to 2 years, the center of the epiphyseal nucleus is used as the point of intersection instead of the center of the femoral head.
Hi   Hilgenreiner's line (line connecting the Y-grooves).
H_1/D_1 Distance from midmetaphysis to Hilgenreiner line/sacrum (Yamamuro–Chene). Pathological if: ♀ > 12 mm, ♂ > 13 mm.
D_2 Distance from the top of the medial femoral neck to the sacrum (Erlacher). Pathological if: >7.5 mm.
H_3 Diaphyseal height = distance from the upper metaphyseal pole to the Hilgenreiner line. Pathological if <6 mm.

Normal measurements of the acetabular angle
(After Petterson and Ringertz (1991).)

Age (months)	Girls (degrees) Right	Girls (degrees) Left	Boys (degrees) Right	Boys (degrees) Left
0	18.3–38.1	19.5–39.8	16.0–33.4	17.6–35.4
1	16.9–35.9	18.0–37.7	14.6–31.9	16.3–33.8
2	16.3–35.0	17.4–36.8	14.0–31.2	15.8–33.1
3	15.8–34.4	16.9–30.7	13.6–30.7	15.4–32.6
4	15.4–33.8	16.5–35.6	13.2–30.3	15.0–32.2
5	15.0–33.3	16.2–35.1	12.9–30.0	14.7–31.8
6	14.7–32.8	15.8–34.6	12.6–29.6	14.4–31.5
7	14.4–32.4	15.5–34.2	12.3–29.3	14.2–31.1
8	14.2–32.0	15.3–33.8	12.0–29.1	13.9–30.8
9	13.9–31.6	15.0–33.5	11.8–28.8	13.7–30.6
10	13.7–31.2	14.8–33.1	11.6–28.5	13.5–30.3
11	13.5–30.9	14.5–32.8	11.3–28.3	13.3–30.1
12	13.2–30.6	14.3–32.5	11.1–28.1	13.1–29.8
18	12.1–28.9	13.1–30.8	10.0–26.9	12.1–28.6
24	11.1–27.5	12.1–29.5	9.1–25.9	11.2–27.5
30	10.3–26.2	11.3–28.2	8.3–25.0	10.5–26.6
36	9.5–25.1	10.5–27.1	7.6–24.2	9.8–25.7
42	8.8–24.0	9.8–26.1	6.9–23.4	9.2–24.9
48	8.1–23.0	9.1–25.2	6.3–22.8	8.6–24.2
54	7.5–22.1	8.5–24.3	5.7–22.1	8.0–23.5
60	6.9–21.3	7.9–23.4	5.1–21.5	7.5–22.9
66	6.4–20.4	7.3–22.6	4.6–20.9	7.0–22.3
72	5.8–19.7	6.7–21.9	4.1–20.4	6.5–21.7

PEDIATRIC SURGERY/ORTHOPEDICS

Diagnosis: hip joint dysplasia/pes adductus

Degrees of dislocation of the hip joint

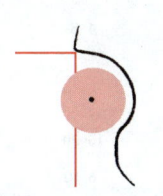

Grade 1
Head nucleus medial to Ombrédanne–Perkins line (vertical line through the acetabular roof bay)

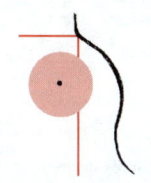

Grade 2
Head nucleus lateral to Ombrédanne–Perkins line and below acetabular roof bay

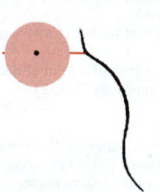

Grade 3
Head nucleus at the level of the acetabular roof bay

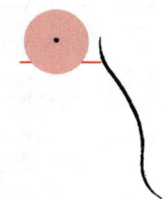

Grade 4
Head nucleus clearly above acetabular roof bay

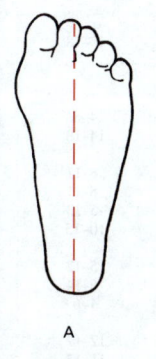

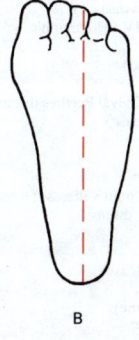

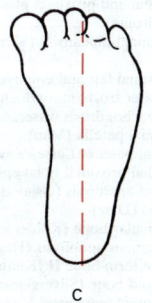

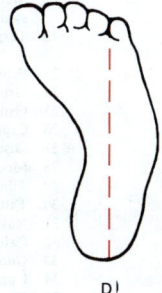

Degrees of pes adductus: Lay the child on its back. Imagine a perpendicular line through the middle of the heel. Normally this passes through the lateral side of the second toe (A); (B) = mild grade pes adductus; C = medium grade; D = marked sickle foot.

MEMORIX PEDIATRICS

Aseptic osteochondronecrosis

		Site	Age of manifestation (years)
Spinal column:	1	Vertebral epiphysis, vertebral apophysis (Scheuermann's disease)	10–16
	2	Vertebral bodies (Calvé's disease)	4–8
Thorax:	3	Sternoclavicular joint (Friedrich)	
	4	Rib epiphyses (Tietze)	
Pelvis:	5	Ilium	
	6	Anterior superior iliac spine	16–20
	7	Symphysis pubis (Pierson)	
	8	Ischiopubic synchondrosis (van Neck's disease)	6–10
	9	Ischial tuberosities	
Arms:	10	Proximal humeral epiphysis (Haas)	
	11	Medial lateral humeral condyle (Frölich's syndrome)	
	12	Humeral capitellum (Panner's disease)	5–12
	13	Olecranon	
	14	Head of radius	
	15	Distal ulnar epiphysis (Burns' disease)	
	16	Distal radial epiphysis	
	17	Lunate bone (Kienböck's disease)	
	18	Scaphoid bone (Preiser)	
	19	Triquetrous and pisiform bones	
	20	Metacarpal heads II–V (Mauclaire's disease)	
	21	Medial and proximal phalanges II–IV (Thiemann's syndrome)	15–18
	22	Terminal phalanx V (Kirner–Schmid)	
Legs:	23	Proximal femoral epiphysis (Legg–Calvé–Perthes disease)	4–8
	24	Greater trochanter (Buchman's disease)	14–18
	25	Osteochondrosis dissecans (König)	
	26	Cranial patella (Mau)	8–11
	27	Distal patella (Larsen's syndrome)	8–11
	28	Medial proximal tibial epiphysis (Blount's disease)	5–13
	29	Tibial apophysis (Osgood–Schlatter disease)	10–15
	30	Talus (Diaz)	
	31	Navicular bone (Köhler's disease)	5–12
	32	Calcaneus apophysis (Haglund's disease)	5–14
	33	Cuneiform bone II (Küntscher)	4–6
	34	Cuboid bone (Silverskjöld's syndrome)	
	35	Proximal metatarsal V (Iselin)	12–17
	36	Metatarsals II–IV (Freiberg's disease)	11–17
	37	Sesamoid leg (Wiedhopf–Greifenstein)	

PEDIATRIC SURGERY/ORTHOPEDICS

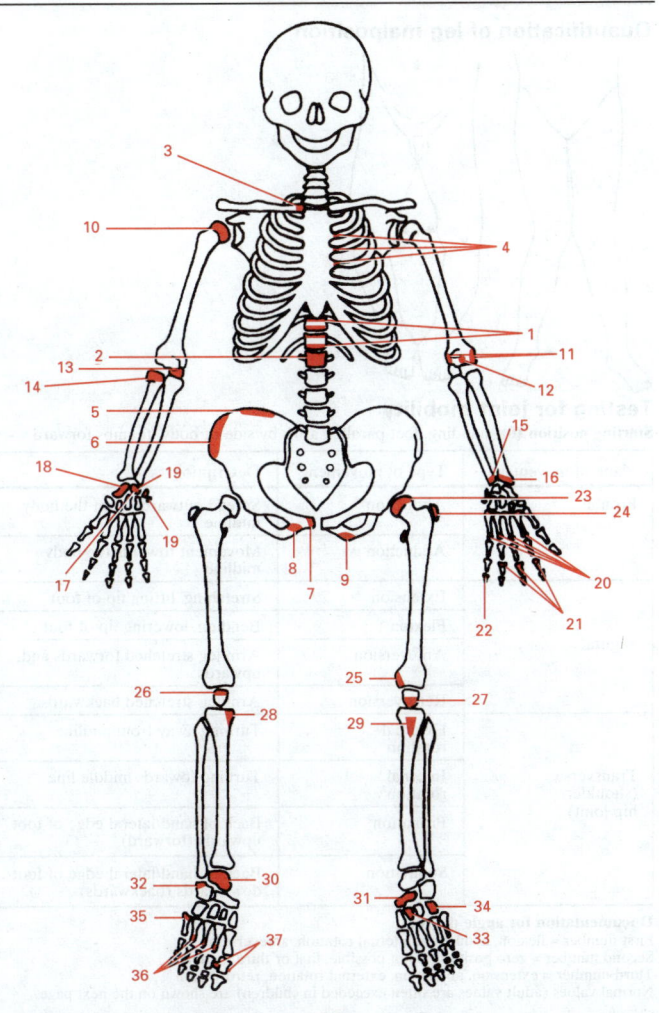

497

MEMORIX PEDIATRICS

Quantification of leg malposition

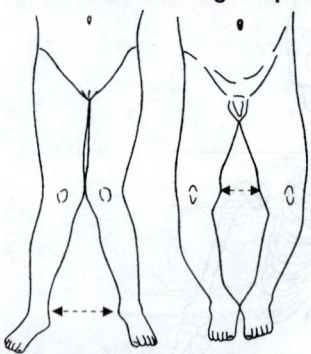

Testing for joint mobility

Starting position (0): standing, feet parallel, arms by side of body, thumbs forward

Plane of movement	Type of movement	Description
Frontal	Abduction	Spread outwards from the body midline
	Adduction	Movement towards the body midline
Sagittal	Extension	Stretching, lifting tip of foot
	Flexion	Bending, lowering tip of foot
	Anteversion	Arm/leg stretched forwards and upwards
	Retroversion	Arm/leg stretched backwards
Transverse (shoulder, hip joint)	External rotation	Turning away from midline
	Internal rotation	Turning towards middle line
	Pronation	Back of hand/lateral edge of foot upwards (forward)
	Supination	Back of hand/lateral edge of foot downwards (backwards)

Documentation for angle degrees:
First number = flexion, adduction, internal rotation, anteversion
Second number = zero position: if not possible, first or third number
Third number = extension, abduction, external rotation, retroversion
Normal values (adult values are often exceeded in children) are shown on the next page

PEDIATRIC SURGERY/ORTHOPEDICS

Neutral-zero method of testing joint mobility

Normal values for shoulder joint
Adduction/abduction 20–40/0/180
Anteversion/retroversion 150–170/0/40

Internal rotation/external rotation
(upper arm adjacent to body) 40–60/0/95
Internal rotation/external rotation
(upper arm abducted 90°) 70/0/70

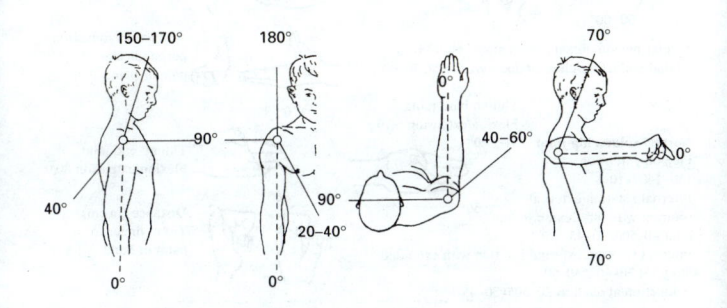

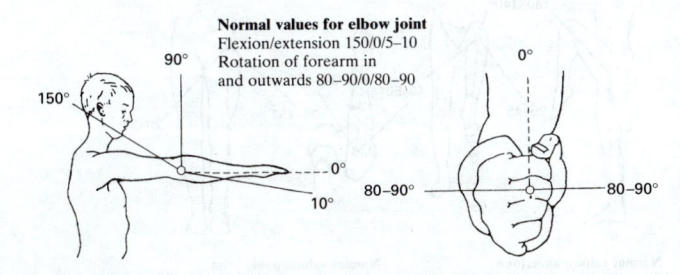

Normal values for elbow joint
Flexion/extension 150/0/5–10
Rotation of forearm in
and outwards 80–90/0/80–90

MEMORIX PEDIATRICS

Normal values: wrist joint

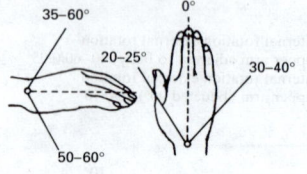

Palmar flexion/dorsal extension 50–60/0/35–60
Radial abduction/ulnar abduction 25–30/0/30–40

Finger 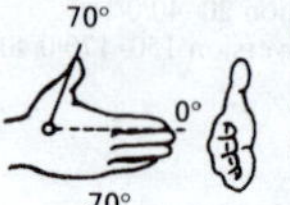
Thumb saddle joint
Abduction/adduction in palmar plane 70/0

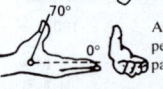

Abduction/adduction perpendicular to palmar plane 70/0

Thumb base joint
Flexion/extension 50/0

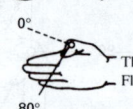

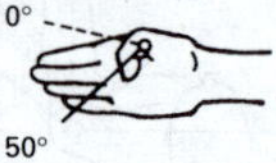

Thumb end joint
Flexion/extension 80/0

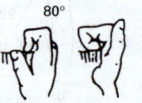

Distance (in cm)
Tip of finger to palm of hand

Normal values: hip joint
Flexion/extension 130–140/0/10
Internal rotation/external rotation with 90° flexion in hip joint 40–50/0/30–45
Internal rotation/external rotation with extended hip joint 30–40/0/40–50
Adduction/abduction 20–30/0/30–45

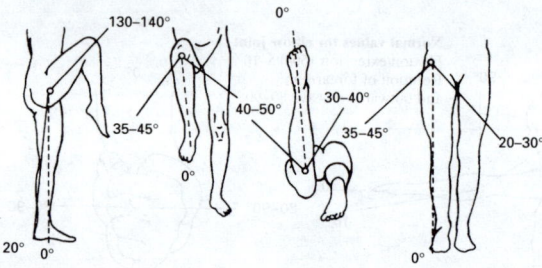

Normal values: knee joint
Flexion/extension 120–150/0/5–10

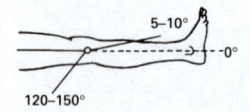

Normal values: ankle joint
Plantar flexion/dorsal extension 40–50/0/20–30
Pronation/supination (calcaneus fixed) 15/0/35
Eversion/inversion (total) 30/0/60

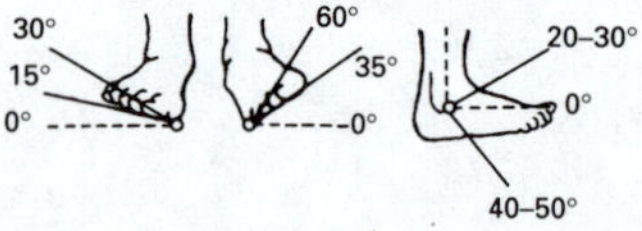

OPHTHALMOLOGY/OTOLOGY

Measurement of visual acuity

This is carried out using special visual charts as a preliminary test.

$$\text{Visual acuity} = \frac{\text{actual distance (m)}}{\text{normal distance (m)}}$$

(m = meters)

Normal function of the ocular muscles

	Right		Straight ahead		Left	
Upwards	Inferior oblique muscle	Superior rectus muscle	Superior rectus muscle + inferior oblique muscle	Superior rectus muscle + inferior oblique muscle	Superior rectus muscle	Inferior oblique muscle
Horizontal	External rectus muscle	Internal rectus muscle	Orthostatic		Internal rectus muscle	External rectus muscle
Downwards	Superior oblique muscle	Inferior rectus muscle	Inferior rectus muscle + superior oblique muscle	Inferior rectus muscle + superior oblique muscle	Inferior rectus muscle	Superior oblique muscle

Strabismus

Measurement of the angle of squint
Primary squint angle: testing when fixing with the normal eye
Secondary squint angle: testing when fixing with the paretic eye, deviation of the healthy eye in the direction of the paretic muscle
Compensatory positioning of the head to avoid the double image = compulsory turning in the direction of the paretic muscle = looking away from the paretic muscle.

Nystagmus

Definitions
Rhythmical oscillation of the eyeballs which can be either pendular or jerky.

Pendular nystagmus: the speed and amplitude of the oscillations are equal in all directions (always ocular-conditioned)

Jerky nystagmus: a slow movement of the eyes in one direction, followed by a rapid recovery movement in the opposite direction (always defined by the rapid component)

fine   amplitude to 5°
medium   amplitude 5–15°
coarse   amplitude >15°

Degrees of intensity

Grade I   Nystagmus only when looking in the direction of the rapid component

Grade II   Spontaneous occurrence and exacerbation when looking in the direction of the rapid component; disappears when looking in the direction of the slow component

Grade III   Nystagmus also when looking in the direction of the slow component

Latent nystagmus: occurs when one eye is covered

OPHTHALMOLOGY/OTOLOGY

Types of nystagmus

Type (N = nystagmus)	Occurrence	Movement J = jerky nystagmus P = pendular nystagmus
Physiological		
Optokinetic N	e.g. rail travel	J Slow phase in the direction of the fixed image; rapid phase = jerking return of the eye to the new fixation
Labyrinthine–vestibular N	Turntable	J Rapid phase in the direction of turning; after stopping, opposite direction
	Caloric stimulus	J Heat stimulus = to the excited side; cold stimulus = to the opposite side
Pathological		
Labyrinthine–vestibular N	Meningitis, otitis media, tumors, trauma	J Horizontal + rotatory components Labyrinthine stimulation = N → in direction of gaze Labyrinthine defect = N → opposite side
Ocular N	Prenatal CNS damage (optokinetic type), cataract, corneal opacity (absent fixation reflex)	P/J Increases with monocular or intended fixation
Central N	Lesion in pons/cerebellum/medulla oblongata	J horizontal + rotatory when direction of gaze changes
Cerebellar N	Any focal cerebellar damage	J Rapid phase in the direction of gaze; when looking to side of focal damage, N frequency ↓ + N amplitude ↑; opposite results when looking to other side
Vertical N	Damage in the region of the quadrigeminal bodies	
Downbeat N	Damage in the region of the quadrigeminal bodies	Only directed downwards

MEMORIX PEDIATRICS

Types of nystagmus (continued)

Type (N = nystagmus)	Occurrence	Movement J = jerky nystagmus P = pendular nystagmus
Rotatory N	Tumors of the medulla oblongata	Changing direction
Gaze paretic N	At the onset or regression of visual paresis	J N in direction of gaze paralysis
Muscular paretic N	Regression phase of an ocular muscle paresis	J Rapid phase in the direction in which the muscle moved before the paresis
Nodding spasm	Origin unknown	P Horizontal

Diseases associated with congenital cataracts

Primary infections

Rubella
Cytomegalovirus
Varicella
Herpes simplex

Metabolic defects

Galactosemia
Hypoparathyroidism
Pseudohypoparathyroidism
Mannosidosis
Refsum's disease (phytanic acid ↑)
Hyperornithinemia
Mevalonic acidemia
Punctate chondrodysplasia

Hereditary

AD, AR, XR

Syndrome

Numerous + other ocular dysplasias

Chromosomal aberrations

OPHTHALMOLOGY/OTOLOGY

Gaze paresis

Type	Gaze paralysis	Site of damage
Conjugated	Vertical (mostly upwards)	Midbrain
	Horizontal to side of lesion (conjugated deviation to side opposite lesion)	Pontine gaze center
	Horizontal opposite-sided (conjugated deviation to side of lesion)	Cortical gaze center or frontopontine pathway
Dissociated	Convergence paresis	Midbrain (perlia nucleus)
	Divergence paresis	Unknown

Pharmacodynamics of pupil size

Stimulation of pupillary dilator muscle → Mydriasis ← **Inhibition of pupillary sphincter muscle and ciliary muscle**

Sympathomimetics
Phenylephrine
Adrenaline tartrate
and others
Cocaine

Parasympatholytics
Atropine
Homatropine
Scopolamine
Tropicamide
Cyclopentolate

Inhibition of pupillary dilator muscle → Miosis ← **Stimulation of pupillary Sphincter muscle**

Sympatholytics
Ergotamine

Parasympathomimetics
Pilocarpine
Physostigmine

International classification of retinopathy of prematurity (retrolental fibroplasia)

Stage	Characteristics
1	Fine, bright demarcation line between vascularized and still avascular retina. Abnormal vascular branching pattern up to the demarcation line.
2	The demarcation line is a pale red or white border raised above the level of the retina. Isolated vascular tufts (excess angiogenesis) appear on the vascularized side (behind the raised border).
3	Extraretinal fibrovascular proliferation in the area of, or close behind, the raised border. Neovascularization leaves the retina in the direction of the vitreous body. Rough subdivision of stage 3 into mild, moderate or marked according to the extent of fibrovascular proliferation along the raised border.
4a	No partial retinal detachment in the macular region.
4b	Partial retinal detachment including the macula.
5	Total retinal detachment, residual fixation of retina in the region of the optic nerve papilla and ora serrata makes detached retina look like a funnel. Additional description of the funnel width anteriorly (near the lens) and posteriorly.
	Additional findings in stages 1–3, usually in 3:
+	'Plus disease': venous dilatation, arteriolar coiling, increasing opacity of the vitreous body, congestion of the iris vessels and rigidity of pupillary movement.

Classification of the cicatrization stages of retinopathy of prematurity
(After Werry and Honegger (1982).)

Stage	
I	Few peripheral tissue changes without detachment: pale fundus, narrow vessels, irregular pigmentation, temporal peripheral vitreoretinal membrane. Often myopia (>6 diopters). Vision usually normal with correction.
II	Extensive peripheral connective tissue proliferation, localized detachment, traction on the papilla and large vessels, macular heterotopia. Temporal peripheral vitreoretinal membrane, usually no myopia. Vision 0.1–0.5.
III	Extensive peripheral proliferation of scar tissue, retinal traction folds from the papilla to the periphery. Vision 1/35–0.1.
IV	Incomplete retrolental membrane, partially obstructs the optic pupil. Partial detachment of the retina. Vision: hand movements.
V	Total retrolental gray–white membrane with complete retinal detachment. No pupil reflex. Amaurosis or light perception only.

OPHTHALMOLOGY/OTOLOGY

Normal speech development

Age	Speech acquisition	Sequence of phoneme acquisition

3 months	Cooing, pitch modulation	• Rule of maximal contrast:
		  – a closed vowel follows an open one; example: 'i' comes after 'a'
		  – combination of a closed consonant with an open vowel; example: bilabial 'p' plus open 'a' = pa
		  – the oral 'p' is followed by the nasal 'm'
		  – alveolar consonants 't' and 'd' are followed by velar consonants 'k' and 'g'
		• first formation of open syllable consonant – vowel sequences; example: consonant 'm' plus vowel 'a' = ma, or this pattern repeated = mama
		• substitution of already acquired consonants for those not yet mastered; example: tea instead of key

4	Beginning of vocalization	
6	Babbling, sound iteration	
8	Emotionally varied intonation	
10	Playing with sounds, syllables	
12	First words	
15	One-word sentence	
18	Two-word sentence, 20–50 words	
2 years	Enlargement of sentences	
2½	Three to five-word sentences, uses pronouns	
3	Uses plurals, uses colloquialisms	
4	Grammar largely mature	
6	Learns and imitates style of adult speech	

Babble · Phonemes · Syntax · Grammar · Vocabulary

Effect of hearing impairment on speech development
(After Bauer (1982).)

dB \ kHz	0.06	0.12	0.25	0.5	1	2	4	8	16
10	h								
20	'er'		No speech formation necessary						
30	r	Retarded speech acquisition							
40	v								
50	e	Faulty sound production							
60	r				Hearing aid required				
70	l								
80	u						Predominantly auditory		
90	s	No hearing possible							
100	t						Visual speech acquisition		
110									

Frequency

OPHTHALMOLOGY/OTOLOGY

Assessment of the tympanogram

The position of the peak in relation to:

(a) Ordinate: eardrum mobility (compliance)
(b) Abscissa: pressure equalization between the external auditory canal and the middle ear (pressure gradient: 0). With normal eardrum function, the middle ear pressure can thus be estimated indirectly.
Limitation: In infants up to six months the distensibility of the external auditory meatus is too high for measurement.
Interpretation: Only combined with eardrum inspection and hearing test (colloquial talk and/or audiogram).

Absent peak (rounded curve) + low compliance + negative pressure: effusion.

Positive pressure: suspicion of effusion in acute otitis media.

Increased compliance + hearing loss: disconnection of the ossicular chain.

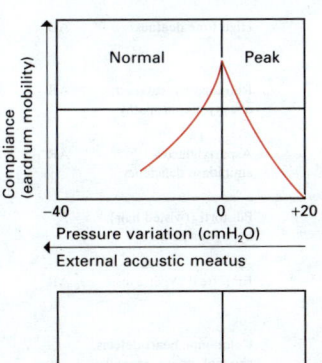

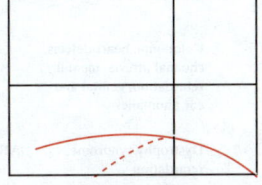

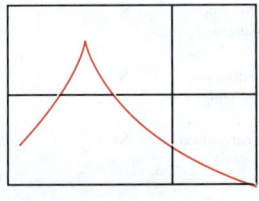

Normal Peak
Compliance (eardrum mobility)
Pressure variation (cmH$_2$O)
External acoustic meatus

Negative pressure
Example: tubal dysfunction

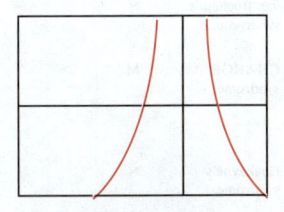

Low compliance
Examples: effusion
perforated eardrum
thickened eardrum
fixation of ossicles
wax ↑

Compliance increased or too high
Examples: slack eardrum
disruption of the ossicular chain

MEMORIX PEDIATRICS

Congenital hearing disorders

Disease or syndrome	Type of hearing disorder (S = sound transmission, N = neurosensory, M = N + S)	Prognosis (C = congenital, P = progressive)	Additional findings, remarks	Mode of inheritance
Achondroplasia	S/N	P	Disproportionate short stature	AD
Albinism–deafness syndrome	N	C	Iris heterochromia	XR
Albinism–deafness syndrome	N	P	Ocular albinism	XR
Albrecht's syndrome	N	P	High tone deafness	AD
Alström's syndrome	N	P	Retinopathy, cataract, obesity, nephropathy	AR
Aspartylglucosaminuria	N	P	Aspartylglucosaminidase deficiency	AR
Björnstad's syndrome	N	C	Pili torti (twisted hair), hypogonadism	?
van Buchem's syndrome	N	P	Endosteal hyperostosis	AR
CHARGE syndrome	M	C	Coloboma, heart defects, choanal atresia, mental retardation, genital and ear anomalies	
Cockayne's syndrome	N	P	Dystrophy syndrome, retardation	AR
DOR (S) syndrome	N	C	Deafness, oncho/osteodystrophy, mental retardation, seizures	AR
Eldridge's syndrome	N	P	Myopia	AR

510

OPHTHALMOLOGY/OTOLOGY

Congenital hearing disorders (continued)

Disease or syndrome	Type of hearing disorder (S = sound transmission, N = neurosensory, M = N + S)	Prognosis (C = congenital, P = progressive)	Additional findings, remarks	Mode of inheritance
Epstein's syndrome	N	C	Macrothrombocytopathy, nephritis	AD
Progressive erythrokeratodermia	M	P	Burns type, (KID syndrome: keratitis, ichthyosis, deafness)	AD
Familial dystonia	N	P	Degeneration, dementia	AR
Flynn–Aird syndrome	N	P	Brain atrophy, myopia, cataract	AD?
Forney's syndrome	S	C	Stapes fixation, mitral insufficiency	AD
Franceschetti's syndrome	S	C	Mandibulofacial dysostosis	AD
Cleft palate	S	P	Associated with other defects	
Goldenhar's syndrome	S	C	Unilateral deafness	AD/AR
Goltz's syndrome	S	C	Multiple ectomesodermal anomalies	XD
Hallgren's syndrome	N	C	Tapetoretinal degeneration	AR
Groll–Hirschowitz syndrome	N	P	Demyelinization of peripheral nervous system, intestinal diverticulitis	AR
Hyperprolinemia I	N	C	Prolinoxidase deficiency, mental retardation, ichthyosis	AD?
Keutel's syndrome	M	C	Brachytelephalangia, peripheral pulmonary stenosis, craniofacial dysmorphism	AR

Congenital hearing disorders (continued)

Disease or syndrome	Type of hearing disorder (S = sound transmission, N = neurosensory, M = N + S)	Prognosis (C = congenital, P = progressive)	Additional findings, remarks	Mode of inheritance
Königsmark–Hollander syndrome	N	C	Atopic dermatitis	AR
Laurence–Moon–Biedl syndrome	N	C	Tapetoretinal degeneration, genital hypoplasia, hexadactyly	AR
LEOPARD syndrome	N	C	Lentigines, ECG changes, ocular hypertelorism, pulmonary stenosis, genital anomalies, retarded growth, deafness	AD
Cleft lip, maxilla, palate	S	P	Sound transmission deafness due to cephalic and facial dysmorphism	
Mannosidosis	N	P	α-Mannosidase deficiency	AR
Marshall's syndrome	N	C	Hypertelorism, saddle nose, cataract, myopia	AD
Möbius' syndrome	M	C	Aplasia or hypoplasia of cranial nerves VI–IX	AD
Mucopolysaccharidosis I	M	P	Hurler's syndrome (α-iduronidase deficiency)	AR
Mucopolysaccharidosis II	M	P	Hunter's syndrome (iduronate sulfatase deficiency)	XR
Mucopolysaccharidosis III	N	P	Sanfilippo's syndrome (4 enzyme defects)	AR
Mucopolysaccharidosis IV	M?	P	Morquio's syndrome (2 enzyme defects)	AR
Mucosulfatidosis	N	P	Neurodegeneration	

OPHTHALMOLOGY/OTOLOGY

Congenital hearing disorders (continued)

Disease or syndrome	Type of hearing disorder (S = sound transmission, N = neurosensory, M = N + S)	Prognosis (C = congenital, P = progressive)	Additional findings, remarks	Mode of inheritance
Nance–Insley syndrome	N/M	C	Otospondylo-megaepiphyseal dysplasia	AR
Nathalie's syndrome	N	C	Oto-oculomusculoskeletal syndrome, cataract, spinal muscle atrophy	AR
Neurofibromatosis	N	P	Acoustic neurinoma	AD
Norrie's syndrome	N	P	Amaurosis, mental retardation	XR
Ear muscle dysplasia	M	P	Mental retardation	AR
Ear auricle dysplasia	S	C	Cryptorchidism, mental retardation	AR
Optic atrophy	N	P	High-grade deafness	AD
Osteogenesis imperfecta I	S/M	P	Deformation of the ossicles	AD
Osteopetrosis	M	P	Albers–Schönberg disease	AR
Otodental dysplasia	N	C	Enlarged molars	AD
Otopalatal-digital syndrome	S	C	See: cleft lip, maxilla, palate	X
Pendred's syndrome	N	C	Hypothyroidism	AR
Pfeiffer's syndrome	S	P	Acrocephalodactyly type V, mild deafness	AD
Photosensitive epilepsy	N	P	Dementia, diabetes mellitus, nephritis	AD?
Polyneuropathic optic atrophy	N	P	Polyneuropathy as in HSMN I (see p. 438)	AR?
Renal tubular acidosis	N	C	Carboanhydrase-B deficiency	AR

Congenital hearing disorders (continued)

Disease or syndrome	Type of hearing disorder (S = sound transmission, N = neurosensory, M = N + S)	Prognosis (C = congenital, P = progressive)	Additional findings, remarks	Mode of inheritance
Renal tubular acidosis	N	P	Hypercalciuria	AD
Richards–Rundle syndrome	N	C	Cerebellar ataxia, mental retardation, hypogonadism	AR
Deafness	M	P	Perilymph pressure ↑, stapes fixation	XR
Deafness (Pfändler type)	N	C	Mental retardation	AR?
Neurosensory deafness	N	C		AR
Neurosensory deafness	N	P	Hair cell degeneration	AR
Stilling–Türk–Duane syndrome	S	C	Eye muscle aplasia	AR
Turner's syndrome	N	C	Short stature, gonadodysgenesis	
Usher's syndrome	N	C,P	Retinitis pigmentosa, retardation	AR
Vitiligo muscle atrophy	N	C	Achalasia	AR?
Vohwinkel's syndrome	N	C	Palmoplantar keratosis	AD
Waardenburg's syndrome	N	C	Ectodermal dysplasia, blue iris, eye-angle dysplasia	AD
Wildervanck's syndrome	M	C	Ear auricle dysplasia, facial asymmetry	XD/AD

CLINICAL PHARMACOLOGY

Drugs during lactation

Properties that facilitate transfer: fat solubility, protein binding ↓, alkalinity (pH of breast milk: 6.8–7.1), molecular weight ↓.

Drug groupings
(Partly after Committee on Drugs, American Academy of Pediatrics (1983) and Bennett (1988).)

Effects on lactation (↑ galactorrhea; ↓ suppression)

Bromocriptine (↓, lactation suppressor), lysuride (↓), methylergometrine (↓), bendrofluazide (↓, diuretic) nicotine (↓).
Neuroleptics (chlorpromazine, methyldopa, metoclopramide, etc.) (↑).

① **Contraindicated during lactation**

Analgesics: indomethacin, metamizol, propyphenazone.
Anesthetics: prilocaine.
Antiarrhythmics: amiodarone, disopyramide, procainamide.
Antibiotics: chloramphenicol, gyrase inhibitors, mefloquine, sulfonamides.
Antidiabetics: oral biguanides and sulfonamide derivatives.
Antihistamines: clemastine.
Antirheumatics: all gold salts.
Antitussives: codeine, pentoxyverine.
β-adrenergics (blockers): acebutolol, atenolol, metoprolol, nadolol, sotalol.
Diuretics: chlorthalidone.
Ergot alkaloids: bromocriptine, ergotamine, methylergometrine.
Thyrostatics: except prophylthiouracil.
Cytostatics: all.
Others: bromides, potassium iodide.

② **Temporarily contraindicated drugs**

Metronizadole (discontinue for 24 h); radiopharmaceuticals, gallium-69 (discontinue for at least two weeks); [125]iodine (discontinue for at least 12 days); [131]iodine (discontinue for two weeks); [99m]technetium (discontinue for three days).

Comparative pharmacological data for glucocorticoids
(After Reinhardt and Griese (1989).)

Corticoid	Clinical equivalent dose (mg)	Relative anti-inflammatory effect	Relative mineral-corticoid effect (Na retention)	Biological half-life (h)	Dose limit/day (excess → suppression of pituitary) (mg)
Cortisol	~30	1	1	8–12	12
Cortisone	25	0.8	0.8	8–12	14
Prednisone	~6	3.5	0.6		
Prednisolone	~6	4	0.6		
6-Methyl-prednisolone	5	5	0	18–36	9
Triamcinolone	5	5	0		
Dexamethasone	1	30	0	36–54	0.6

CLINICAL PHARMACOLOGY

Action of the glucocorticoids

Therapeutically useful action	Indications	Unfavorable side-effects
Anti-inflammatory Antiedematous (endothelial permeability ↓)	Inflammations Cerebral edema Anaphylaxis	Tendency to infection
Catabolic	Suppression of cell-mediated immunity	Gluconeogenesis Growth inhibition Myopathy Increase in lipolysis caused by adrenaline (Triglycerides ↑)
Anabolic (Surfactant synthesis via administration to mother)	Fetal lung maturation	Fat redistribution (Cushing's syndrome)
	Stimulation of toxic/allergic damaged leukopoiesis	
Anticalcemic Renal calcium excretion Intestinal calcium absorption	Hypercalcemia	Negative calcium balance: Osteoporosis
Promotes clotting, inhibits angiogenesis	Simple capillary hemangioma	Thrombosis
		Hypertension
		Acne, skin atrophy, distension striae
		Posterior subcapsular lens opacification, glaucoma
		Mucosal damage: stomach, duodenum (minor)
		Psychosis

517

References

American Academy of Pediatrics (1983) The transfer of drugs and other chemicals into human breast milk. *Pediatrics*, **72**, 375–83.

American Academy of Pediatrics (1992) Statement on cholesterol. *Pediatrics*, **90**, 469–73.

American Heart Association, Council on rheumatic fever and congenital heart disease (1984) *Circulation*, **69**, 204–8.

Apgar, V. (1953) A proposal for a new method of evaluation of the newborn infant. *Anesth. Analg.*, **32**, 260.

Arbeitsgemeinschaft für pädiatrische Endokrinologie (1991) Zur Therapie des Hodenhochstands. Endokrinologie – Informationen No 1.

Arbeitsgemeinschaft für pädiatrische Endokrinologie (1992) Pränatale Diagnostik und Therapie des adrenogenitalen Syndroms mit 21-Hydroxylase-Defekt. *Monatsschr. Kinderheilkd.*, **140**, 661–63.

Arbeitsgemeinschaft für Pädiatrische Nephrologie (APN) (1993) *Eur. J. Pediatr.*, **152**, 357–61.

Arnett, F.C. (1990) *EULAR Bulletin*, **2**, 49–54.

Böhles, H. (1991) Differentialdiagnose der Hypoglykämien im Kindesalter. *Pädiat. Prax.*, **42**, 255–70.

Bachmann, C. (1987) Hyperammonämie: Überlegungen zum diagnostischen und therapeutischen Vorgehen. In *Stoffwechselerkrankungen im Kindesalter* (ed H.J. Böhles), Perimed, Erlangen.

Ball, F. (1990) Untersuchungstechnik und Röntgenanatomie der Thoraxorgane. In *Kinderradiologie 2*. (ed W. Schuster) Springer, Berlin, Heidelberg and New York.

Ballard, J.L., Novak, K. and Driver, M. (1979) A simplified score for assessment of fetal maturation of newly born infants. *J. Pediatr.*, **95**, 769–74.

Barnes, P.D. and Mulkern, R.V. (1992) Physical and biological principles of magnetic resonance imaging. In *MRI in Pediatric Neuroradiology* (eds M.S. Wolpert and P.D. Barnes), Mosby, Baltimore.

Bauer, H. (1982) In Phonoatrie–Pädaudiologie (eds P. Bielsalski and F. Frank) Thieme, Stuttgart.

Bayley, N. and Pinneau, S. (1952) Tables for predicting adult height from skeletal age: revised for use with the Greulich-Pyle hand standards. *J. Pediatr.*, **40**, 423–41.

Bennet, J.M., Catovsky, D. and Daniel, M.T. (1981) French-American-British-Cooperative Group: The morphological classification of the acute leukemias. *Br. J. Hematol.*, **47**, 553–61.

Bennet, J.M., Catovsky, D., Daniel, M.T. and Sultan, C. (1985) Proposed revised criteria for the classification of acute myeloid leukemia. *Ann. Intern. Med.*, **103**, 626–9.

Bennett, P.N. (1988) *Drugs and Human Lactation*. Elsevier, Amsterdam.

Bohnhof, K. (1991) *MR-Tomographie des Skeletts und der peripheren Weichteile*. Springer, Berlin and Heidelberg.

REFERENCES

Bors, E. and Comarr, A.E. (1971) *Neurological Urology*. Karger, Basel.

Brandt, I. (1980) *Der Kinderarzt*, **11**, 43–51.

Brandt, I. (1983) *Griffiths Entwicklungsskalen (GES) zur Beurteilung der Entwicklung in den ersten 2 Lebensjahren*. Beltz Verlag, Weinheim.

Brandt, I. (1983) In *Human Growth. A comprehensive treatise*, 2nd edn, Vol 1, (eds F. Falkner and J.M. Tanner) Plenum Press, New York.

Brandt, I. and Reinken, L. (1988) *Klin. Pädiat.*, **200**, 451–6.

Broedehl, J. (1991) The treatment of minimal change nephrotic syndrome. *Eur. J. Pediatr.*, **150**, 380–7.

Bundesgesundheitsamt (BGA) (1993) Erweiterung der AIDS-Falldefinitionen in Europa. *Bundesgesundheitsblatt*, **8**, 342–44.

Butenandt, I. and Coerdt, I. (1979) *Verbrennungen im Kindesalter*. Enke, Stuttgart.

Centers for Disease Control (1987) Classification system for human immunodeficiency virus (HIV) infection in children 13 years of age. *Morbidity and Mortality Weekly Report*, **36**, 225–30

Chávez la lama, M., Lentze, M.J. and Versmoldt, H.T. (1980) Der Silastic-Katheter nach Shaw zur parenteralen Ernährung des Neugeborenen. *Pädiat. Prax.*, **23**, 205–10.

Chan, J.C.M. (1983) Renal tubular acidosis. *J. Pediatr.*, **102**, 327–40.

Chatburn, R.L. and Lough, M.D. (1990) *Handbook of Respiratory Care*, 2nd edn, Year Book Medical Publishers, Chicago, p. 143.

Crawford, J.D., Terry, M.E. and Rourke, M. (1950) Simplification of drug dosage calculation by application of the surface area principle. *Pediatrics*, **5**, 783–9.

Dörner, K. (1990) Ausgewählte allgemeine Referenzwerte. In: Pädiatrie in Praxis und Klinik, 2nd edn, Volume 4 (eds K.-D. Bachmann, H. Ewerbeck, E. Kleihauer, E. Rossi and G. Stalder), Fischer-Thieme, Stuttgart.

Dinkel, E., Ertel, M., Dittrich, M., Peter, H., Berres, M. and Schulte-Wissermann, H. (1985) Kidney size in childhood. Sonographic growth charts for kidney length and volume. *Pediatr. Radiol.*, **15**, 38–43.

Dittrich, M., Milde, S., Dinkel, E., Baumann, W. and Weitzel, D. (1983) Sonographic biometry of liver and spleen size in childhood. *Pediatr. Radiol.*, **13**, 206–11.

Dost, F.H. (1968) *Klin. Wschr.*, **46**, 503–5.

Droste, C. and von Planta, M. (1989) *Memorix Clinical Medicine*. VCH, Weinheim.

Dubowitz, L.M.S. and Dubowitz, V. (1977) *Gestational Age of the Newborn*. Addison-Wesley Publishing Company, London.

Dummermuth, G. (1965) *Elektroenzephalographie im Kindesalter*. Thieme, Stuttgart, p57.

Dunn, P.M. (1966) *Arch. Dis. Child.*, **41**, 69.

DVV (1986) *Dt. Ärztebl.*, **83**, 3208–9.

Ehrich, J.H.H. *et al.* (1993) Proteinurie und Enzymurie als Leitsymptom renaler und extrarenaler Erkrankuungen im Kindesalter Monatsschr. *Kinderheilkd*, **141**, 59–69.

Empfehlung der Ges. für Pädiatrische Gastroenterologie und Ernährung (1992) *Dt. Ärztebl.*, **89**, 39–45.

Empfehlungen der AG 'Endokarditis'. Paul-Ehrlich-Gesellschaft für Chemotherapie.

Ergäntze Empfehglungen der Arbeitsgemeinschaft 'Meningitis' der Paul-Erhlich-Gesellschaft.

Federation Dentaire Internationale (1971) *Zahnärztliche Weltreform (ZWR)*, **80**, 259.

Finnström, O. (1977) Studies on maturity in newborn infants, IV. *Acta Paediatr. Scand.*, **66**, 601–4.

Flehmig, I. (1971) Statisch-motorische Entwicklung des Säuglings und Kleinkindes. In *Handbuch der Kinderheilkunde*, Vol 1, (eds H. Opitz and F. Schmid) Springer, Berlin, p1 S129.

Foon, K.A. and Todd, R.F. (1986) Immunologic classification of leukemia and lymphoma. *Blood*, **68**, 1–21.

Fox, W.W. (1988) In *Assisted Ventilation of the Neonate* (eds J. Goldsmith and E. Karotkin), W.B. Saunders, Philadelphia.

Garson, A. (1987) Electrocardiography. In *Pediatric Cardiology*, (eds R.H. Anderson, E.A. Shinebourne, F.J. Macartney and M. Tynan) Churchill Livingstone, Edinburgh.

Garson, A., Gillette, P.C. and McNamara, D.G. (1980) *A Guide to Cardiac Dysrhythmias in children*, Grune and Stratton, New York.

Gell, P.G.H. and Coombs, R.R.A. (1963) *Clinical Aspects of Immunology*. Davies, Philadelphia.

Gesellschaft für pädiatrische Gastroenterologie und Ernährung (1992) Orale Rehydratation im Kindesalter. *Dr. Ärztebl.*, **89**, 39–45.

Gillette, P.C. and Garson, A. (1990) *Pediatric Arrhythmias: Electrophysiology and Pacing*, W.B. Saunders, Philadelphia and London.

Girard, J. (1990) Endokrine Labordiagnostik. In *Pädiatrie in Praxis und Klinik*, 2nd edn, Vol III (eds K.-D. Bachmann, H. Ewerbeck, E. Kleihauer, E. Rossi and G. Stalder), Fischer–Thieme, Stuttgart, pp. 495–502.

Graf, R. (1989) *Sonographie der Säuglingshüfte: Bücherei des Orthopäden*. 3rd edn, Vol 42, Enke, Stuttgart.

Gross, R. (1953) *The Surgery of Infancy and Childhood*, W.B. Saunders, Philadelphia.

Gutheil, H. (1989) *Kinder-EKG*, 4th edn, Thieme, Stuttgart.

Gutheil, H. and Singer, H. (1982) *Herzrythmusstörungen im Kindesalter*, Thieme, Stuttgart.

Gutjahr, P. (1987) *Krebs bei Kindern und Jugendlichen*, 2nd edn. Deutscher Ärzteverlag, Cologne.

Harisiadis, L. and Chang, C.H. (1977) Medulloblastoma in children: a correlation of staging with results of treatment. *Int. J. Radiat. Oncol. Biol. Phys.*, **9**, 833–42.

Harnden, D.A. and Klinger, H.P. (1985) *An International System for Human Cytogenetic Nomenclature*. Karger, Basle.

Heinecker, R. (1986) *EKG in Praxis und Klinik*, 12th edn, Thieme, Stuttgart.

Heinze, E. and Holl, R. (1991) Diabetes mellitus. In *Therapie der Krankheiten des Kindesalters*, 4th edn (eds D. Reinhardt, G.-A. Von Harnack), Springer, Berlin, Heidelberg and New York.

Hinrichsen, K.H. (1990) *Humanembryologie*, Springer, Berlin and Heidelberg.

REFERENCES

International League against Epilepsy (1981) *Epilepsia*, **22**, 489–501.

International League against Epilepsy (1985) *Epilepsia*, **26**, 268–78.

International system of radiographic grading of vesicoureteric reflux. (1985) *Pediatr. Radiol.*, **15**, 105–9.

Jüngst, B.-K. (1990) Beurteilung der körperlichen Belastbarkeit. In *Herz-Kreislauf-Erkrankungen im Kindes- und Jugendalter*, (ed H. Gutheil), Thieme, Stuttgart.

Keutel, J. (1979) Echokardiographie im Kindesalter. In *Echokardiographie*, (eds S. Effert, P. Hanrath, and W. Bleifeld), Springer, Berlin.

Klimt, F. and Rutenfranz, J. (1976) Standardisierung von Tests zur Prüfung der orthostatischen Regulationen im Kindes- und Jugendalter. *Cardiology*, **61**, Suppl. 1, 199–212A.

Koch, G. and Wendel, H. (1968) Adjustment of arterial blood gases and acid–base balance in the normal infant during the first week of life. *Biol. Neonate*, **12**, 136.

Largo, R.H. and Prader, A. (1983) Pubertal development in Swiss boys and girls. *Helv. Paediatr. Acta*, **38**, 211 and 229.

Laurent, J.P., Chang, C.H. and Cohen, M.E. (1985) A classification system for primitive neuroectodermal tumors (medulloblastoma) of the posterior fossa. *Cancer*, **56**, 1807–9.

Leiber, B. (1981) *Die klinischen Syndrome*, 6th edn, Urban-Schwarzenberg, Munich.

Leichsenring, M., Bussmann, H. and Bremer, H.J. (1991) *Monatsschr. Kinderheilkd*, **139**, 482–6.

Lindinger, A. (1990). In *Herz-Kreislauf-Erkrankungen im Kindes- und Jugendalter* (ed H. Gutheil), Thieme, Stuttgart.

Lipid Research Clinics Program (1980) *NIH publication no. 80-1527*, National Institutes of Health, Bethesda, MD, USA.

Lubchenco, L.O., Hansman, Ch., Dressler, M. and Boyd, E. (1963) Intrauterine growth as estimated from liveborn birth-weight data of 24–42 weeks of gestation. *Pediatrics*, **32**, 793–800.

Lund, C.C. and Browder, N.C. (1944) The estimation of areas of burns. *Surg. Gynec. Obstetr.*, **79**, 352.

MacDonald et al. (1986) *Semin. Perinatol.*, **10**, 224.

Macpherson, T.A. et al. (1988). In *Neonatal Intensive Care* (ed R.D. Guthrie), Churchill Livingstone, New York.

Melnick, J.L. (1982) Enteroviruses. In *Viral Infections of Humans* (ed A.S. Evans), Plenum, New York.

Michaelis, R. and Krägeloh-Mann, I. and Haas, G. (1989) Beurteilung der motorischen Entwicklung im frühen Kindesalter. In *Normale und gestörte Entwicklung* (eds D. Karch, R. Michaelis, B. Renne-Allhoff and H.G. Schlack), Springer, Heidelberg.

Moore, K.L. and Lütjen-Drecoll, E. (1990) *Embryologie*. Schattauer, Stuttgart.

Moser, H. (1992) *Erbliche neuromuskuläre Erkrankungen beim Kind*, Fischer, Stuttgart.

Nathan, D.G. and Oski, F.A. (1981) *Hematology of Infancy and Childhood. Part II*, 2nd edn., W.B. Saunders, London.

Nora, J.J. (1989) Etiologic aspects of heart diseases. In *Heart Disease in Infants, Children and Adolescents.* 4th edn (eds F.H. Adams, G.C. Emmanoulides and T.A. Riemenschneider), Williams and Wilkins, Baltimore, pp. 15–23.

Osathanondh, V. and Potter, E.L. (1964) Pathogenesis of polycystic kidneys. *Arch. Pathol.*, **77**, 459–512.

Pagtakhan, R.D. and Pasterkamp, H. (1990) Intensive care for respiratory disorders. In *Disorders of the Respiratory Tract in Children*, 5th edn (ed V. Chernick), W.B. Saunders, Philadelphia, p. 207.

Pak, C.Y.C., Nicar, M. and Northcutt, C. (1982) The definition of the mechanism of hypercalcuria is necessary for the treatment of recurrent stone formers. *Contr. Nephrol.*, **33**, 136–51.

Pediatric Brain Tumour Workshop (1985) *Cancer*, **56**, 1869–86.

Perelman (1986) *Semin. Perinatol.*, **10**, 217.

Peters, H., Deeg, K.-H. and Weitzel, D. (1987) *Die Ultraschalluntersuchung des Kindes.* Springer, Berlin and Heidelberg.

Petterson, H. and Ringertz, H. (1991) *Measurements in Pediatric Radiology.* Springer, Berlin, Heidelberg and New York.

Prader, A. (1986) Growth and development. In *Clinical Endocrinology*, 2nd edn (ed. A. Labhart), 1013–59.

Reese, A.B. (1976) *Tumors of the Eye*, Harper and Row, Hagerstown.

Reiber, H. (1980) The discrimination between different blood–CSF barrier dysfunctions and inflammatory reactions of the CNS by a recent evaluation graph for the protein profile of CSF. *J. Neurol.*, **224**, 89–99.

Reinhardt, D. (1991) Therapie des Asthma bronchiale im Kindesalter. *Der Kinderarzt*, **222**, 959.

Reinhardt, D. and Berdel, D. (1990) Asthma bronchiale und obstruktive Bronchitis. In *Therapie der Krankheiten des Kindesalters*, 4th edn (eds D. Reinhardt and G.-A. von Harnack), Springer, Berlin, Heidelberg and New York, p523.

Reinhardt, D. and Griese, M. (1989) Glucocorticoids in childhood. *Ergebnisse Inn. Med. Kinderheilkd*, **58**, 24–54.

Reinken, L. *et al.* (1980) *Klin. pädiat.*, **192**, 25–33.

Rogers, M.C. (1987) *Textbook of Pediatric Intensive Care*, Williams & Wilkins, Baltimore.

Schmid, F. (1973) *Pädiatrische Radiologie*, Vol 1, Springer, Berlin, Heidelberg and New York, p22.

Schöch, G., Chahda, C. and Kersting, M. (1988) Alternative Säuglingsernährung im Vergleich. *Ernährungsumschau*, **35**, 239–44.

Schulte, F.J. (1989) Neurologische Erkrankungen des Neugeborenen. In *Pädiatrie in Praxis und Klinik* (eds K.-DF. Bachmann, H. Ewerbeck, E. Kleihauer, E. Rossi and G. Stalder), 2nd edn, Vol 1, Fischer–Thieme, Stuttgart.

Schumacher, G. and Bühlmeyer, K. (1989) Diagnostik angeborener Herzfehler. In *Beiträge zur Kardiologie*, 2nd edn. Vol 13 (ed K.A. Zölch), Perimed, Erlangen.

REFERENCES

Schumacher, G., Schreiber, R., Niebel, J., Genz, T. and Adam, D. (1989/90) Aktuelle Empfehlungen zur Endokarditis-Prophylaxe bei Kindern mit Herz- und Gefässfehlern. *Pädiat. Prax.*, **39**, 641–6.

Schutgens, R.B.H., Heymann, H.S.A., Wanders, R.J.A., v d Bosch, H and Tager, J.M. (1986) Peroxisomal disorders: a newly recognized group of genetic diseases. *Eur. J. Pediatr.*, **144**, 430–40.

Second Task Force on Blood Pressure Control in Children (1987) *Pediatrics*, **79**, 1–25.

Simon, C. and Stille, W. (1989) *Antibiotika-Therapie*, 7th edn, Schattauer, Stuttgart.

Singer, H. (1988) Das Kind mit angeborenem (operiertem oder nicht operiertem) Herzvitium. *Anaesth. Intensivmed.*, **205**, 362.

Singer, H. (1989) *Herzerkrankungen im Kindes- und Jugendalter*, Perimed, Erlangen.

Sitzmann, F.C. (1976) *Normalwerte*, Marseille, Munich.

Speiss, H. (1987) *Impfkompendium*, Thieme, Stuttgart.

Spranger, J. *et al.* (1982) Errors of morphogenesis: concepts and terms. *J. Pediatr.*, **100**, 160–5.

Stiehm, E.R. and Wara, D.W. (1991) Immunology of HIV. In *Pediatric AIDS* (eds P.A. Pizzo and C.M. Wilfert), Williams and Wilkins, Baltimore.

Stoermer, J. and Heck, W. (1971) *Pädiatrischer EKG–Atlas*, 2nd edn, Thieme, Stuttgart.

Tanner, J.M. (1962) *Growth at Adolescence*, 2nd edn, Blackwell, Oxford.

Teasdale, G., Jennet, B. and Jakobi, G., cited in Yager, J.Y., Johnston, B. and Seshia, S.S. (1990) Coma scales in pediatric practice. *Amer. J. Dis. Child.*, **144**, 1088–91.

Teilweise nach Committee on drugs, American Academy of Pediatrics (1983) *Pediatrics*, **72**, 375–83.

Thoenes, W. (1979) Aktuelle Pathologie der Glomerulonephritis. *Klin. Wochenschr.*, **57**, 799–814.

Thomas, L. (1988) *Labor und Diagnose*, 3rd edn Medizinische Verlagsgesellschaft, Marburg.

Toro-Figueroa, Morriss, F.C. and Levin, D.L. (1990) *Essentials of Pediatric Intensive Care*, Quality Medical Publishing Inc., St Louis.

Trompeter, R.S. (1987) *Pediatr. Nephrol.*, **1**, 183–94.

Union internationale contre le cancer, UICC (1989) *TNM-Atlas*, Springer, Berlin.

Vogt, E.G. (1929) *Amer. J. Roentgenol.*, **22**, 1–163.

Von der Hardt (1989) Asthma bronchiale. In *Pädiatrie in Praxis und Klinik*, 2nd edn, Vol 1 (eds K.D. Bachmann, H. Ewerbeck, E. Kleihauer, E. Rossi and G. Stalder), Fischer–Thieme, Stuttgart, p. 637.

Warner, J.O., Götz, M., Landau, L.I., Levison, H., Milner, A.D., Pedersen, S. and Silverman, M. (1989) Management of asthma: a consensus statement. *Arch. Dis. Childh.*, **64**, 1065–79.

Werry, W. and Honegger, H. (1982) Stadieneinteilung und Seitenvergleich der retrolentalen Fibroplasie. In *Retrolentale Fibroplasie* (eds H. Metze and W.D. Schäfer), Enke, Stuttgart.

Wiegand, R. (1992) Nachwies von Virusinfektionen des Menschen. In *Mikrobiologische Diagnostik* (ed F. Burkhardt) Thieme, Stuttgart, pp. 330–3.

Winkel, K. (1990) *Nuklearmedizin*, 2nd edn, Springer, Heidelberg.

Wiss. Beirat der Bundesärztekammer (1991) Kriterien des Hirntodes. *Dt. Ärzteblatt*, **88**, 2855–60.

World Health Organization (1984) WHO expert commitee on rabies. *WHO Technical Report Series*, **709**, 1–104.

Yared, A., Foose, J. and Ichikawa, J. (1990) Disorders of osmoregulation. In *Pediatric Textbook of Fluids and Electrolytes* (ed I. Ichikawa) Williams and Wilkins, Baltimore.

Zapletal, A., Samanek, P. and Paul, T. (1987) Lung function in children and adolescents. *Progress in respiration research*, Vol **22**, Karger, Basle.

Index

Abdominal cavity puncture 46
Acetazolamide 451
Achrondroplasia 510
Acid–base balance 205
Acid–base disorders 206
Acid–base equilibrium, causes of disorders 207
Acidosis 205
Actinomycin D 392
Acute respiratory failure 458
Acylaminopenicillins 351
Adenoviruses 325
 types 19/37 326
 types 40/41 326
Adrenal cortex, congenital lipoid hyperplasia 265
Adrenocorticotropic hormone (ACTH) test 276
Adrenogenital syndrome 253, 264, 265
β$_2$-Adrenoreceptor stimulants 174
Airway infection, viruses causing 325
Alanine loading test 226
Albinism–deafness syndrome 510
Albrecht's syndrome 510
Alkaloids 393
Alkalosis 205
Alkylating agents 392
Allergic reactions 336
Alström's syndrome 510
Aminobenxylpenicillins 351
Aminoglycosides 350
Amiodarone 133
Anderson's disease 221
Anemia
 diagnosis 356
 Fanconi's 389
 morphological differentation 359
 pathophysiological differentiation 360
Angiosarcoma (neoplastic angioendotheliosis) 384
Anglo-American units conversion to metric system/SI units 20
Anion gap 208
Anti-arrhythmic drugs 132–3
Anti-asthma drugs 174–5
Antibiotics 347–52, 393
 against rarer organisms 349
 treatment 350–2
Antifungal drugs 352
Antihypertensive treatment 149–51
 hypertensive crises 150
 long-term 151
Antimetabolites 391, 393
Antituberculous drugs 352
Antiviral drugs 352
Aortic coarctation 93, 96–7
Aortic regurgitation 98–9
Aortic stenosis 96
Aortic valve stenosis 92
Apgar score 395
Apo-C-II deficiency 237
Apolipoprotein-B deficiency (A-β-lipoproteinemia, Bassen–Kornzweig disease) 238
Apoproteins 234
Appendicitis, diagnosis 489
Arachnoid cyst 385
Arginine–LHRH–TRH test 277
Arterial puncture/catheterization 44
Arthralgia, viruses causing 325

Aseptic osteochondronecrosis 496–7
Asparaginase 393
Aspartylglucosaminuria 510
Asthma 172–3
 drug treatment 173, 174–5
 grading 172
 symptom scores 172
Astrocytoma 380
 anaplastic 380
Astrovirus 326
Ataxia telangiectasia 337
Atrial fibrillation 128
Atrial flutter 128
Atrial septal defect 94, 106–7
Atrioventricular septal defect 110
Automatic blood cell analysis 358

Bacterial cell structure 301
Bacterial microscopy 302–3
 Gram staining 303
 Ziehl–Neelsen staining 303
Bassen–Kornzweig disease (A-β-lipoproteinemia, apolipoprotein-B deficiency 238
Beckwith–Wiedemann syndrome 389
Beclomethasone 175
Benign reversible infantile mitochondrial myopathy 215
Biliary atresia 284
Bilirubin, conversion table 3
Biot's respiration 159
Björnstadt's syndrome 510
Bladder function schema 196

INDEX

Bleomycin 392
Blood, reference values 8–17
Blood gases, normal levels 204
Blood presure 141
  high normal 141
  indirect measurement 141
  Korotkoff sounds 141
  normal 141
  percentiles 142–4
Blood transfusion 362–4
  exchange transfusions 362
  reactions 363–4
Bloom's syndrome 389
Blue rubber nevus syndrome 389
Bombesin 280
Bone-age determination 245
Bornholm's disease, virus causing 327
Bradyarrythmias 129
Brain death 51
Brain tumors 380–7
  choroid plexus 381
  classification 380–6
  ependymal 380
  germ cell 384–5
  glial 380
  glioblastoma 381
  malformation tumors 385
  medullary epithelioma 382
  meningeal sarcomatous 383
  meningioma 383
  mixed glioma 381
  nerve sheath 384
  neuroendocrine 385–6
  neuronal 381
  oligodendroglial 380
  pineal cell 383
  primary malignant lymphoma 384
  primary melanocytic 384
  'primitive' neuroectodermal 382
  vascular tissues 384
  see also specific tumors
Breast development 255
Breast milk, nutrition in prematures 297–8
Breathing rate at rest 158
Bronchial segments 162
Bronchogenic cyst 385
Budesonide 175
Buffering 204
Burkitt's lymphoma 375
Burns 467–8
Busulphan 392

Cabrera circle 117, 118
Calcitonin 241
Calcium loading test 201
Calcium phosphate 43, 244
Calicivirus 326
Carbamazine 450
Cardiac cycle 86
Cardiac failure, treatment 156
Cardiomyopathies 139–40
  idiopathic 140
  primary 139
  secondary 139–40
    dilated forms 139, 140
    hypertrophic forms 139, 140
Cardiomyopathy (histiocytoid cardiomyopathy of infancy) 215
Cardiovascular presures, normal values 87
Cataracts, congenital, associated diseases 504
Catheter sizes 18
Cell–cell interactions 344
Central hyperventilation 171
Cephalosporins 350
Cerebral gigantism 253
Cerebral gliomatosis 381
Cerebrospinal fluid (CSF)
  blood barriers 444
  reference values 8–17

CHARGE syndrome 510
Cheyne–Stokes breathing 159, 171
Chlorambucil 392
Cholecystokinin 280
Cholelithiasis 285
Cholesterol, conversion table 4
Choriocarcinoma 385
Choroid plexus papilloma 381
  anaplastic 381
Chromosomes
  analysis indications 31
  group classification 31
Cisplatin 393
Cleft lip 512
Cleft maxilla 512
Cleft palate 511, 512
Clonazepam 450
Coagulation disorders, differential diagnosis 354
Coagulation system 353
Coarctation syndrome 96
Cockayne's syndrome 510
Colloid cyst 385
Colonic polyposis 388
Common arterial trunk 104–5
Complement activation 341
Complement defects 340
  associated diseases 340
Complete AV canal 94
Computed tomography (CT) 58–64
  characteristics 59
  imaging topography 59–64
    abdominal space-occupying structures 64
    mediastinal space-occupying structures 63
  window technique 58
Congenital hearing disorders 510–14

INDEX

Congenital heart defects
  hemodynamic assessment of operative results 113
  hemodynamic degrees of severity 112
  shunt-dependent 115
Conjunctivitis, viruses causing 326, 327
Consciousness disorders 463–4
  investigations 463, 464
  pupillary reaction 463
Conversion tables 3–4
Copper malabsorption (trichopoliodystrophy, Menkes' syndrome, kinky-hair disease) 215
Cori's disease 221
Coronaviruses 325
Cortisol 516
Cortisone 516
Cowden's disease 388
Coxsackievirus A 326, 327, 328
Coxsackievirus A16 325
Coxsackievirus B 326, 327, 328
Craniopharyngioma 385
Creatine 177
Creatinine, conversion table 3
Crohn's colitis 388
Cryptorchidism 266
Cyanosis, differential diagnosis 161
Cyclophosphamide 392
Cytarabine 393
Cytogenetic nomenclature 34–39
Cytokines 344
Cytomegalovirus 325, 326
Cytostatic agents 391, 392–3

Dacarbazine 392
Daunorubicin 392
Deafness 514
  neurosensory 514
  Pfändler type 514
  see also Congenital hearing disorders
Dehydration 290
Deletion 14 syndrome 390
Dental chart, double-digit 25
Dentition sequence 26
2-Deoxyglucose test 226
Dermoid cyst 385
1,20-Desmolase deficiency 265
Desmopressin (vasopressin) test 278–9
Developmental disorders, morphological terminology 24
Dexamethasone 516
  test 275
Diabetes mellitus 222–30
  blood test 222
  coma 475
  daily energy requirements 226
  tests 226–30
  diagnosis 222–3
  gestational 222
  insulin 223–5
    biphasic 225
    intermediate 224
    long-acting 224
    soluble 224
  insulin-dependent 222
  latent 222
  maturity onset, of the young 222
  non-insulin dependent 222
  pre-diabetes 222
  virus causing 327
  White's classification 222
Diagnostic tests assessment 28
Diarrhea, viruses causing 328
DiGeorge syndrome 337
Digitalis 134
  poisoning 135
  treatment 136–7
Digoxin 133
Dihydrolipolyhydrogenase deficiency 212
Diphtheria immunization 314
Disaccharide loading test 288
Disopyramide 132
DNA
  analysis by blot technique 22–3
  restriction fragment length polymorphism 40
DOR(S) syndrome 510
Down's syndrome 389
Doxorubicin 392
Drug doses in impaired renal function 485–6
Drug overdose antidotes 478
Dwarfism 246
Dysbetalipoproteinemia 237
Dysmaturity, definitions 394

Ear auricle dysplasia 513
Ear muscle dysplasia 513
Early summer meningoencephalitis (ESME) immunization 313, 324
ECHO virus 326, 327, 328
Echocardiogram, M-mode 84
  one-dimensional 85
Eldridge's syndrome 510
Electrocardiogram (ECG) 116–129
  age-dependent normal ranges 119
  Cabrera circle (hexaxial reference system) 117, 118
  cardiac arrythmias, sequence in diagnosis 126
  electrode positions 116

INDEX

electrolyte disorders 138
hypertrophy signs 122–4
  atrial 125
  left-sided 124
  right-sided 123
  normal values for R:S ratio, R and S amplitudes 121
  relative/rate-corrected QT interval 120
  RS patterns of electrical axis positions/derivations 117
Electroencephalogram (EEG) 427–32
  electrode positions 427
  evoked potentials 431
  pathological patterns 430
  pathological variations 429
  sleep stages 428
  visual evoked potential 432
Electrolyte disturbances 138, 202
Electromyography 436
Electrophysiological differences between neuropathies and myopathies 437
Electroretinogram 434
ELISA (enzyme-linked immunosorbent assay) 21
Embryonic carcinoma 385
Embryopathies, viruses causing 325
EMG syndrome 388
Encephalitis, viruses causing 326, 327
Encephalofacial angiomatosis (Sturge–Weber syndrome) 443

Encephalomyopathy of childhood and adolescence (Kearns–Sayre syndrome) 214
Endocarditis prophylaxis 153
  antibacterial doses 154–71
Endodermal sinus tumor 385
Endotracheal aspiration complications 459
Endotracheal intubation complications 459
Energy, conversion table 3
Energy metabolism, congenital defects 212
Enterogenic cyst 385
Enteroglucagon 280
Enteroviruses 325, 326, 327, 328
Enzyme defects 212
Ependymoastrocytoma 381
Ependymoma 380
  anaplastic 380
  myxopapillary 380
Epidemiological definitions 27
Epidermoid cyst 385
Epilepsy 445–51
  absences 445
    atypical 445
  atonic seizures 446
  clonic seizures 445
  complex focal (partial) seizures 445
  febrile convulsions 448
  focal seizures 445
    with subsequent generalization 445
  international classification 446–7
  myoclonic seizures 445
  photosensitive 513
  single focal seizures 445
  status epilepticus 469
  tonic–clonic seizures (grand mal) 446

tonic seizures 445
treatment 449
  antiepileptics 450–1
Epstein–Barr virus 325, 326
Epstein's syndrome 511
Erythrocytes 356–7
  blood smear forms 356
  staining variants 357
Escherichia coli 289
Esophageal atresia types 491
Ethosuximide 450
Etoposide 393
Evoked potentials 431–3
  acoustic 432
  somatosensory 435
  visual 432–3
Exanthemata, viruses causing 325, 328
External cardiac massage 460–1

Fabry's disease 233
Familial dystonia 511
Familiar disposition dermatomyositis 388
Fanconi's anemia 389
Farber's disease (lipogranulomatosis) 24
Fasting test 227
Febrile convulsions 448
Feces, reference values 8–17
Fenoterol 174
Fernandes' disease 221
Fetal infantile encephalomyopathy (progressive infantile poliodystrophy) 214
Fever + influenza, summer flu, viruses causing 327
Fever types 300
Fibrosarcoma 383
Fibroxanthosarcoma 383
Flecainide 132
Fluorouracil 393

528

INDEX

Flynn–Aird syndrome 511
Foot-and-mouth disease, virus causing 328
Forney's syndrome 511
Franceschetti's syndrome 511
Fructose tolerance test 227
Fukuhara's syndrome (MERRF) 514
Fumarase deficiency 212

Galactose stress test 227
Gangliocytoma 381
  anaplastic 381
Ganglioglioma 381
  anaplastic 381
Gardner's syndrome 388
Gasping respiration 159
Gastric inhibitory polypeptide 280
Gastric lavage 477
Gastrin 280
Gastroenteritis, viruses causing 326
Gaucher's disease 233
Gaze paresis 505
Genitalia development (boy) 256
Germinoma 384
Giant cell glioma 380
Glasgow Coma Scale 465
Glioblastoma
  giant cell 381
  multiform 381
  with sarcomatous components 381
Gliofibroma 381
Globoid cell leukodystrophy (Krabbe's disease) 233
Glomerulonephritis 189
Glomerulosclerosis, focal segmental 189
Glucagon test 228
Glucocorticoids 175, 516
  action 517
Glucose
  abnormal tolerance 223
  conversion table 3
  impaired tolerance 222, 223
  requirement 230
Glucose loading test 228
Glucose tolerance test 25–6
Glycerine loading test 230
Glycogen metabolic defects 221
Glycogen storage defects 221
Glycopeptides 350
GM_1-gangliosidosis 233
Goiter stages 270
Goldenhar's syndrome 511
Goltz's syndrome 511
Great vessels, congenital defects 90–1
  recurrence risk 95
Groll–Hirschowitz syndrome 511
Growth 245
  catch-up 245, 253
Growth function tests 271–3
  clonidine test (oral) 272
  HGH secretion profile during sleep 272
  HGH secretion suppression test 273
  hypoglycemia test, insulin-induced 271
Growth hormone deficiency 253
Growth velocity percentiles (boys 0–18 years) 252
Growth velocity percentiles (girls 0–18 years) 250
Growth and weight percentile curves (boys 0–18 years) 251
Growth and weight percentile curves (girls 0–18 years) 248

Hallgen's syndrome 511
Hamartoma 385
  glial 385
  neuronal 385
  neuronoglial 385
Hand radiograph 247
HbA from HbF distinguishing test 407
Head circumference percentile growth curves (boys 0–6 years) 440
Head circumference percentile growth curves (girls 0–6 years) 441
Heart
  ausculation points in congenital heart lesions 89
  congenital defects 90–5
    oxygen saturation 92–5
    pressures 92–5
    recurrence risks 95
  causes of arrhythmias 127
  congenital defects *see* congenital heart defects
  cycle 86
  murmurs 89
  normal rate 88
  pulse types 88
Hemangioblastoma 384
Hemangiopericytoma 384
Hematopoiesis 369
Hematuria 185, 187
Hemoglobin development 361
Hepatitis, viruses causing 326, 327
Hepatitis A
  immunization 313
  serology course 323
Hepatitis A virus 326

INDEX

Hepatitis B 325
  immunization 313, 322
  infectivity assessment by antigen–antibody pattern 323
  prophylaxis 319
  serology course in acute/chronic hepatitis B 322
Hepatitis B virus 323, 325
Hepatitis C virus 326
Hereditary sensorimotor neuropathies 438
Hereditary sensory neuropathies 439
Hermaphrodism, true 261
Herpangioma, virus causing 327
Herpes simplex virus 325, 326
Herpes viruses, classification 324
Hers' disease 221
Hip joint 492–4
  dysplasia 495
  sonography 492–3
  X-ray 494
Histiocytoid cardiomyopathy of infancy (cardiomyopathy) 215
Histiocytoses 367
HIV infection 331–4
  classification 333–4
  immunological findings 331
Hodgkin's disease, stages 376
Human chorionic gonadotrophin test 274
Human herpes virus-6 325, 326
Hunter's disease 231
17-Hydroxylase deficiency 265
3β-Hydroxysteroid-dehydrogenase isomerase deficiency 265

Hyperalphalipoproteinemia 237
Hyperammonemia 216–7
Hyperbilirubinemia 284, 403
Hypercalcemia, ECG 138
Hypercalciuria 201
Hypercholesterolemia 235, 237
  heterozygous 237
  homozygous 237
Hyperkalemia 202
  ECG 138
Hyperparathyroidism 242
Hyperlipoproteinemia, familial 237–8
Hyperprolinemia I 511
Hypertension 46–53
  age-related classificaion 145
  algorithm for diagnosis, children/adolescents 145
  definition 141
  diagnosis 147
  diagnostic investigations 147–8
  treatment see Antihypertensive treatment
  underlying diseases 146
Hyperthyroidism 128
Hypertriglyceridemia 237
Hypetrophic pyloric stenosis 281
Hyperventilation 171
  central 171
Hypoaldosteronism 265
Hypocalcemia, ECG 138
Hypoglycemia 218–20
  diagnostic substances 220
  tests 220
Hypokalemia 203
  ECG 138
Hypoparathyroidism 242
Hypotension, active orthostatic test 152

Hypothyroidism 276–9
  aftercare program in congenital hypothyroidism 269
  causes 267
  screening 268
Hypoventilation 171
Hypopoxemic atack 157
Ifosfamide 392
Ileus 490
Immune defects
  diagnosis 343
  primary 338–9, 342
  secondary 342
Immunization 312–24
  in allergy/suspected allergy combined immunization 321
  incomplete 314
  indications 313
  in pregnancy 315
  rabies 317
  schedule 317
  special indications 316
  travellers 320
Immunodeficiency syndrome, associated diseases 337
Immunoglobulins, biological properties 335
Indigestion (malabsorption) function tests 288
Infant(s), neurological investigation see Neurological investigation, neonates/infants
Infant respiratory distress syndrome 401
Infectious diseases, notification 310–11
Influenza vaccination 313
Influenza virus 325, 326
Infusions, drip speed calculation 19
Insulin–LHRH–TRH test 277
Intestinal innervation 282

INDEX

Intracranial pressure 466–7

Joint mobility testing 498–500
   neutral zone method 499–500
   ankle 500
   elbow 499
   hip 500
   knee 500
   shoulder 499
   wrist 500
Juvenile chronic arthritis 345

Kawasaki's syndrome 330
Kearns–Sayre syndrome (encephalomyopathy of childhood and adolescence) 214
Keratitis, viruses causing 326
Ketoacidosis, diagnosis 211
17-Ketosteroid reductase deficiency 265
Keutel's syndrome 511
Kidney *see* Renal
Kinky-hair disease (trichopoliodystrophy, Menkes' syndrome, copper malabsorption) 215
Klinefelter's disease 389
Königsmark–Hollander syndrome 512
Krabbe's disease (globoid cell leukodystrophy) 233

Lactoacidosis, congenital 209
Lactate dehydrogenase deficiency 212
Lactation, drugs during 515
Leg malposition 498
Laurence–Moon–Biedl syndrome 512

Leigh's disease (subacute necrotizing encephalomyelopathy) 214
LEOPARD syndrome 512
Lesch–Nyhan syndrome 200
Leucine loading test 230
Leukemia 364–7, 389
   acute nonlymphocytic 366–7, 369
   diagnosis 364
   FAB classification 365–7
   phenotypical classification 368
Leukocytes, normal/neoplastic, CD antigens on 370–1
Lewis' disease 221
Lignocaine 132
Lipid(s), normal levels 236
Lipid storage diseases 232–3
Lipogranulomatosis (Farber's disease) 233
Lipoma, cerebral 385
Lipoprotein, serum 234, 236
   normal levels 236
Lipoproteinemia
   A-α- 238
   A-β- (apolipoprotein-β-deficiency, Bassen–Kornzweig disease) 238
   hypo-α- 238
   hypo-β- 238
Lipoprotein lipase deficiency 237
Lomustine 392
Louis–Bar syndrome 389
Lungs
   bronchial segments 162
   development morphology 158
   flow–volume curve 170
   function diagnosis 170
   normal volumes 169

O_2 treatment 169
   parameters of function 168
   dynamic volumes 168
   static volumes 168
   ventilation disorder 171
   X-ray diagnosis 163–6
   lobar atelectasis 164
   pleurisy 164
   pulmonary vessels 165
   thymus hyperplasia 166
Luteinizing hormone releasing hormone test 274
Lymphocytic choriomeningitis virus 326
Lymphocytopoiesis 368
Lymphoma 375, 389
   B cell 375
   non-Hodgkin, stages 376
   primary malignant 384

Macrocephaly 442
Macrolides 350–1
Magnetic resonance imaging 67–69
   indications 68
   interpretations 68
   intracranial 69
   signal intensity of tissues/fluids 67
Malabsorption (indigestion) function tests 288
Malaria, prophylaxis 329
Malignant lymphoma, primary 384
Malignant melanoma 384
Mannosidosis 512
Maroteaux–Lamy disease 231
Marshall's syndrome 512
Masculine differentiation/development disorders 262
McArdle's disease 221

INDEX

Mean target size 245
Measles virus 325, 326
Medulloblastomas 386–7
Medulloepithelioma 382
Megacolon 282
Megaloencephaly 442
Melanocytic tumor 384
Melanoma, malignant 384
Melanomatosis 384
MELAS 214
Melphalan 392
Meningeal sarcoma 383
Meningioma 383
  anaplastic 383
  papillary 383
Meningitis 304–5
  bacterial, treatment 305
  cerebrospinal fluid 304
  serous, viruses causing 327
  viruses causing 326
Meningoangio-neurinomtosis 385
Menkes' syndrome (trichopoliodystrophy, kinky-hair disease, copper malabsorption) 215
Mercaptopurine 393
MERRF (Fukuhara's syndrome) 514
Mesenchymal chondrosarcoma 383
Methotrexate 393
6-Methyl-prednisolone 516
Metyrapone test 276
Metyrapone–TRH–arginine–LHRH test 277
Mexiletine 132
Metabolic acidosis 205, 206, 210
Metabolic alkalosis 205, 206
Metachromatic leukodystrophy 233

Micturition disorders 198
  neurogenic 198
  pharmacological treatment 197
Midfacial fracture 492
Milk feeds, ready-made 296
Miller's syndrome 389
Mitochondrial respiratory chain enzyme complex 203
Mitoxantrone 393
Mitral stenosis 100–1
Mitral valve prolapse 127
Mixed germ cell tumors 385
MMN syndrome 388
Mobius' syndrome 512
Morquio's disease 231
Motilin 280
Motor development 424–6
  erect gait 424–5
  grasp 426
  milestones 423
  timetable 414
Mucopolysaccharidoses 231, 512
Mucosulfatidosis 512
Mucoviscidosis disease 283
Multiple exostoses 389
Mumps virus 326
Myasthenia gravis 437
Mycocarditis, viruses causing 326, 327
Myopathy 215

Nance–Insley syndrome 513
Nasogastric tube 287
Nathalie's syndrome 513
Neonates
  antibiotics for 413
  assessment of fetal maturity 396
  drug doses 412
  endotracheal tubes 406
  feeding tube 407
  Finnström method of calculating fetal maturity 399
  jaundice, differential diagnosis 402
  laryngoscope 406
  mask 406
  neurological investigation *see* neurological investigation, neonates/infants
  neuromuscular signs of maturity 397, 398
  seizures 408
  ventilation 457
  viral infection 325
Neoplastic angioendotheliosis (angiosarcoma) 384
Nephritic syndrome 188
Nephroblastoma *see* Wilm's tumor
Nephrotic syndrome 190
  causes 191
  'minimal change' 189
  treatment 192–3
Neurilemmoma 384
  anaplastic 384
Neuroblastoma 377–8
  classification 372
  stages 377
Neurocutaneous melanosis 390
Neurofibroma 384
  anaplastic 384
Neurofibromatosis 443, 513
Neurological investigation, neonates/infants 415–22
  abdominal skin reflex 416
  Achilles' tendon reflex 422
  anal reflex 416
  asymmetrical tonic neck reflex 419
  automatic reaction 415
  axillary suspension reaction 420
  Babinski's sign 418
  Bauer reaction 418

INDEX

biceps tendon reflex 422
blink reflex 417
body position to head reflex 420
checking head control 418
Chvostek's sign 417
Collis reactions (horizontal, vertical) 421
corneal reflex 417
cremasteric reflex 416
doll's eye test 417
foot clonus 418
Galant's (infantile) reflex 416
glabella reflex 416
grasping reflex 418
head-hanging reaction (Peiper–Isbert reflex) 420
labyrinth positions reflex 420
Landau reaction 421
lip reflex 415
magnet reflex 418
Moro reflex 419
neck position reflex 420
oblique position reaction 421
oral sucking reflex 416
patella tendon reflex 422
placing reaction 419
recoil of arms 417
ready to jump 422
rotation test 417
side tilting reaction 421
step reaction 419
sucking reflex 416
symmetrical tonic neck reflex 419
tonic labyrinth reflex 415
traction reaction 420
Neurotensin 280
Niemann–Pick disease 233
Non-Hodgkin's lymphoma 376

Norris' syndrome 513
Norwalk virus 326
Nuclear medicine diagnosis 65–6
Nutrition 293–9
 first year of life 293
 nutritional energy 294
 parenteral 295
 special, in metabolic defects 299
 vitamin requirements 296
Nystagmus 502–4

O_2 saturation, normal values 87
Ocular muscles, normal function 501
Oldfield's syndrome 388
Oligoastrocytoma 381
Oligoastroependymoma 381
Oligodendroglioma 380
 anaplastic 380
Oligoependymoma 381
Ollier's disease 389
Optic atrophy 513
 polyneuropathic 513
Organ development, sensitive periods 41
Orogastric tube 287
Osteogenesis imperfecta I 513
Osteopetrosis 513
Otodental dysplasia 513
Otopalatal digital syndrome 513
Ovarian tumors 379
Oxyhemoglobin binding 160

Pain 487–8
 treatment 488
Pancreatic polypeptide 280
Pancreatitis, viruses causing 326, 327
Parainfluenza virus, types 2–5, 325

Paralysis, viruses causing 327
Parathormone 241, 242
Parenteral nutrition 410–11
Partial albinism 337
Parvovirus B19 325
Pendred's syndrome 388, 513
Penicillin(s) 351
Penicillinase 351
Peptide hormones in gastrointestinal tract 280
Peptide Y 280
Pericarditis, viruses causing 327
Peroxisomal diseases 240
Peroxisomes 239
Persistent ductus arteriosus 93, 104
Pes adductus 495
Peutz–Jeghers syndrome 388
Pfaunder–Hurler diseases 231
Pfeiffer's syndrome 513
Phenobarbitone 450
Phenytoin 132, 450
Phosphorus, conversion table 4
Pineal cell tumor 383
Pineoblastoma 383
Pineocytoma 383
Pituitary adenocarcinoma 385
Pituitary adenoma 385
Pituitary function tests 277
Plasma, reference values 8–17
Pleural puncture 46
Pleurodynia, viruses causing 327
Pleuromediastinal lines in chest film 166
Pneumococci, immunization 313
Poisoning 476–9
 antidotes 478–9
 elimination 476–7
 gastric lavage 477

INDEX

information services, UK/Republic of Ireland 479
Poland's syndrome 389
Polio immunization 314
Polio virus 327
Polyarthritis, chronic 346
Polymerase chain reaction 24
Pompe's disease 221
Potassium imbalance estimation 294
Pre-diabetes mellitus 222
Prednisolone 175
Prednisone 516
Pressure, conversion table 3
Prefixes for multiplication/ division of decimal units 20
Premature infant, nutrition 409
Prenatal development, early 42–3
Primidone 450
'Primitive' neuroectodermal tumor 382
Procarbizine 392
Progressive erythrokeratodermia 511
Progresive infantile poliodystrophy (fetal infantile encephalomyopathy) 214
Propafenone 132
Propranolol 133
Protein, analysis by blot technique 22–3
Proteinuria 186, 187
Pseudohemaphrodism 261, 262
Puberty 257–60
  age of onset 257
  delayed 289
  development 257
  onset 259
  phenotypical course 258
  premature 260

Pubic hair development 256
Pulmonary edema 473
Pulmonary regurgitation 102
Pulmonary stenosis 100
Pulmonary valve stenosis 93
Pupil size, pharmacodynamics 505
Pyruvate carboxylase deficiency 212
Pyruvate dehydrogenase deficiency 212
Pyruvate metabolism model 213

Quinidine 132

Rabies immunization 317
Rachitogenic disorders 243
Radioiodine uptake changes 66
Rathke's pouch cyst 385
Recklinghausen's disease type 1 389
Rehydration 201–2
  oral 291
  parenteral 292
Renal biopsy 187
Renal cystic diseases 182–4
  dysontogenetic cyst 184
  medullary cystic disease (juvenile nephrothiasis) 183
  medullary cystic nephropathy 183
  polycystic neuropathy 183
  Potter's classification 182
  pseudocysts ('urinomas') 184
  pyelogenic cyst 184
Renal diagnostic methods 187
Renal failure, acute 481–4
  treatment 483–4
    of complications 484

Renal function 176–8
  distal tubular function tests 178
  glomerular filtration rate 177
  impaired, drug doses 485–6
  osmolality values 176
  tubular 177
  urine production 176
Renal tubular acidosis 179–81, 513, 514
  causes 181
  diagnostic plan 180
Retinopathies 435
Reproterol 174
Respiration
  Biot's 159
  Cheyne–Stokes 159, 171
  gasping 159, 171
  Kussmaul's 159
  partial pressure profile 160
  resting respiratory rate 158
  rhythmic, differential diagnosis 159
  true spontaneous 453
Respiratory acidosis 205, 206
Respiratory alkalosis 205, 206
Respiratory chain defects 214–15
Respiratory syncitial virus 325
Resuscitation 452, 460–2
  external cardiac massage 406–1
  medication 452
  treatment in postresuscitation phase 462
Retinoblastomas 390
Retinopathy of prematurity (retrolental fibroplasia) 506
Reye's syndrome 480
Rhabdomyosarcoma 383

INDEX

Rhinovirus 325
Richards–Rundle syndrome 514
Rifampicin 351
RNA, analysis by blot technique 22–3
Rotaviruses 326
Rubella virus 325, 326

Salbutamol 174
Sandhoff's disease 233
Sanfillipo's disease 231
Sarcoma 389
Scheie's disease 231
School sports, children with heart disease 114
Secondary sex characteristics, developmental stages 255–6
Secretin 280
Serum, reference values 7–18
Sexual development, normal 261
Shock 470–2
 anaphylactic 471
 cardiogenic 471
 hypovolemic 470
Short stature 245, 254
Sipple's syndrome 388
SI units 5–7
Skeletal development 247
Sly's disease 231
Sodium cromoglycate 174
Sodium valproate 451
Soft tissue sarcoma, classification 374
Sotalol 133
Sotos' syndrome 389
Speech 507–8
 effect of hearing impairment on development 508
 normal development 507
Status asthmaticus 474
Status epilepticus 469

Steroid biosynthesis
 congenital disorders 263
 enzyme defects 265
Stilling–Türk–Duane syndrome 514
Stomatitis, viruses causing 326
Strabismus 502
Stridor, differential diagnosis 167
Sturge–Weber syndrome (encephalofacial angiomatosis) 443
Subacute necrotizing encephalomyelopathy (Leigh's disease) 214
Subependymal giant cell tumor 380
Subependymoma– subependymal astrocytoma 381
Sulfonamides 351
Supraventricular tachycardia 127–8
Sweat, reference values 8–17
Symbols for documentation of family tree 30
Sympathomimetics 130–1
13q Syndrome 390
Syphilis 309

Tall stature 245, 254
Tangier disease 238
Tarui's disease 221
Tay–Sachs disease 233
Tenoposide 393
Teratocarcinoma 385
Teratoma 385
Terbulatine 175
Testicular tumors 379
Tetanus immunization 314
Tetracyclines 352
Tetralogy of Fallot 102–3
 O_2 saturation 94
 pressures 94
Theophylline 175
Thoracic puncture 45

Thoracic suction drainage 44
Thrombocytosis 354
Thrombophilia 355
Thymus hyperplasia 166
TNM classification 371
Tolbuterol 175
Total anomalar pulmonary venous connection 110–11
Toxoplasmosis 307–8
Transcobalamin-2 deficiency 337
Transposition of great arteries 106
 O_2 saturation 95
 pressures 95
TRH test (TSH-releasing hormone) 273
Triamcinolone 516
Trichopoliodystrophy (Menkes' syndrome; kinky-hair disease, copper malabsorption) 215
Triglyceride, conversion table 4
Tuberculosis 306
 immunization 313
Tumors as complications of diseases/ syndromes 388–90
Turcot's syndrome 388
Turner's syndrome 253, 388, 514
Tympanogram 509

Ulcerative colitis 388
Ultrasound diagnosis 70–83
 Doppler 80–2
 flow velocities in heart/ great vessels 82
 intracranial hemorrhage 79
 normal values
  kidney 77–8
  spleen 77
 organs 71–6
Umbilical artery catheter 405

INDEX

Umbilical vein catheter 404
Undescended testis, treatment 266
Urea, conversion table 4
Uric acid, conversion table 4
Urinary stones 199–200
Urinary tract infection 195–6
Urine
  bacterial count 196
  reference values 7–16
Usher's syndrome 514

Vaccines 318
Van Buchem's syndrome 510
Varicella immunization 313
Varicella zoster virus 325
Vasoactive intestinal polypeptide 280
Vasopressin (desmopressin) test 278–9
Venepuncture
  central venous catheter 47–8
  epicutaneous catheter 49
Ventilation 453–9
  abbreviations 453
  complications of assisted ventilation 459
  endotracheal aspiration 459
  endotracheal intubation 459
  controlled 453
  continuous positive airway pressure 454
  guidelines for initial setting of ventilator 456
  intermittent mandatory ventilation 454
  intermittent positive pressure ventilation 454
  mechanical 455, 456
  neonatal 457
  parameters 454
  positive end-expiratory pressure 454
  complications 455
Ventricular fibrillation 129
Ventricular flutter 129
Ventricular septal defect 108–9
  O_2 saturation 92
  pressures 92
Ventricular tachycardia 128–9
Verapamil 133
Vesicoureteral reflux grading 194
Vigabatrin 451
Vinblastine 393
Vincristine 393
Vindesine 393
Viral diseases, commonest, diagnostic survey 325–8
Visual acuity measurement 501

Vitamin, requirements 296
Vitamin D 241, 243
Vitiligo muscle atrophy 514
Vohwinkel's syndrome 514
Vomiting, differential diagnosis 286–7
von Gierke's disease 221
von Willebrand's disease 355

Waardenburg's syndrome 514
Werner's syndrome 388
Wildervanck's syndrome 514
Wilms' tumor (nephroblastoma) 389
  classification 373
  postoperative stages 379
  staging 378
Wiskott–Aldrich syndrome 337, 389
Wolff–Parkinson–White syndrome 127

Xanthosarcoma 383
X-chromosomal inherited disorders 32–3
Xeroderma, pigmented 390
X-ray
  diagnosis 54–6
  investigations 52–3
  thoracic imaging 57